Neuroliterature 2
Biography, Semiology, Miscellany

Further literary perspectives on
disorders of the nervous system

AJ LARNER

AJ Larner MD DHMSA PhD FRCP(UK)

Consultant Neurologist, Walton Centre for Neurology and Neurosurgery, Liverpool, L9 7LJ, United Kingdom

Formerly Society of Apothecaries' Honorary Lecturer in the History of Medicine, University of Liverpool, United Kingdom.

e-mail: andrew.larner2@nhs.net

CP
THE CHOIR PRESS

First published in the United Kingdom in 2023 by
The Choir Press

ISBN 978–1–78963–369–6

Contents

Foreword

Dr Andrew Larner's earlier book of fascinating ephemera titled *Neuroliterature: Patients, Doctors, Diseases,* published in 2019, set out his thoughts gathered over twenty years as a highly experienced neurologist practising at The Walton Centre in Liverpool. The subtitle to that book *Literary perspectives on disorders of the nervous system* is now complemented here in his new book by a new set of papers. He is an avid reader and once described himself to this reviewer as a scribbler but even if that were so then he is a worthy successor to the earlier Dr Johnson.

This collection of papers is truly eclectic and teaches those in medicine that the wider literature embeds our medical biography. Larner's interests and wide reading in Dickens and Gaskell remind us of the poverty of older days and of how far medicine has progressed, to a large extent through the medium of public health and providing for the needs of daily living, sometimes considered reduction in poverty. Larner's vast experience over many years qualifies him for writing these many reviews of literature and medicine. His specialty is about persons and their predicaments, and the measures that help analyse these and suggest solutions. That is what medicine is about, reducing disability without increasing overall distress.

Larner's thoughts on biography relate more widely than the persons named in the chapter headings, and his examples of semiology provide us with many signs of disorders to be met with in his patients and the meanings they convey to a busy but enquiring practitioner. Curiously-named disorders, many of Greek root, illustrate the phenomena on the one hand of the borderlands of understandable physical processes in the nervous system and on the other hand of complicated cognitive processes. A glance at the index will show the range of such disorders but the understanding will rest in the reading of each chapter.

What's in a name, asks the author? We reply that we find some answers here but for each answer to a neurological problem there arise more questions, requiring more answers and so on – hence the impatient wait for this author's next and third volume of literary and medical thoughts. In the meantime let us explore the significance of the shape of our heads, and whether mirror phenomena (mirror-writing being a favourite of Leonardo and of Agatha Christie) has some embryological significance: we can turn arguments, turn our perception of our surroundings, but can we use these inversions to our developmental advantage? On the other hand, we do not understand sufficient of lassitude, that difficult-to-define state where we feel obtunded (rather than acute) in our everyday ability to cope, a phenomenon well-described in the aftermath of the Covid-19 pandemic so recently current around the time of publication of this volume.

Lest this writer suffer from a medic's variation on dysphonia clericorum, too many words akin to Mozart's alleged too many notes, the time has come to stand aside from obstructing readers from getting to the meat of the issues this author introduces into our diet and to say read on, with surprises and enjoyment ahead.

Christopher Gardner-Thorpe

President, History of Medicine Society, Royal Society of Medicine

Introduction

As a pleasure, writing has great limitations; as an outlet, none.[1]

The Nightingale Silenced

Thus Margiad Evans (1909–58), the Anglo-Welsh writer afflicted in her later years with epilepsy, of which she wrote two book-length accounts, only one published in her lifetime. I echo her sentiments about writing, but find it impossible to desist from it entirely, perhaps as a mechanism for trying to enhance my own understanding of the world I encounter. But with what success? I find myself largely in agreement with another clinician-writer, Richard Asher (1912–69):

Writing is done more by toil than by gift. Is it worth it? I don't really think it is.[2]

However, as some readers have apparently enjoyed items included in a previous volume of my occasional pieces, *Neuroliterature. Patients, doctors, diseases,*[3] I have gathered some further material here, most published but some unable to find a home in print. I have categorised these pieces as biography, semiology (which supplements a previous volume, *A dictionary of neurological signs*[4]) and miscellany, an arrangement which may pretend to more cohesion than the pieces actually possess. *Ars sine scientia nihil est.*

AJ Larner

References

1. Pratt J (ed.). *The Nightingale Silenced and other late unpublished writings by Margiad Evans.* Dinas Powys: Honno (Welsh Women's Classics), 2020, p.xviii, 156.
2. Avery Jones F (ed.). *Richard Asher talking sense.* Edinburgh: Churchill Livingstone, 1986, p.101.
3. Larner AJ. *Neuroliterature. Patients, doctors, diseases.* Gloucester: Choir Press, 2019.
4. Larner AJ. *A dictionary of neurological signs* (4th edition). London: Springer, 2016.

Biography

Thoughts on medical biography

1.

Even a cursory reading of Hermione Lee's book on biography[1] will give some pause for thought about the nature of the discipline of biography in general, much of it equally applicable in the medical sphere. Biography is an unstable genre, an artificial cultural construct, which is always to some extent an index of its time. Clearly some factors, such as authenticity and verification, remain touchstones of good biography but interpretations change – there is no such thing as a definitive biography, all are temporary, partial, contingent. Medical lives and practices may be reappraised in each succeeding generation, with different emphases as biography and its methods evolve.

Muriel Spark (1918–2006), no stranger to medical issues of a psychiatric nature, as revealed in her work,[2] drew a distinction in 1950 between the "sort of biographical writing that adheres relentlessly to fact" and the "approach in which the author's imagination rampages across history",[3] obviously detecting problems with both styles. The same may also be true of medical biography. Clearly factual accuracy is an inviolable necessity, but much will be absent in any documentary historical record, necessitating some type of post-hoc inter-pretation which may be coloured by many factors and which may change over time. This constitutes much of the fascination of biography and explains why no account can be regarded as definitive.

Acknowledgement

Adapted from: Larner AJ. Editorial. *J Med Biogr* 2015;23:1 and 2017;25:1.

References

1. Lee H. *Biography. A very short introduction.* Oxford: Oxford University Press, 2009.
2. Beveridge AW. The secular and the supernatural: madness and psychiatry in the short stories of Muriel Spark. *J R Coll Physicians Edinb* 2015;45:305–312.
3. Spark M. Pensée: Biography. In: Jardine P (ed.). *The informed air. Essays by Muriel Spark.* New York: New Directions, 2014: 95.

2.

In AS Byatt's novel *The biographer's tale*, two of the characters discuss the nature of biography:

> "The art of biography is a despised art because it is an art of things, of facts, of arranged facts."

> "... Tales told by those incapable of true invention, simple stories for those incapable of true critical insight."[1]

These viewpoints set me thinking once again[2] about the nature of the biographical enterprise.

Having spent much of the past 30 years attempting to deliver professional health care, it was a new, involuntary, and salutary experience in late 2016 to be on the receiving side of the equation. I had to recount my clinical narrative, initially to those clinicians caring for me, and later to friends and family. The events, largely unremarkable and clinically commonplace, have, willy-nilly, become part of my biography.

Most of the contributions to the *Journal of Medical Biogrpahy* (*JMB*) relate to the deliverers of health care, be they physicians, surgeons, or practitioners of professions allied to medicine, but rather fewer give us the perspective of the receiver, what might be termed patient biographies, pathographies, or autopathographies.[3] A brief examination of the first 10 issues published during my stint as *JMB* editor (February 2015 to May 2017) suggests that, of 141 substantive articles, those which might be classified as doctor biographies (120) outnumber patient biographies (13) by a ratio of almost 10:1.

Why should this be? Professionals are more likely to write, publish, and leave the kinds of archival material beloved of biographers, as well as having profile, renown, presence, celebrity even, and hence of potential general interest, factors which may be lacking for many patients.

Nevertheless, there is something to be learned from patient narratives, from "hearing the patient voice", which may present a perspective on illness and medical practice different from that presented by members of the faculty. The interpretation of patient narrative is a core activity of medical practice.[4] We should therefore value patient biographies and ensure that they remain an integral component of "medical biography".

Acknowledgement

Adapted from: Larner AJ. Editorial. *J Med Biogr* 2018;26:1.

References

1.   Byatt AS. *The biographer's tale*. London: Chatto & Windus, 2000: 5.
2.   Larner AJ. Editorial. *J Med Biogr* 2017;25:1.
3.   Bou Khalil R, Jayatunge R. Pathography and autopathography: the case of Nikolai Gogol (1809–1852). *J Med Biogr* 2018;26:145–146
4.   Larner AJ. Neurology and literature. *Neurosciences and History* 2017;5:47–51.

3.

In her very readable book *History's people. Personalities and the past*, the Canadian historian Margaret MacMillan eloquently addresses the tension sometimes evident between biography and history:

> … the relationship between historians and biographers is often an uneasy one, marked by mutual suspicions. Historians complain that biographers do not properly understand or short change the context while biographers feel that historians miss out the individuals who help to make history.

Speaking of Thomas Carlyle, she notes that, notwithstanding his work on "heroes", he understood that:

> … the secret of good biography – and indeed of much good history – is to understand that relationship between individuals and their societies … we must always locate people in their times and also remind ourselves that we cannot expect them to think things that hadn't yet been discovered or articulated.[1]

Escaping from, or resisting, our own subjectivity, be that in historical or biomedical contexts, remains a challenging task, indeed a necessity of which we may be totally unaware.

Acknowledgement

Adapted from: Larner AJ. Editorial. *J Med Biogr* 2018;26:217.

References

1.   MacMillan M. *History's people. Personalities and the past*. London: Profile Books, 2017: xiii, 4–5.

4. On Anthony Powell

Amongst the calvacade of characters who populate the twelve volumes of Anthony Powell's (1905–2000) sequence of novels entitled, after the painting by Nicolas Poussin, *A Dance to the Music of Time* (published 1951–1975), one, Russell Gwinnett, who appears in the last two novels, undertakes a biography of the writer X. Trapnel.[1] Reflecting on this, the books' narrator, Nicholas Jenkins, reports (in the eleventh book of the series, *Temporary Kings*):

> Gwinnett's approach, not uncommon among biographers, seemed to be to see himself, at greater or lesser range, as projection of his subject. He aimed, anyway to some extent, at reconstructing in himself Trapnel's life, getting into Trapnel's skin, "becoming" Trapnel.

We also have, in the final book of the series, *Hearing Secret Harmonies*, Trapnel's views on biography:

> Biography and memoirs can never be wholly true, since they can't include every conceivable circumstance of what happened. The novel can do that. The novelist himself lays it down. His decision is binding. The biographer, even at his highest and best, can be only tentative, empirical.

This interplay between biography and fiction is further illustrated by the interrelationship of Powell as novelist and Nicholas Jenkins as fictional narrator. Powell himself was also a biographer, of John Aubrey (1626–1697),[2] himself one of the first biographers. Nicholas Jenkins, like Powell an author, produces one (fictional) work of non-fiction, entitled *Borage and Hellebore*, a study of Robert Burton (1577–1640), the author of *The Anatomy of Melancholy*, a work which informs particularly the tenth book in the *Dance* sequence, *Books do furnish a room*, and also the penultimate paragraph of the whole novel sequence.

Amongst the calvacade of characters who populate Anthony Powell's own biography,[3] most were writers, journalists, or artists, but at least one was a doctor: Wyndham Edward Buckley Lloyd. He was best man at Powell's wedding to Violet Pakenham in 1934. The firm for which Powell then worked, Duckworth's, published a number of books under the title of the "100 years series", one of which was by Lloyd, *A hundred years of medicine*.[4] It first appeared in 1936, with a revised edition in 1939. An American edition, co-authored with Cushman Davis Haagensen, appeared in 1943 (New York: Sheridan House), to somewhat mixed reviews.[5–7] One review describes Lloyd as a specialist in public health.[6] The epigraph of the book is from Burton's *Anatomy of Melancholy*, presumably a shared interest of Powell/Jenkins and Lloyd.

Acknowledgement

Adapted from: Larner AJ. Editorial. *J Med Biogr* 2019;27:1.

References

1. Spurling H. *Invitation to the dance. A handbook to Anthony Powell's A Dance to the Music of Time*. London: Arrow Books, 2005 [1977]: 82–4; 177–9, 254–5.
2. Powell A. *John Aubrey and his friends*. London: Eyre & Spottiswoode, 1948.
3. Spurling H. *Anthony Powell. Dancing to the music of time*. London: Hamish Hamilton, 2017.
4. Lloyd WEB. *A hundred years of medicine*. London: Duckworth, 1936.
5. Baumgartner L. *American Journal of Public Health* 1944;34:906.
6. Clapesattle H. *American Historical Review* 1944;49:455.
7. [Anonymous]. *Science Education* 1946;30:166.

5. Retrospective diagnosis: pitfalls and purposes

There are many arguments against the practice of retrospective diagnosis, also known as posthumous diagnosis or retrodiagnosis. These include the nature of the sources used (general absence of physical evidence; reliance on second hand evidence) and the context (historically contingent diagnostic categories; the subject's different cognitive world), not to mention potential ethical issues (lack of "patient" consent), all of which render any conclusions speculative, even presumptuous. The clinical skill of pattern recognition may involuntarily suggest diagnosis, without sufficient attention to sources and context. Yet both clinicians and historians still attempt retrospective diagnosis (in the interests of full disclosure, I must admit to being a serial offender, using both patient and literary narratives[1]), and pathography constitutes a well-recognised genre within medical biography. Lane Fox devotes a chapter to retrospective diagnosis in his investigation of certain books (*Epidemics* 1 and 3) in the Hippocratic corpus, acknowledging it to be a "fragile business".[2] The matter is rendered urgent by Karenberg's recommendation to journal editors to reject such papers when submitted for publication.[3]

The issues involved have been carefully formulated by Muramoto,[4] who identified two challenges: the ontological and the epistemic. The ontological challenge questions whether disease entities persist over time. Evidently, diseases may come and go (e.g. epidemics) even though there is probably little change in human biology over historical time and culture (i.e. transhistorical and transcultural), albeit some predispositions or vulnerabilities to disease may vary between times and places. But if it be accepted, as seems likely to clinicians, that many disease entities did exist before their clinical description and incorporation into evolving nosologies,[5] the central question is therefore the epistemic challenge: how can diagnosis be empirically verified retrospectively?

This is, of course, rarely possible, although molecular genetic diagnosis using fortuitously preserved tissue ("molecular biography"[6]) or archaeological findings (paleopathology[7]) may sometimes occur. However, Muramoto argues that since all diagnoses are cultural constructs, hence liable to change over time, and based on hypothesis-making and hypothesis-evaluation following iterative probabilistic Bayesian reasoning in circumstances of uncertainty, retrospective syndromic diagnosis based on history alone is permissible as an explanatory device (as in day-to-day clinical practice) provided that overspecification is avoided. This approach, based on the reasoning originally developed by Thomas Bayes (1701?–1761), is a clear intersection with current clinical practice in the evaluation of testing procedures.[8]

Retrospective diagnosis does have purpose: to better understand an individual's life and work and to correct or amend previous interpretations. Occasionally an author may specifically indicate their writing is intended for scrutiny by clinicians (autopathography, e.g. Margiad Evans' "desire to put into physician's [sic] hands … clues to the feelings of such a sufferer [from epilepsy] as myself"[9]), an invitation which should be accepted.

Hence, pace Karenberg,[3] this editor will continue to consider papers suggesting retrospective diagnoses, applying the guidance suggested by Muramoto.[4] A good example of this approach has already appeared.[10]

Acknowledgement

Adapted from: Larner AJ. Editorial. *J Med Biogr* 2019;27:127–8.

References

1. Larner AJ. *Neuroliterature. Patients, doctors, diseases.* Gloucester: The Choir Press, 2019.
2. Lane Fox R. *The invention of medicine. From Homer to Hippocrates.* London: Allen Lane, 2020:236–51,277.
3. Karenberg A. Retrospective diagnosis: use and abuse in medical historiography. *Prague Med Rep* 2009;110:140–5.
4. Muramoto O. Retrospective diagnosis of a famous historical figure: ontological, epistemic, and ethical considerations. *Philosophy, Ethics, and Humanities in Medicine* 2014;9:10.
5. Larner AJ. Neurology and literature. *Neurosciences and History* 2017;5:47–51.
6. Hunt DM, Dulai KS, Bowmaker JK, Mollon JD. The chemistry of John Dalton's color blindness. *Science* 1995;267:984–8.

7. Shaw B, Burrell CL, Green D et al. Molecular insights into an ancient form of Paget's disease of bone. *Proc Natl Acad Sci USA* 2019;116:10463–72.
8. Larner AJ. *Diagnostic test accuracy studies in dementia: a pragmatic approach.* (2nd edition). London: Springer; 2019.
9. Larner AJ. Margiad Evans (1909–1958): a history of epilepsy in a creative writer. *Epilepsy Behav* 2009;16:596–8.
10. Goldman AS,. Goldman DA. *Prisoners of time. The misdiagnosis of FDR's 1921 paralytic illness.* EHDP Press, 2017.

6. Valedictory

… we must not forget that the writing of history – however dryly it is done and however sincere the desire for objectivity – remains literature. History's third dimension is always fiction.

"To study history one must know in advance that one is attempting something fundamentally impossible, yet necessary and highly important. To study history means submitting to chaos and nevertheless retaining faith in order and meaning."

Hermann Hesse[1]

History … is not what happens when it happens, but what seems to people to have happened when they look back on it.

Michael Frayn[2]

One of the purposes of medical biography is to document the lives and works of those practitioners in the sphere of medicine and allied professions in various times and cultures who have preceded us. This endeavour is predicated, at least in part, on the notion that their actions have generally been a worthy pursuit in the cause of good, for human benefit, and against those afflictions to which the human condition is involuntarily prey. Ill health, illness, is usually regarded as accidental, beyond personal control, a misfortune, with no fault attached to the sufferer. But what if these parameters were changed? What if ill-health were deemed culpable, criminal?

This is the situation described in Samuel Butler's (1835–1902) novel of imaginary travels, *Erewhon, or Over the Range* (1872, revised 1901).[3] The traveller, named as Higgs in the sequel *Erewhon Revisited Twenty Years Later, Both by the Original Discoverer of the Country and by His Son* (1901), discovers that:

… illness of any sort was considered in Erewhon to be highly criminal and immoral; and that I was liable, even for catching a cold, to be had up before the magistrates and imprisoned for a considerable period (p.90) thus explaining the thorough physical inspection before a magistrate which he undergoes on arrival in the kingdom (pp.80–81).

> ... if a man falls into ill health or catches any disorder, or fails bodily in any way before he is seventy years old, he is tried before a jury of his country-men, and if convicted is held up to public scorn and sentenced more or less severely as the case may be. There are subdivisions of illnesses into crimes and misdemeanours as with offences amongst ourselves ... (p.102)

As an example, having typhus fever is deemed a particularly heinous offence (pp.87,97).

A consequence is that the Erewhonians "conceal ill health by every cunning and hypocrisy and artifice which they can devise" (pp.104–105) perhaps because the law "consists in the sternest repression of all diseases whatsoever" (p.117). This may also partially explain why headaches "were not very preva-lent, for the people were the healthiest ... imaginable, owing to the severity with which ill health was treated" (p.136).

Butler is quoted approvingly by a character in the classic American novel of medicine, Sinclair Lewis's (1885–1951) *Arrowsmith* (1925):

> As Butler shows in *Erewhon* – the swine stole that idea from me ... maybe thirty years before I ever got it – the only crime for w'ich [sic] we should hang people is having toobercoolosis [sic].[4]

It has also been said that "Like many people (E.M. Forster among them) [Alan Turing] found a special pleasure in discovering Samuel Butler's *Erewhon*. Here was a Victorian writer ... exchanging the associations of 'sin' with those of 'sickness'".[5]

A somewhat similar state of affairs is described in Ursula Le Guin's (1929–2018) novel *The Dispossessed* (1974), affecting the inhabitants of the settler colony of Anarres:

> Most young Anarresti felt that it was shameful to be ill; a result of their society's very successful prophylaxy, and also perhaps a confusion arising from the analogic use of the words "healthy" and "sick". They felt illness to be a crime, if an involuntary one.[6]

Of course, Butler's purpose is satire, not logic, and Le Guin's idiom is "sci-fi" not "sci-fact". But that is not to say that these imagined things cannot or will not come to pass: "the influence of Erewhon had made me begin to see things in a new light" (p.179). Indeed, it may be all too easy to envisage that the exist-ing consensus on the non-culpability of illness could break down.

Anthropologists distinguish "guilt culture," typical of Western nations, from "shame culture". In the former the focus is on individual culpability rather than shared responsibility. In such a context, in a society where competitive individualism triumphs over collectivism, it is conceivable that illness might come to be equated with wrongdoing, abetted by clinicians, and laid at the door of the individual. This might perhaps occur under the perceived pressure of escalating health care costs and/or a belief that many common ailments (heart attack, stroke, dementia) are at least partially preventable. If this paradigm shift were to occur, it may be for posterity to judge whether those biographized in the pages of this Journal are to be seen as benefactors or criminals, heroes or villains.

Acknowledgement

Adapted from: Larner AJ. Editorial: valedictory. *J Med Biogr* 2020;28:1–2.

References

1. Hesse H. *The glass bead game.* London: Vintage Books [1943] 1970:39, 156–157.
2. Frayn M. *Copenhagen.* London: Bloomsbury [1998] 2009:148.
3. Butler S. *Erewhon.* Harmondsworth: Penguin Books [1872,1901] 1970. All page references cited in the text refer to this edition.
4. Lewis S. *Arrowsmith.* New York: Signet Classics [1925] 2008:180.
5. Hodges A. *Alan Turing: the enigma.* London: Vintage [1983] 2014:95, 480–481.
6. Le Guin, U. *The Dispossessed.* London: Orion Books [1974], 2002:100–101.

7. Valedictory 2 (or "The long goodbye")

Karl Pearson (1857–1936) claimed, in his biography of Francis Galton (1822–1911), that biography is the richest form of history.[1] But what is the "richest" form of biography? Or the most appropriate?

Thomas Söderqvist[2] suggested a fourfold typology of science biography:

- Existential biography: this is an attempt to reconstruct the subject's life from the inside, "to narrate the development of his [sic] life 'as it is directly experienced by the biographical subject'". This approach, Söderqvist's preferred option, contrasts with the other three categories, all of which are "external to the experiencing individual confronted with his [sic!] existential choices".

- Social biography: in which the individual is contextualised with reference to his [*sic*!!] "situatedness" in a certain time, a certain culture.
- Psychobiography: in which certain traits of the subject's personality or his [*sic*!!!] achievements are explained with reference to psychological theory.
- Biographical case histories: aimed to generalise about genius, creativity or the life cycle.

One might argue that "science biography" is different to "medical biography", in that not all practitioners of medicine or allied professions are, or aspire to be, scientists, and hence this classification is not applicable or transferable.

However, putting this caveat to one side, I think it would be fair to say that most contributions to medical biography fall within the latter category, namely biographical case histories, hopefully with some overlap with social biography such that the individual life and work is contextualised. It may be that this is the best one can do in writing medical biography. Attempts at psychobiography, for example, as described by Söderqvist, must be vulnerable to shifts in psychological theory.

Those committed to the theory of mind, that is the ability to attribute or impute mental states to others, a faculty which appears to be an innate aspect of mental development in most individuals, will no doubt endorse Söderqvist's idea of existential biography. As a neurologist I remain sceptical about such an approach (as previously expressed: *Medical Historian* 2018;28:75–76). Can a biographer legitimately claim to know the mind states of contemporaries ("I know what you're thinking" = "I think I know what you're thinking"), even those intimately known, let alone recapitulate the direct experiences of those long dead?

This is surely not objective, unless contemporary primary source(s) exist(s), which can be referenced, in which the protagonist specifically states "I decided" or "I thought" or "I recognised". Even then such sources are often written in retrospect, and hence susceptible to Kierkegaard's dictum: "Life can only be understood backwards; but it must be lived forwards". I fear that the existential biographer might become confused with the omniscient narrator. We surely wish to avoid the situation where "Even great historians write down what the actors should have said, rather than what they did".[3]

Acknowledgement

Adapted from: Larner AJ. Editorial: valedictory 2. *J Med Biogr* 2020;28:67.

References

1. Porter TM. *Karl Pearson. The scientific life in a statistical age.* Princeton and Oxford: Princeton University Press 2004:91.
2. Söderqvist T. Existential projects and existential choice in science: science biography as an edifying genre. In: Shortland M, Yeo R (eds.). *Telling lives in science. Essays on scientific biography.* Cambridge: Cambridge University Press 1996:45–84 [at 73].
3. Pears I. *An instance of the fingerpost.* London: Vintage, 1998:364.

Richard Lower (1631–1691)

Richard Lower was a distinguished member of the scientific community which flourished in Oxford in the 1650s and 1660s, most of whose members later migrated to London to form the nucleus of the newly established Royal Society.[1] He made notable contributions to the study of both anatomy and physiology and was also a practising physician. Despite his achievements, being the first Englishman to carry out a successful transfusion of the blood between animals and from an animal to man, he remains largely unknown, being overshadowed by his illustrious contemporaries, amongst whom were Thomas Willis, Robert Boyle, John Locke, and Robert Hooke.

Early life

Richard Lower was born in St Tudy, near Bodmin in Cornwall, in 1631. Little information concerning his early life survives, but it is known that his parents were prominent members of the Cornish gentry. Accordingly, at the age of 12, Lower was sent to Westminster School in London where he fell under the tutelage of Richard Busby, the redoubtable headmaster who ruled the school from 1638 to 1695. Lower was a King's Scholar and in 1649 proceeded to a Studentship at Christ Church, one of the largest of the Oxford colleges. Busby had established close connections between Westminster School and Christ Church,[2] and in the space of the decade from the mid-1640s to the mid-1650s he sent many of his ablest pupils there: Nathaniel Hodges in 1648, Henry Stubbe (1649), John Locke (1652), and Robert Hooke (1653). Other Westminsters were admitted to other Oxford colleges: Christopher Wren went to the recently founded Wadham College in 1649, and Thomas Millington to All Souls in the same year; the occasional pupil went to Cambridge, such as Walter Needham who entered Trinity in 1650. Many of these individuals were to become part of the scientific community based in Oxford in the following two decades and some made important contributions in the fields of anatomy, physiology, chemistry, astronomy, and mathematics.

Oxford

Lower arrived in Oxford at a time when the University was undergoing a period of transition in terms of both attitudes and personnel. The factors underlying the growth of experimental science in Oxford during the seventeenth century have been admirably delineated in the monograph by Frank.[3] From the end of the sixteenth century onwards the University underwent a general expansion: there was a dramatic increase in the number of students admitted to Oxford, concomitant with a building programme which saw the founding of several new colleges (Trinity, St John's, Jesus, Wadham, Pembroke) and the refurbishment of others. There was a doubling in the number of endowed teaching positions in the sciences, including the foundation of the Sedleian Professorship in Natural Philosophy and the Tomlins Readership in Anatomy, and library facilities were improved under the guidance of Sir Thomas Bodley. Thus by 1640 Oxford was one of the best equipped universities in Europe for scholars in the sciences. This was the situation at the outbreak of the Civil War when Oxford became a garrison town for Royalist troops, thereby causing an almost total cessation of normal University life. However, the War was to bring to Oxford one further vital ingredient for the beginning of scientific study in earnest: William Harvey.

In October 1642, King Charles I and his retinue arrived in Oxford after the battle of Edgehill. Among this contingent was the king's senior physician-in-ordinary, William Harvey, now some 64 years old, and known throughout Europe for his discovery of the circulation of the blood. Harvey was to remain in Oxford for some three and a half years, the last eighteen months (January 1645 to June 1646) as Warden of Merton College. Information about his life and work during this period is scanty,[4-6] but it is known that, his duties to the monarch being few, he became associated with a group of natural philosophers based at Trinity College, which included George Bathurst and Nathaniel Highmore. By early 1643 these men were involved in a study of the embryology of the chick, a broody hen being used to incubate eggs for various periods before they were opened in Bathurst's chambers. Many of the observations were subsequently recorded in 14 of the 72 chapters of Harvey's book *De generatione*, published in 1651, detailing the day-to-day development of the chick in the egg. Highmore also published a book, *The History of Generation*, in 1651 which features observations on the development of the chick, but he is better known for his *Corporis Humani disquisitio Anatomica*, dedicated to Harvey, in which he gave a description of the maxillary antrum which now bears his name, albeit described by Leonardo da Vinci 150 years prior to this.

Although ill-recorded, it seems that Harvey's presence in Oxford attracted a circle of followers who were able to witness at first hand the Harveian method of vivisectional experimental investigation, predominantly in the study of the embryology of the chick, although it is possible that he gave a practical demonstration of his experiments on the circulation whilst in Oxford. The intellectual community thus formed readily adopted the Harveian methodology to tackle the set of problems in physiology and chemistry which had been delineated by the discovery of the circulation. Furthermore, following Harvey's sudden departure in 1646 his Oxford protégés were able to reframe many of the outstanding Harveain problems in terms not of the the Aristotelian philosophy so dear to Harvey but of the newer atomistic and mechanical philosophy emanating from the Continent in the works of such men as Descartes, Gassendi, and Mersenne. This allowed them to escape more fully from the Galenic system of physiology, doomed as it was by the discovery of the circulation, and therby to complete the intellectual revolution begun by Harvey. The expansion in scientific knowledge resulting from the coming together of these multifarious influences was just beginning when Lower arrived in Oxford in 1649.

Thomas Willis

At Christ Church, Lower became assistant to Thomas Willis, whose eminence as both doctor and scientist was growing at this time. He was to be a life-long influence, despite the fact that he originated from a very different background to Lower. Born in 1621, the son of a farm steward, Willis entered Christ Church in 1638 as servitor to one of the Canons, Dr Thomas Isles, from which lowly position he had gradually worked his way up, receiving his MA in 1642. During the Civil War he served in one of the Royalist auxiliary regiments recruited from members of the University to defend Oxford.[7] Six months after the War ended he gained his BM and a licence to practice medicine. It is unlikely that he ever met Harvey.

Although a staunch Royalist, Willis survived the purges of the Parliamentary Visitors in 1648, and around this time it is known that he was an active member of the group of natural philosophers meeting at Trinity College. Other members included Ralph Bathurst (the younger brother of George), Richard Highmore (the younger brother of Nathaniel), John Lydall, and John Aubrey, the antiquarian, who referred to Willis in his letters as "our chymist". In 1650, Willis is known to have been part of another philosophical club which shared the expense of running a laboratory at Wadham in space provided by the Master of the College, John Wilkins, who took an active part in scientific debate and through whom Willis came into regular contact with the chemist Robert Boyle. It was here that Willis, as part of his ongoing studies of various aspects of combustion, analysed, amongst other things, blood and urine. Besides this, Willis was also a member of a less well-defined group which met at Christ Church to carry out experiments and dissections, and which included Lower and Hooke. At Christ Church, Lower kindled Locke's interest in medicine, as evidenced by receipts and observations recorded in Locke's notebooks dating from the mid-1650s.

Medical training at Oxford was then, as now [1986], a somewhat haphazard affair. Students attached themselves as apprentices to more established practitioners and learned clinical medicine largely by imitation of their master, theoretical questions being covered by the reading of approved medical texts. Physicians and medical students also regularly met to learn anatomy by means of the dissection of executed criminals, and it is possible that Lower was present on 14th December 1650 when Willis and the anatomist William Petty met at the latter's lodgings in the High Street to dissect the body of Anne Green, a young woman hanged for infanticide. Although she had been pronounced dead by the under-sherriff, the woman was heard to breathe with a rattling noise when the coffin was opened prior to the dissection, whereupon Willis and Petty undertook by various means to resuscitate her,[8] in which attempt they were eventually successful. So great was the public interest generated by this remarkable episode that Anne Green was displayed in her coffin and a charge made for the privilege of seeing her, all of which did much to enhance Willis's reputation and thereby his medical practice. Likewise for Petty, who some two weeks later was appointed to the Tomlins Readership in Anatomy.

Although still a student, Richard Lower frequently treated patients including his close friend and drinking chum Anthony Wood, an historian from Merton College. Furthermore, in the early 1650s, he accompanied Willis on the regular trips to local market towns where poor patients were seen in order to build up the practice. The small size of the practice left Willis with plenty of time for research and by 1656 he had completed his first chemical work, *De fermentatione*, in which he set forth his doctrine of fermentation. This, along with his treatise on fevers, *De febribus*, was published in 1658–9 as the *Diatribae duae medico-philosophicae*.

Cerebri anatome (1664)

The first research Richard Lower undertook, under the guidance of Thomas Willis, was an investigation of the anatomy of the nervous system. In 1660, Willis was appointed to the Sedleian Professorship in Natural Philosophy, the tenure of which required him to expound Aristotle. However, from the start Wills neglected ths injunction, preferring instead to concentrate on more recent anatomical questions. His views were eagerly transcribed by Lower, copies of whose notes later passed to Robert Boyle and Locke.[7] However, Willis became increasingly dissatisfied with the highly speculative nature of some of his own teaching, particularly with regard to the functions of the cerebrum and cerebellum and the pathogenesis of dysfunctions of the nervous system such as paralysis, insomnia, epilepsy, hysteria, and convulsions. Being a man inculcated with the experimental philosophy of Harvey, he determined to undertake a new programme of research to resolve these questions by means of dissection of the brain.

By January 1662, Lower was reporting to Boyle that the work was underway, and in the ensuing months large numbers of animals were slain and their brains examined. In addition to human cadavers, horses, sheep, dogs, calves, goats, foxes, hares, geese, turkeys, fishes, and even a monkey were dissected. It is clear that much of the work was actually performed by Lower, who was an extremely skilled dissector. Other philosophers such as Christopher Wren and Thomas Millington were frequently in attendance. By November 1662 the anatomical investigation was adjudged complete, and the following spring Wren drew a series of plates to illustrate the work that Willis was then preparing. *Cerebri anatome cui accessit nervorum* appeared in early 1664 and represented the most advanced text on neuroanatomy produced to that time.

Cerebri anatome is chiefly remembered for the first complete description of the arterial circle at the base of the brain which now bears Willis's name. Although Willis did not discover the anastomosis, and indeed never claimed any priority,[9] his interpretation of it in terms of physiology and pathology retains its importance and thus merits the eponymous description.[10] Although many of the discoveries concerning the cranial nerves detailed in *Cerebri anatome* were anticipated by Eustachius in his Anatomical Tables of 1552, these were only published by Lancisi in 1714, and it seems that Willis reached his conclusions independently of any knowledge of Eustachius's work.[9] The classification of the cranial nerves introduced by Willis was retained until 1778 when Sommerring produced the system which is still in use today. *Cerebri anatome* also contained the first description and illustration of the spinal accessory (XI) nerve. This discovery was almost certainly made by Lower, for in the preface to the book, Willis, in acknowledging his debt to Lower's skill as an anatomist, states that:

> ... when we were entering upon a much more difficult task, the dissection of the nerves, the really wonderful dexterity of this worker and his untiring perseverance were conspicuous in the extreme and no obstacle could withstand his effort ...

Indeed, Lower is almost always alluded to by his contemporaries as "that expert anatomist".

The exact mechanics of the cooperation between Willis and Lower in this seminal work on neuroanatomy has occasioned considerable speculation ever since, with one faction protesting that *Cerebri anatome* in fact represents the work of Richard Lower which the more senior Willis appropriated as his own.

This belief stems from a damning comment made by Anthony Wood on the subject of *Cerebri anatome* in his 1691–2 sketch of the life and work of Thomas Willis:

> Whatever is anatomical in that book, the glory thereof belongs to the said R Lower, whose indefatigable industry at Oxon produced that elaborate piece.

This bald statement subsequently gained wide acceptance and was propagated by a number of authors, the most eminent of whom was Michael Foster, the founder of the Cambridge Physiological Laboratory and a Fellow of Trinity College, who incorporated it in his influential monograph[11] entitled *Lectures on the History of Physiology* published in 1901. He described Lower as:

> … a singularly able man, the henchman of the fashionable Willis whose false fame in large measure rested on Lower's careful, unacknowledged work.

Franklin, Lower's biographer, also seems to have accepted this conclusion.[12] However, the validity of Wood's judgment is called into question when one remembers that Wood and Lower were close friends and, as evidenced by Wood's extensive diaries, frequent drinking companions in the taverns of Oxford. Furthermore, both Symonds[10] and Dewhurst[13] present evidence that there was a long-standing quarrel between the families of Wood and Willis, who were neighbours, and that this dispute gave rise to an antipathy which provoked Wood's unsubstantiated remarks. Additionally,[10] it has been shown that Wood's words were in fact taken verbatim from another book entitled *Legends No Histories* written in 1670 by Henry Stubbe. This book was written, allegedly at the behest of the physician Hamey, with the sole aim of discrediting the Royal Society whose growing influence threatened that of the Royal College of Physicians. A closer reading of Stubbe's book, however, shows that in the postscript he recants his criticisms of Willis, lest he be seen as unduly partial to his old school-fellow Lower. There are no other known sources to support the contention that Lower's work was stolen by Willis, most notably no accusations made by Lower himself. Indeed, Lower's letters to Boyle describing the progress of the anatomical work indicate that Willis planned, directed, and checked all the research himself, albeit that Lower did much of the initial knife work.[13] It is possible that Willis made a number of a priori hypotheses, discussing such conjectures and speculations especially with Thomas Millington, which he then turned over to Lower for him to see by actual investigation if nature agreed.

Vindicatio (1665)

The research pursued by the members of the Oxford scientific community in the 1650s and 1660s represented a fusion of a number of disparate strands. The problems investigated related to the discovery of the circulation by Harvey and the implications this had for the understanding of cardiac and pulmonary physiology. The answers to these questions were to be reached by means of experiment, putting nature to the test. The conclusions were to be framed in terms of the recently acquired corpuscular philosophy.

The centrality of these axioms to the Oxonians meant that an attack on one of their number represented an attack on all, and thus when in 1665 the elderly Bristol physician Edmund Meara published an unsympathetic attack on Willis's beliefs on the blood and fevers, it was Lower who sprang to his defence. (Incidentally, this is another indication that Lower was in no way aggrieved with Willis over the authorship of *Cerebri anatome*.[1,14]) During the early months of 1665, Lower, in great haste, wrote his first book, the *Vindicatio* of Willis's *Diatribae duae*, dedicating it to Robert Boyle. This work, part polemic part physiological text, was published in May 1665. Its theme was the primacy of the blood, and Lower reiterated the theory that blood absorbed a nitrous food during the pulmonary transit which caused a fermentation of the blood in the left ventricle which was in turn responsible for bringing out the heat of the blood ("ascension") and causing it to change colour. In his haste, and without experimental proof, he even stated that the blood in the pulmonary veins was identical to that in the lungs. The problem of the change in the colour of the blood was to recur in Lower's later researches.

Injection and transfusion

Richard Busby, the headmaster of Westminster School, was best known for his teaching of Latin and Greek, though he also took an interest in natural philosophy and mathematics. Thus his pupils were well versed in classical literature before going up to Oxford where its study formed part of most subjects, including natural philosophy. Lower, for instance, was Praelector in Greek at Christ Church from 1656–7, before becoming Censor in Natural Philosophy for the next three years.[3] Thus Lower and his contemporaries would all have been familiar with the story of Aeson, the father of Jason, to be found in the seventh book of Ovid's *Metamorphoses*. Jason requests his wife, the barbarian princess Medea, to prolong the life of his ageing father, which she does by drainng out Aeson's blood and refilling his veins with a magic concoction containing such rejuvenating ingredients as "the scaly skin of a scraggy Cinyphian water-snake, a stag's liver (for stags survive to a great age), and the head and beak of a crow more than nine generations old", plus "a thousand other nameless ingredients". This potent brew had the desired effect, Aeson's hair and beard losing their whiteness, and "the shrivelled, neglected look of old age was dissipated".[15]

A number of men reflecting on this legend had conceived the idea of transfusing blood from one man to another in order to effect rejuvenation or cure disease. The discovery of the circulation and the experimental bent of the Oxford natural philosophers combined to provide a new impetus for an attempt at transfusion of blood from one animal to another. The feasibility of the procedure had certainly been discussed at Oxford as early as 1651–2. It is recorded by John Aubrey in his *Brief Lives* that Franics Potter, a fellow of Trinity College (until he was ejected by the Visitors in 1648), first thought of transfusion around 1639 and actually attempted the procedure at his rectory in Wiltshre in 1652. He attempted to collect blood from hens and transfer it by means of a pullet's crop and ivory tubes to another hen, apparently with no success.[3,4] However, more recently his claim to be the first successful English transfuseur has been upheld by Webster.[16]

In March 1656, Boyle, Wilkins, and Wren were discussing the question of how a serpent's venom could so quickly kill a man when bitten, an observation cited by Harvey as further proof of the existence of the circulation. Prompted by the conversation, Wren conceived a way to infuse liquid poisons into the circulation of a dog. Assisted by a number of physicians, including Thomas Willis, he isolated and ligatured the crural vein of a dog which was then incised proximal to the ligature and the pipe of a syringe inserted. Through this Wren infused a solution of opium which quickly stupefied the dog. In further experiments a bladder attached to a quill was found to be better for the purposes of infusion. Injections of wine and ale rendered dogs extremely drunk before promoting a brisk diuresis, and the emetic *crocus metallorum* also had the expected effect. The success of these experiments was well publicised amongst the Oxford scientists.

The departure of Wren in 1657 to take up the Gresham Professorship of Astronomy in London left Willis and Lower as the most enthusiastic proponents of the technique of infusion in Oxford. Its use may be observed in *Cerebri anatome*, where injections of ink were used to trace blood flow in the brain, for example in the dura and pia mater, and to confirm the functional significance ascribed by Willis to the arterial circle. In 1663 Lower and Willis disproved Franciscus Sylvius's conjecture that liquids fell from the brain into the throat and palate: ink or milk injected as a tracer into the cerebral circulation was never observed to emerge into the mouth. By 1664 Lower was increasingly undertaking experimental work alone as Willis's extensive and expanding private medical practice began to prove increasingly time consuming. He attempted to feed a dog intravenously by infusing warm milk into a vein, but the dog died within an hour. An autopsy showed the milk to be mixed with the blood, as if curdled.

Soon after taking his DM in August 1665, Lower, working with Boyle, attempted to convey blood from one dog's jugular vein by means of pipes to the jugular vein of another dog. The experiment was a complete failure because of the tendency of the blood to coagulate in the pipes. Although Boyle was moderately optimistic about these trials, they came to an abrupt halt by the end of the month, for Lower had other things on his mind. With the assistance of Anthony Wood he had been purusing a mysterious widow in nearby Garsington, known only as Mrs H, and when she declined Lower's suit, he resolved to return to Cornwall to seek a wife there. Experimental work came to a temporary cessation.

Upon returning to Oxford in February 1666, Lower took up the experiments again, this time working alone. He modified hs experimental procedure and attempted transfusion from artery to vein, rather than from vein to vein as before, thus utilising the higher arterial pressure to obviate the problem of blood clotting in the tubing. Within a short time he was able to conduct blood from the cervical artery of a large dog to the jugular vein of a smaller dog which had been previously bled. Eventually, after repeated bleedings and transfusions, the donor dog died whereas the recipient lived, showing few signs of "discomfort or displeasure". By the end of the month Lower was repeating the experiment for the benefit of Thomas Millington and other Oxford physicians, and a detailed protocol was sent to the Royal Society. However, the letter miscarried, and it was not until some nine months later, in November of 1666, that Edmund King was able to replicate Lower's results at Gresham.

The experiments on transfusion reached a spectacular zenith the following year when Lower, in collaboration with Edmund King, performed the first human transfusion in England, just five months after Jean Denis in Paris had performed the first ever successful human transfusion.[17–19] Lower managed to persuade one Arthur Coga to undergo a transfusion of sheep's blood for the princely remuneration of twenty shillings. The trial was conducted successfully on 23rd November 1667 at Arundel House in London. Less than one month later, 19th Decemeber, it was repeated for the benefit of the Fellows of the Royal Society, and Coga himself described the effects of the procedure. The Fellows were suitably impressed by this demonstration, and in the ensuing discussion a Dr Terne proposed that chronically sick patients in the hospitals of London should be transfused. However, Thomas Willis, on one of his rare visitis to the Royal Society, demurred, suggesting that the procedure be tried first on "rotten sheep".[20]

The success of the human blood transfusion experiment had a similar effect on Lower's fortunes as had the revival of Anne Green on Willis's some 17 years before; it ensured a rapid expansion of his London practice and that he was a physician sought after by the richer clientele. Meantime, the success of transfusion was assiduously promoted by Henry Oldenburg who published an account of it in the *Philosophical Transactions of the Royal Society* and corresponded on the topic with other investigators throughout Europe. Furthermore, it was to Oldenburg that Denis wrote in February 1668 when one of his subjects was taken ill and died following a transfusion, which served to forewarn Lower of the potential risks of transfusion and brought an end to his experiments before such a disaster could dent his growing reputation. Indeed, it was not to be until the early years of the 20th century that blood transfusion became a viable clinical proposition.[17]

The function of respiration

Lower's marriage in November 1666 to the widow who possessed the neighbouring manor to his in Cornwall shifted the focus of his life away from the bounds of Thames and Cherwell to London. Perhaps mindful of having to provide for a wife, he set up practice in Hatton Gardens in March 1667. He was followed to London later that year by both Locke and Willis. Locke came in April as personal physician to the Earl of Shaftesbury and lived at Exeter House in the Strand. Willis brought his family later that summer to a house in St Martin's Lane, at the urging of Gilbert Sheldon, Archbishop of Canterbury, who ensured that Willis's practice was patronised by the upper echelons of society and was therefore extremely lucrative. However, it was also extremely time consuming, and this, along with family sickness and bereavements, conspired to keep Willis from attending the Royal Society on more than a few occasions.[7] Lower, however, soon visited Boyle and Hooke in London, and in May was introduced to the Royal Society by Boyle.

The problems of respiration had stimulated the interest and research efforts of Boyle, Hooke, and others for a number of years, both in Oxford and London,[3] and it was to these that Lower now turned his attention. Some philosophers, such as Locke, believed the primary function of respiration to be chemical, in that it conveyed a nitrous substance from the air to the heart which fermented with the blood in the left ventricle to produce heat, motion, and change of colour of the blood. Indeed, this was Lower's position as stated in the *Vindicatio*. However, in November 1664 Hooke had shown, in an experiment with a dog whose thorax had been opened, that the reciprocal movements of the lungs, performed artificially with a pair of bellows, were essential to life; if they were stopped the dog went into convulsions and died.

This implied that respiration had a mechanical function. Furthermore, anatomists were unable to demonstrate any channel whereby the air in the lungs could reach the left ventricle. The resolution of this issue, either for the mechanical theory or for the chemical theory, was planned by Boyle and Hooke in 1667; they would repeat the open thorax experiment of 1664 with the added innovation of making an incision in the dog's lungs to let air out as fast as it was pumped in, so circumventing the criticism that air became unfit for respiration in the closed system. However, although carefully planned, Hooke was unwilling to perform the trial because of his distaste for the extreme pain inflicted on the experimental animal. He procrastinated for several months in the hope of gaining Lower's assistance in the execution of the experiment, even trying to procure for Lower the post of assistant curator of experiments at the Royal Society, but without success. Meantime, Walter Needham had published *Disquisitio anatomica de formato foetu* which argued strongly for the mechanical theory, utilising a number of Lower's ideas and experiments in so doing, even though Lower supported the chemical theory. Thus, Lower was challenged to uphold his views expressed in the *Vindicatio*.

On 10th October 1667, Lower and Hooke performed the open thorax experiment at the Royal Society. Firstly they exposed the heart and lungs of a dog and showed that, as in 1664, the animal could be kept alive by blowing air into the lungs with bellows. If the movement of the lungs was stopped the dog went into convulsions which ceased as soon as the bellows were once again worked. Next, a second pair of bellows was attached to the first in such a way that a constant stream of air could be pumped into the lungs, and the pleural membranes were nicked so that the air could escape as fast as it was forced in. Thus, the lungs could be kept continuously inflated with fresh air without the reciprocal movements. The dog's heart was seen to beat regularly, but when the stream of air was stopped it went into convulsive motions. This pulmonary insufflation experiment conclusively showed that movement of the lungs per se was not necessary for life, thereby refuting the mechanical theory. A week later, Lower was elected a Fellow of the Royal Society, and over the next five months he performed a wide variety of experiments before the Fellows, including the transfusion of blood to Arthur Coga and the demonstration that foodstuffs entered the veins only via the thoracic duct.

The colour of the blood

Lower next turned to the vexed question of how the change in the colour of the blood was related to respiration. It is known from Locke's notebooks that Lower had toyed with the problem of why arterial blood was a florid red and venous blood a darker colour as early as 1664–5. In the *Vindicatio* he had tied this colour change unequivocally to the left ventricle, but subsequent experimental work was to convince him otherwise.

It had been known for many years that dark venous blood if left to stand in a dish became florid red on its exposed surface. This "separation" of the blood had been cited, with varying explanations, in Harvey's *De generatione* (1651), Highmore's *Corporis humani disquisitio anatomica* (1651), Willis's *Diatribae duae* (1659), and Lower's *Vindicatio* (1665). However, the clue to the true cause of "separation" was not forthcoming until 1667 when Oldenburg by chance came upon the work of the Bolognese anatomist Carlo Fracassati, in which he stated that the dark colour of venous blood resulted solely from its not being exposed to the air. Both Lower and Willis believed that something entered the blood in respiration but they believed this to be effected by fermentation in the left ventricle and one can imagine the lateral thinking required of Lower to recognise that air might have a direct effect on blood. Lower submitted this proposition to experimental investigation. At Hooke's urging he repeated the open thorax experiment with pulmonary insufflation, then identified and cut the pulmonary vein. Florid red blood came out, indicating that the colour change took place in the lungs, not the left ventricle. Furthermore, if the animal was asphyxiated, by putting a cork into the trachea, the pulmonary vein blood remained purple, showing that whatever it was that entered the blood in the pulmonary transit was also essential to life. Thus Lower was the first man to explain the cause of the change of colour of the blood.

Tractatus de corde (1669)

Lower ceased to attend the Royal Society in March 1668, for reasons which are not clear, and spent the rest of the year compiling his *Tractatus de corde*, which he dedicated to Thomas Millington. The book represents a summary of Lower's finest anatomical and physiological achievements and clearly reflects the legacy of Harvey, Lower's stated objective being to add to the description of the circulation those points which Harvey had promised but never actually published.

The long first chapter concentrated on the anatomy of the heart: its position, its relation to the pericardium, the origins of the blood vessels, its innervation, its internal strucuture (including the description of the intervenous tubercle in the right atrium which now bears Lower's name), and most particularly the arrangement of the cardiac musculature. From specimens of boiled hearts, Lower was able to trace the layered helical pattern of the muscle fibres, from which he inferred that when the heart contracted the walls of the ventricles were squeezed together to eject the contained blood. From this understanding of the functional anatomy, Lower moved on, in the second chapter, to more physiological questions such as the cause of the heart beat. He refuted Descartes and Hooghelande who believed that the heart was put into motion by the blood which when mixed with the ferment in the left ventricle resulted in an ebullition or effervescence which lightened the blood and caused it to rise into the aorta. Lower marshalled a number of arguments against this ebullition theory, the most telling of which was an experiment in which he drew off about half a dog's total blood volume from the jugular vein and replaced it with an equal volume of beer infused into the crural vein. The strength of the heart beat diminished only slightly during this procedure, indicating that the heart moved by virtue of its own structure rather than any contained ebullition. Next the dependence of the muscular movements on the nerve supply were described, including an account of the effects of ligature and section of the vagus nerve. The chapter concluded with details of various pathological conditions which could affect the heart's motion or interfere with blood flow in arteries or veins, including the mechanism of oedema formation.

The third chapter tackled the question of the colour of the blood. Lower, admitting his mistake in the *Vindicatio*, showed that the red colour of arterial blood is due to mixture with the air and is in no way dependent on its heat – arterial blood left to cool retains its florid red colour. Loss of air during its passage through the body renders the blood dark. The final chapters of the book detail Lower's experimental work on transfusion and give a description of the passage of chyle into the blood. As in the *Vindicatio*, the blood is identified as the principal locus of human physiology, continuously supplying heat and nutriment to all organs of the body.

Later life

In the early 1670s, Lower was principally concerned with building up his London practice, although he did have time to revise his *Tractatus de corde*. The third edition, published in 1671, contains a *Dissertatio de origine catarrh* which disproves Galen's theory that nasal secretions originate in the pituitary gland. When Willis died of pneumonia in 1675 it was Lower who inherited the bulk of his practice, thereby becoming the most pre-eminent physician in London which allowed him to move successively to more fashionable addresses. In the same year he became a Fellow of the Royal College of Physicians. However, during the years of Charles II's absolute power, the outbreak of the "Popish Plot" in 1678 saw a decline in Lower's fortunes as a result of his Whig politics (the same reason that Locke was expelled from Christ Church in 1684[2]). This culminated with the loss of his court appointment at the accession of James II in 1685, which also signalled the loss of his wealthy patients, most of whom went to Dr Thomas Short. Nonetheless, Lower was amongst the many physicians called to attend Charles II on his deathbed, and after the 1688 Revolution he was once again in favour, giving advice to the Crown on the organisation of naval medical services. He died in January 1691 at his house in King Street, Covent Garden, and was buried in his native town of St Tudy, Cornwall, although his final resting place is unknown.[12]

Dr Thomas Short died in 1685 and his practice in turn devolved largely to another physician who was to have a great influence on Oxford medicine, Dr John Radcliffe.[21]

Postscript

Despite his notable achievements in anatomical and physiological research, Richard Lower remains relatively unknown. There are probably a number of reasons for this. Firstly, scanty details of his life are available. He always seems to have lived in the shadow of his more illustrious contemporaries, especially Thomas Willis, being his assistant in anatomical research and eventually inheriting his considerable London practice.[22] The eponymous immortality afforded to Willis by the arterial circle at the base of the brain did not come to Lower: the tubercle that bears his name, one of his minor anatomical discoveries, has been a subject of dispute, inasmuch as it is apt to disappear when the pericardium is incised between the venae cavae. Furthermore, it is more evident in lower anmals than it is in man, and merits only a short paragraph in *Gray's Anatomy* in which Lower's name is not mentioned.[23] Franklin believed that some of the discredit attached to this structure stems from the subsequent divergence in meaning of the Latin *tuberculum*, a swelling, from the English *tubercle*, which has a more precise anatomical and physiological connotation.[12]

Of Lower's physiological achievements, both the transfusion of blood and the explanation of the differing colour of arterial and venous blood had to wait a considerable time for their full implications to be realised. Lower suggested that since the blood of an asphyxiated animal remained purple, whatever it was in the air that changed the colour of the blood in its pulmonary transit was also responsible for keeping the animal alive. Although John Mayow, the last of the great Oxford physiologists of the 17th century,[3] had discovered oxygen in all but name in his researches (*Tractatus de respiratione*, 1668), it had to await Lavoisier's explanation of the nature of air in 1779 for the significance of Lower's observations to become fully apparent. In the case of transfusion, it was not until some two and half centuries later, in 1900, that Karl Landsteiner discovered the existence of different types of human blood which enabled the procedure to be used safely and widely as a therapeutic manoeuvre.

Acknowledgements

This, with minor amendments, is the text which won the John Friend Prize in Medical History for 1986 at the University of Oxford Medical School, when I was a medical student. Keen to have it published, I consulted with Dr. Charles Webster and he advised the journal *Endeavour*, but the editor would only agree to publish a shortened version (Larner AJ. A portrait of Richard Lower. *Endeavour* 1987;11:205–208; other material from the essay also appeared in Larner AJ. Richard Lower (1631–1691): a pioneer of cardiologic research. *Am J Cardiol* 1992;69:565). I felt somewhat aggrieved by the requirement for abridgement, but as a medical student was hardly in a position to argue. Hence, I take this opportunity to present the full text here, along with a few extra footnotes.

References

1. Gotch F. *Two Oxford physiologists, Richard Lower 1631 to 1691, John Mayow 1643 to 1679*. Oxford: Clarendon Press, 1908.
2. Trevor-Roper H. *Christ Church Oxford. The portrait of a college*. Oxford: Oxford University Press, 1973.
3. Frank RG Jr. *Harvey and the Oxford physiologists. A study of scientific ideas and social interaction*. Berkeley: University of California Press, 1980.
4. Robb-Smith AHT. Harvey at Oxford. *Oxf Med Sch Gaz* 1957;9:70–6.
5. Keynes G. *The life of William Harvey*. Oxford: Clarendon Press, 1966.
6. Cooke AM. William Harvey at Oxford. *J R Coll Physicians Lond* 1975;9: 181–8.
7. Dewhurst K (ed.). *Thomas Willis's Oxford lectures*. Oxford: Sandford Publications, 1980.
8. Hughes JT. Miraculous deliverance of Anne Green: an Oxford case of resuscitation in the seventeenth century. *BMJ* 1982;285:1792–3.
9. Hierons R, Meyer A. Some priority questions arising from Thomas Willis' work on the brain. *Proc R Soc Med* 1962;55:287–92.
10. Symonds C. The circle of Willis. *BMJ* 1955;i:119–24.
11. Foster M. *Lectures on the history of physiology in the 16th, 17th, and 18th centuries*. Cambridge: Cambridge University Press, 1901.
12. Franklin KJ. The work of Richard Lower. *Proc R Soc Med* 1931;25:113–8.
13. Dewhurst K. An Oxford medical quartet: Sydenham, Willis, Locke and Lower. In: Dewhurst K (ed.). *Oxford medicine. Essays on the evolution of the Oxford Clinical School 1770–1970*. Oxford: Sandford Publications, 1970.
14. Fulton JF. *A bibliography of two Oxford physiologists, Richard Lower 1631–1691, John Mayow 1643–1679*. Oxford: Oxford University Press, 1935.
15. I missed a significant reference opportunity here. At the time of writing, 1986, the only Shakespeare play with which I had any familiarity was *The Merchant*

of Venice, wherein (Act 5, scene 1) Jessica, speaking with Lorenzo, refers to this legend: "In such a night/Medea gathered the enchanted herbs/That did renew old Æson".

16. Webster C. The origins of blood transfusion: a reassessment. *Med Hist* 1971;15:387–92.
17. Keynes G. *Blood transfusion*. London: H Froude, 1922.
18. Maluf NSR. History of blood transfusion. *J Hist Med* 1954;9:59–107.
19. Hoff HE, Guillemin R. The first experiments on transfusion in France. *J Hist Med* 1963;18:103–24.
20. Young blood as a treatment for the diseases of ageing remains a topic of interest in the 21st century. Following animal studies suggesting that aged mice exposed to young blood plasma had improved ("rejuvenated") synaptic plasticity and cognitive function (Villeda et al., *Nat Med* 2014;20:659–63), a trial of young fresh frozen plasma in AD patients ("parabiosis") has now been reported (Sha et al., *JAMA Neurol* 2019;76:35–40).
21. Quinton A. Dr John Radcliffe, the benefactor and his benefactions. *J R Soc Med* 1986;79:380–6.
22. Wittingly or not, a novel set in late 17th century Oxford, *An instance of the fingerpost* (London: Vintage, 1998) by Iain Pears, features Lower and his work but entirely omits Willis.
23. Williams PL, Warwick R. *Gray's Anatomy* (36th edition). London: Churchill Livingstone, 1980.

Edward Tyson (1650–1708) and
The Anatomy of a Pygmie, 1699

Orang-Outang, sive Homo Sylvestris: or, the Anatomy of a Pygmie Compared with that of a Monkey, an Ape and a Man, a seminal work in the history of comparative anatomy, published in 1699, has been suggested as one of the key works in the development of Western thought, ranking alongside those of Copernicus, Vesalius, and Newton. Yet despite these accolades, few may have heard of either the book or its author, Dr Edward Tyson, even though he was a celebrated anatomist. Since his most thorough biography appeared over 50 years ago and is difficult to obtain,[1] it seems appropriate to offer this brief sketch.

Biography

Edward Tyson was born in Bristol in 1650, the second son of a wealthy merchant who twice served as the Mayor of Bristol. After being educated locally, Tyson proceeded in 1667 to Magdalen Hall at Oxford, an exciting time to be at the University, which in the previous decade had witnessed an incredible growth in the study of natural philosophy by the virtuosi, men such as John Wilkins, Robert Boyle, Robert Hooke, John Locke and Christopher Wren.[2] Natural history was not the least among the interests of these men, many of whom later migrated to London to form the nucleus of the Royal Society. Thomas Willis had recently (1664) published his seminal work on neuroanatomy, *Cerebri anatome cui accessit nervorum*, illustrated by Christopher Wren and based largely upon the expert dissections of Richard Lower, with whose anatomical skills Tyson's subsequent studies readily merit comparison.[3]

At Magdalen Hall, later part of Hertford College, Tyson came under the influence of one of the virtuosi, Robert Plot, who encouraged his interests in natural philosophy. Plot's *The Natural History of Oxfordshire* (1677) records Tyson's anatomical dissections of the scent galnds of various mammals, the first comprehensive account of these structures, and also alludes to his eminence in botany. By the time of this publication, Tyson had gained his medical degree and, after 10 years in Oxford, moved to London to develop his medical practice, following in the footsteps of Willis and Lower.

In London, Tyson quickly established contact with Robert Hooke, then Curator of Experiments at the Royal Society, and began to attend meetings of the Royal Society held at Gresham College. In the following year, 1678, his first publications in the *Philosophical Transactions of the Royal Society* appeared: morbid anatomies reporting a horseshoe kidney and, in a human embryo, double ureters and the greater relative size of the adrenal glands compared with those of adults. In December 1679, following Hooke's nomination, Tyson was elected a Fellow of the Royal Society. A brief foray to Corpus Christi College in Cambridge in 1680 to supplicate for the degree of doctor of medicine (MD) was successful but disappointed Tyson, who found that Cambridge dons seemed more interested in having his money rather than questioning his learning.

Returning to London, Tyson continued his programme of anatomical dissections, which was to stretch over nearly 30 years. These works, many published in the *Philosophical Transactions of the Royal Society*,[4] include accounts of the anatomy of the rattlesnake, roundworm, tapeworm, Mexico musk-hog (peccary), and mandrill. There were also monographs devoted to the porpoise (1680), the opossum (1698),[5] and the "Pygmie" (1699; *vide infra*). Other animals dissected, details of which were not published although some were presented at meetings of the Royal Society, included the ostrich, green lizard, bot fly, and, in a comparative study, the lion and the cat. Tyson's philosophy in performing these dissections was the development of a comprehensive natural history of animals, based on the systematic study of single cases, his belief being that careful and accurate descriptions of representative creatures would enlighten the study of related animals.[6]

As a physician, Tyson also made and reported many clinical observations, and had a particular interest in dermoid cysts and stones in the kidney and bladder. As befitting a follower of Hooke, Tyson used the microscope to augment his naked eye observations,[7] and this assisted him in reaching the conclusion that hydatids were in fact a species of worm, and that cochineal was a fly. Yet despite these many contributions of lasting importance, Tyson's eponymous fame (if such it can be called) rests upon his discovery of the mucilaginous or odoriferous glands of the prepuce and corona of the glans penis, an observation published by his colleague William Cowper (1666–1709) in 1694, but never by Tyson himself.[8]

Some of Tyson's dissections were performed in the Anatomical Theatre of the Royal College of Physicians, to which he was elected a Fellow in 1683 and which he served as Censor in 1694. Two further appointments were bestowed in 1684. After the death of Dr William Croone, Tyson succeeded to the Ventera Readership in Anatomy at Chirurgeons' Hall, serving until 1699. Here he continued the tradition, dating back to Dr John Caius (1510–1573) in the mid-sixteenth century, of teaching anatomy through dissection of the human body.[9] He produced a comprehensive (but unpublished) syllabus which amounts to a manual for human dissection.

Also in 1684, Tyson was appointed medical superintendent of the Bethlem Hospital ("Bedlam"), which in 1676 had moved from the site of its original foundation in Bishopsgate to a palatial new building in Moorfields designed by Robert Hooke. Tyson held the post at Bethlem until his death, and was acknowledged to be a humane and caring physician to the mentally ill.[10] Innovations during his tenure included the provision of clean straw for the patients to sleep on, and the employment of female "nurses" to attend the patients in addition to the traditional "basketmen". Feeding of patients with an adequate diet, superintended by the "nurse", was encouraged, and cure of concomitant physical ailments may have accounted at least in part for Tyson's estimate of having cured or relieved two-thirds of the patients admitted to his care over 20 years. A system of aftercare to provide clothes and continuing medication to patients following discharge was also a novel development at this time, somewhat akin to modern day outpatient care. However, this was still a period in which "Bedlam" was a meeting place for sightseers, the fashionable and the curious,[11] and probably little different from the scene illustrated by William Hogarth in the final plate of *A Rake's Progress* (1735).[12]

Orang-Outang, sive Homo Sylvestris

The animal whose dissection Tyson first reported to the Royal Society on 1st June 1698, and which formed the subject of his treatise published the following year,[13] was neither an orang-outang nor a pygmy. The animal had been brought to England from Angola in south-west Africa, probably early in 1698, sustaining an injury during the voyage which was subsequently responsible for its death. There is no doubt from Tyson's description and illustrations (drawn by William Cowper and engraved by Michael van der Gucht) that it was in fact a young male chimpanzee (*Pan troglodytes*). Tyson is explicit about his use of the term "orang-outang" (Malay for "man of the woods") as a general name, reserving "pygmie" as the specific name, in view of the creature's stature and its concordance with the pygmies described in classical literature.

In *Orang-Outang*, Tyson gives a detailed and accurate account of the external appearance, abdominal and thoracic viscera, urogenital system, brain, skeleton, and musculature of his "pygmie" (its skeleton may still be viewed [1999] in the entrance hall of the Natural History Museum in South Kensington, London, as "Tyson's pygmy"). Meritorious though this work is, as the first description of a non-human primate with any pretensions to scientific accuracy, it is the comparative aspect of Tyson's work which renders it of the greatest importance. From the outset, Tyson makes clear his plan of comparing the anatomy of the "pygmie" with that of a man (familiar to Tyson from his clinical work) and of a monkey and of an ape (here he had to rely on the published accounts of others, not having had the opportunity to dissect either; it was not until 1701 that he performed his study of the West African mandrill). This comparative approach allowed Tyson to construct a table of the features in which his "pygmie" most resembled a man (e.g. the hair of the shoulder pointing downwards, that in the arm upwards; the liver not divided into lobes), and those in which it more nearly resembled a monkey or ape (e.g. flat nose, more hirsute). Nearly all of these comparisons still stand, although Tyson did make some errors, for example assuming the "pygmie" walked erect like a man, and had the same number of teeth as an ape (an observational error). As a result of these comparisons, Tyson concluded that his "pygmie" was closely related to man in the "Great Chain of Being" and was in fact an intermediate link in nature's gradation between man and apes. However, he was clear that it was an animal, and not a type of man as the ancients had thought, basing this judgment at least partly upon observations of the animal made during life by the sailors who brought the creature from Africa; they made it a little crib to sleep in but it was "so careless, and so very a Brute, as to do all Nature's Occasions there".

Tyson was not the first anatomist to dissect an ape – certainly Galen had done so centuries before and made errors in his accounts of human anatomy by assuming its equivalence to ape anatomy (as pointed out by Vesalius). Nor was Tyson the first to dissect a chimpanzee, for Nicolas Tulp (Tulpius) had done so in Amsterdam in 1641. Tulp's published account was very brief, but Tyson did borrow from it the title of his own work, *Orang-Outang, sive Homo Sylvestris*.[14] However, Tyson's account was certainly the most detailed study of a non-human primate published up to that time.

Likewise, Tyson was not the first to point out the similarities between man and ape. Forbidden to dissect human corpses, Galen recommended dissecting animals "near to man" in order to understand human anatomy, but included in this category not only Barbary apes but also pigs and dogs.[15] The critical importance of Tyson's work was the demonstration of not merely the resemblance but the profound morphological kinship of man and a "Brute" animal, and hence their relatedness in the gradation of nature. This conceptual development was not readily accepted; almost a century after Tyson's work, James Burnett Lord Monboddo (1714–1799), a Scottish judge, was the object of much contemporary ridicule (not least from Dr Samuel Johnson) for suggesting, in his *Of the Origin and Progress of Language* (1773–1792), a kinship between man and apes, an idea he certainly derived from reading Tyson.[16] However, these ideas were eventually to lead to the theory of evolution as propounded in the works of Charles Darwin and Thomas Henry Huxley in the late nineteenth century. Nevertheless, although Tyson may be Darwin's intellectual forefather, he cannot be envisaged as an unwitting "proto-evolutionist" since, despite delineating a relationship between man and ape, he saw creatures as essentially immutable within the gradation created by God (he was a pious churchman), rather than capable of giving rise to new varieties under evolutionary pressures.

To his work on the "pygmie", Tyson appended a further work, *A Philological Essay Concerning the Pygmies, the Cynocephali, the Satyrs and Sphinges of the Ancients, wherein it will appear that they were all either apes or monkeys; and not men as formerly pretended.*[17] While dissecting his "pygmie", it seems to have occurred to Tyson that this, or a similar, animal might explain the various reports of classical authors of strange man-like creatures, variously named pygmies, satyrs (Tulp called his animal a satyr), sphinges, or cynocephali. He postulated that these reports may have had elements of truth in them rather than being pure fable.

Epilogue

Tyson died suddenly in 1708, while attending a patient. He was buried in the church of St Dionis Backchurch in the City of London, a building probably designed by Robert Hooke in the aftermath of the Great Fire of London.[18] This church was demolished in 1878, and Tyson's memorial, designed by Stanton, was removed to All Hallows Church, Lombard Street, a Wren church, which itself was demolished in 1939. Along with many of the other fixtures and fittings, the Tyson monument was moved to All Hallows Church, Twickenham, where it can now be seen on the internal west wall of the tower.[19] Tyson's portrait by Sir Godfrey Kneller, originally commissioned for Chirurgeons' Hall, now hangs in the Royal College of Physicians, to the right of the entrance to the Council Chamber, facing that of John Radcliffe [1999].[20]

Despite these memorials and the legacy of his works, Tyson remains an obscure figure. Why should it be that Tyson's "name … [is] no longer known to the mouths of mortal men", or almost so?[21] Contemporary references are few: he features not at all in the works of John Aubrey and Samuel Pepys, who certainly knew him through their attendance at the Royal Society, and only glancingly in the diaries of Hooke and John Evelyn. He was noted to be something of a bookworm, opposed to intemperance, and never married.[22] He was remarkable for his taciturnity: during the dispute between the Royal College of Physicians and the Society of Apothecaries (1696–7) over the setting up of a free dispensary by the former, Tyson sided with the apothecaries, which earned him the displeasure of the physician Samuel Garth, in whose mock-epic poem *The Dispensary* Tyson is satirised as "Carus" for his hesitant, deliberating speech.[23] Judging by his multiple publications, Tyson may have been more at ease with the written word than the spoken word, although he did make many oral presentations to the Royal Society. Possibly our ignorance of him is the result of the fact that, as Ashley Montague suggests, during his life few were interested in the kind of work Tyson was doing and fewer still were interested in Tyson.[24]

Acknowledgements

Thanks are due to Ms Ravina Mather for "introducing" me to Tyson and his work in 1987; and to Professor Ian McDonald, Harveian Librarian of the Royal College of Physicians, for permission to view the Tyson folio. Adapted from: Larner AJ. Edward Tyson (1650–1708) and *The Anatomy of a Pygmie, 1699. J Med Biogr* 2000;8:78–82.

References

1. Ashley Montague MF. *Edward Tyson, M.D., F.R.S. 1650–1708 and the Rise of Human and Comparative Anatomy in England. A Study in the History of Science.* Philadelphia: Memoirs of the American Philosophical Society, 1943, volume 20. The author of this work is erroneously given as "Montague MFA" in Morton LT, Moore RJ. *A bibliography of medical and biomedical biography* (2nd edition). Aldershot: Scolar Press, 1994:257. Ashley Montague draws the comparison between Tyson and Copernicus, Vesalius, and Newton, at p.401. Other, succinct, accounts of Tyson's achievements may be found in Munk W. *The Roll of the Royal College of Physicians of London.* London: Royal College of Physicians, 1878, Vol. 1, pp.426–8; and in Lee S (ed.). *Dictionary of National Biography.* London: Smith, Elder & Co., 1899, volume 57, pp.448–9. Neither is without error, as pointed out by Ashley Montague, pp.50 n28, 106, 189 n4, 199, and 200 n90.

2. For a stimulating account of Oxford during this time, see Frank RG Jr. *Harvey and the Oxford physiologists. A study of scientific ideas and social interaction.* Berkeley: University of California Press, 1980.

3. For an account of Richard Lower, see Larner AJ. A portrait of Richard Lower. *Endeavour* 1987;11:205–208. Besides their anatomical expertise and Oxford training, other parallels between Tyson and Lower include their West Country origin, the possession of an eponymous structure of little importance compared with the contribution of their major works, and the almost complete neglect of posterity. Tyson alludes to Lower, in describing the pygmie's heart (p.50): "[he] shewed us the way of dissecting it, and … made it most evident that it is muscular".

4. For a bibliography of Tyson's works, see Ashley Montague MF (op. cit. ref. 1): 462–5. He lists almost 40 publications in all, including 25 communications in the *Philosophical Transactions of the Royal Society*, as well as the three monographs. The Tyson folio of drawings may be viewed at the Royal College of

Physicians of London (MS 618); it comprises 204 sketches, most pasted in, some loose, with a few pages of description, most in Latin. The sketches, not all of which are by Tyson's hand, appear to be in no particular order; few are dated.

5. Tyson's account of a perforated gastric ulcer in the American opossum has attracted some recent attention: Baron JH. Edward Tyson's case of an American with gastric perforation. *J R Coll Physicians Lond* 1998;32:265–7.

6. This is clearly stated in the Preliminary Discourse to *Phocaena, or the Anatomy of a Porpess* ... (1680).

7. Hooke's *Micrographia: or Some Physiological Descriptions of Minute Bodies Made by Magnifying Glasses. With Observations and Inquiries Thereupon* was published in 1665.

8. For Tyson's glands, see Ashley Montague MF (op. cit. ref. 1:206–8). These continue to be referred to by Tyson's name, for example in *Gray's Anatomy*.

9. For John Caius performing anatomies at the Barber-Surgeons' Hall, see O'Malley CD. *English Medical Humanists: Thomas Linacre and John Caius. Logan Clendening Lectures on the History and Philosophy of Medicine, 12th Series*. Lawrence: University of Kansas Press, 1965:32.

10. For Tyson at Bethlem Hospital, see: O'Donoghue EG. *The Story of Bethlehem Hospital from its Foundation in 1247*. London: Unwin, 1914:224–7. Allderidge P. *Bethlem Hospital 1247–1997. A Pictorial Record*. Chichester: Phillimore, 1997:26.

11. See, for example, Silvette H. On insanity in seventeenth-century England. *Bull Hist Med* 1938;6:22–33. O'Donoghue EG (op. cit., ref. 10: 239) mentions a representation to the governors of Bethlem in 1699 regarding public visiting but does not say from whom. Ashley Montague MF (op. cit. ref. 1:348) gives a new regulation instituted at Bethlem in 1699 aiming to exclude "lewd or disorderly persons" and believes this is due to Tyson.

12. Hogarth's 1735 paintings of *A Rake's Progress* may be viewed at Sir John Soane's Museum in London. The print of Bedlam is reproduced in Allderidge P (op. cit., ref. 10:28) and in Bindman D. *Hogarth and his times: serious comedy*. London: British Museum Press, 1997:200 (in its 1763 revision).

13. Tyson E. *Orang-Outang, sive Homo Sylvestris: or, the Anatomy of a Pygmie Compared with that of a Monkey, an Ape and a Man*. London, 1699; 2nd edition 1751.

14. Ashley Montague MF (op. cit. ref. 1:249).

15. Galen. *On the Natural Faculties* III;ii:146–7, cited in Jackson R. *Doctors and diseases in the Roman Empire*. London: British Museum Press, 1988:62. See also Ashley Montague MF. Knowledge of the ancients regarding the ape. *Bull Hist Med* 1941;10:525–43.

16. Charles Dickens refers to the "Monboddo doctrine touching the probability of the human race having once been monkeys" in the final paragraph of the first chapter of his novel *Martin Chuzzlewit* (1843–4).

17. Tyson E. *A Philological Essay Concerning the Pygmies, the Cynocephali, the*

Satyrs and Sphinges of the Ancients, wherein it will appear that they were all either apes or monkeys; and not men as formerly pretended. London: 1699. Reprinted in Windle BCA. *A Philological Essay concerning the Pygmies of the Ancients.* London, 1894.

18. Jeffery P. *The City Churches of Sir Christopher Wren.* London: Hambledon Press, 1996:96.
19. Charles JHA (rev. Stevens GH). *The Parish Church of All Hallows Twickenham.* 1965:16,18. Tyson is erroneously described as a surgeon.
20. Note added in proof: these paintings have now been moved.
21. O'Donoghue EG (op. cit., ref. 10: 25).
22. Contrary to the statement that Edward Tyson was the father of Richard Tyson, which appears in Munk W (op. cit., ref. 1): Vol. 2, p.53, and repeated in the *Dictionary of National Biography* entry for Tyson (op. cit., ref. 1). Richard Tyson was in fact his nephew, and inherited his uncle's extensive library.
23. This is probably an allusion to the Roman poet Lucretius (full name Titus Lucretius Carus, ca. 94–55BCE). His *De Rerum natura* had recently been translated by John Dryden (1685) and would certainly have been known to the literati; Tyson cites it, on the subject of satyrs, in the *Philological Essay* (p.48). Ashley Montague MF (op. cit. ref. 1:322) suggests the use of the name Carus reflects the esteem in which Garth held Tyson, despite his opposition to his stance in the dispensary dispute. However, this may be a double-edged compliment, since there was a tradition that Lucretius was mad (see, for example, Alfred Lord Tennyson's poem "Lucretius" in his 1869 collection *The Holy Grail and Other Poems*), which may have had a greater appeal for Garth.
24. Ashley Montague MF (op. cit. ref. 1:321).

Lord Monboddo (1713–1799) and Charles Dickens

In November 1842, Charles Dickens began his new novel, *Martin Chuzzlewit*, the first number appearing in January 1843. In the final paragraph of the first chapter, "Introductory, concerning the pedigree of the Chuzzlewit family", Dickens wrote:

> … that it may be safely asserted, and yet without implying any direct participation in the Monboddo doctrine touching the probability of the human race having once been monkeys, that men do play very strange and extraordinary tricks.

Although the evolutionary relationship of man and the anthropoid apes is a commonplace today, this passage was written some years before Charles Darwin's publications *On the Origin of Species* (1859) and *The Descent of Man* (1871), and the vigorous public debates on the subject of evolution by natural selection which followed. Thus it is appropriate to ask, what was the "Monboddo doctrine", and what were Dickens's sources for this allusion?[1]

James Burnett, Lord Monboddo (1713–1799), was a Scottish advocate and, from 1767, a judge in the Court of Session.[2] He was an intellectual, devoted to classical literature. As a young man, Walter Scott (1771–1832) encountered him, and speaks of his learning, wit and liberal spirit of hospitality.[3] Monboddo was the author of two multi-volume works, *Of the Origin and Progress of Language* (1773–1792) and *Antient Metaphysics* [sic] (1779–1799). It was in the first of these that he addressed the question of language in apes. His stated belief was that monkeys do not speak not because they are incapable of speech but because they have not been taught to do so.[4]

The stimulus to the development of Monboddo's ideas came largely, if not exclusively, from his reading of the work of the English anatomist and physician Edward Tyson (1650–1708), initially indirectly, via the French naturalist Buffon (1707–1788).[5] In 1699, Tyson had published what may be regarded as the first account of the anatomy of the "Orang-outang" with any scientific pretensions. The creature was in fact a young chimpanzee, which died shortly after being brought from Angola. Tyson performed a careful dissection and noted many morphological similarities between this creature and man. His findings were reported at the Royal Society in London in 1698 and recored in the treatise *Orang-Outang, sive Homo Sylvestris: or, the Anatomy of a Pygmie*

Compared with that of a Monkey, an Ape and a Man published in 1699. Accompanying the anatomical researches, Tyson appended *A Philological Essay Concerning the Pygmies, the Cynocephali, the Satyrs and Sphinges of the Ancients, wherein it will appear that they were all either apes or monkeys; and not men as formerly pretended.* With Monboddo's love of classical literature, this appendix would have been of particular interest.[6]

Although Tyson's work was largely neglected by his contemporaries, Monboddo was "the first person in England [*sic*] upon whose thought Tyson's *Orang-Outang* exercised the greatest traceable influence".[7] He was particularly interested in Tyson's account of the creature's vocal organs, which did not differ from those of man, and also Tyson's (second hand) report that the creature was observed during life to "cry like a child". Hence Monboddo reasoned that, since the animal possessed all the organs necessary for speech, their use for this purpose was simply a matter of appropriate training.[8]

Based on these arguments, the neurologist Lord Brain (1895–1966) labelled Monboddo an evolutionist,[9] but this is not so. Neither Monboddo nor Tyson foreshadowed evolution, since both believed in a divinely ordained chain of being. They had no concept of creatures changing with time, under pressure of evolutionary forces, from one form into another, as postulated by Darwin. The "Monboddo doctrine" was simply, building upon Tyson, that monkeys and men shared many morphological similarities and hence might be considered adjacent in the great chain of being, or of the same stock, without any implication that one developed from or evolved into another.

How Dickens came to know of Monboddo and his doctrine is not known, but the circumstantial evidence suggests that it was second hand. The inventory of Dickens's books from Tavistock House, taken on 27th May 1844, does not include either of Monboddo's major works.[10] Moreover, it is difficult to imagine Dickens wading through the six volumes comprising *Of the Origin and Progress of Language*, which even Monboddo's biographer labels as "heavy, exasperating reading".[11]

The nineteenth century author most significantly influenced by Monboddo was Thomas Love Peacock (1785–1866), the friend of Shelley. In his second novel, *Melincourt*, published in 1817, one of the central characters is an ape who remains speechless throughout. Peacock's footnotes to the novel refer to Monboddo's two major works more than 40 times, although their author is named only once.[12] It is not clear whether Dickens read Peacock: *Melincourt* is not mentioned in the Tavistock House inventory, although in 1837 Dickens apparently requested a complete set of Bentley's Standard Novels which included works by Peacock.[13]

It has been suggested by Lord Brain, himself a student of the medical material in Dickens's novels,[14] that Monboddo is remembered today only because of Samuel Johnson (1709–1784).[15] It would perhaps be more correct to say that Monboddo is remebered because of his fellow Scot, James Boswell (1740–1795), specifically because of his *Life of Johnson*.[16] Like Monboddo, Boswell's father, Alexander Lord Auchinleck, was a judge of the Court of Sessions, appointed thirteen years before Monboddo (1754).[17] Boswell describes Monboddo as "my father's old friend; always very good to me".[18] Monboddo is mentioned several times in the *Life of Johnson*. For example, in a discussion between Johnson and Boswell on the question of the superior happiness of savages, dated 30th September 1769, Johnson asserts that Monboddo "talked a great deal of such nonsense".[19]

More memorable is the meeting between Johnson and Monboddo on the former's visit to Scotland in 1773.[20] On 21st August, travelling between Montrose and Aberdeen, Boswell and Johnson detoured to Monboddo in Kincardineshire where the Lord had his seat. Boswell, knowing of their mutual antipathy, was uneasy about the prospect, and sent a message by his servant to request a meeting, but both Johnson and Monboddo seemed willing to meet, Johnson later observing "the magnetism of his conversation easily drew us out of our way, and the entertainment which we received would have been a sufficient recompence [*sic*] for a much greater deviation".[21] Despite an inauspicious start, when Johnson contradicted his host's opening gambit, Boswell comments that the two men were "liking each other better every hour" and that Johnson was "much pleased with Monboddo". Various topics were discussed, but the nearest they came to the "Monboddo doctrine" was a dispute as to whether savages or shopkeepers enjoyed a better existence, Johnson siding with the shopkeepers largely because Monboddo favoured the savages. However, a few days earlier, whilst in Edinburgh, Boswell and Johnson had talked of "the *Orang-Outang*, and of Lord Monboddo's thinking that he might be taught to speak. Dr Johnson treated this with ridicule".[22] This passage is the clearest exposition of the "Monboddo doctrine" contained in the *Life*. Perhaps not surprisingly, Monboddo was less than happy with his treatment in Boswell's book, subsequently snubbing him in the Advocates' Library in Edinburgh and avoiding any communication with Johnson, even when they subsequently met in London.[23]

Dickens's admiration of Johnson is well attested. He was familiar with Johnson's "opinions and conversation as revealed in Boswell's famous *Life* of 1791",[24] a work whose ten volumes (edited by J.W. Croker, revised T. Wright, 1835) were in his possession according to the inventory from Tavistock House.[25] Parallels have been suggested between Dr Strong, in *David Copperfield* (1850), and Dr Johnson, both lexicographers.[26] Hence, I suggest that Boswell's *Life of Johnson* is the source of Dickens's knowledge of Monboddo and his doctrine, prompting the allusion in *Martin Chuzzlewit*.

A resurgence of interest in Monboddo followed Darwin's publications on evolution in 1859 and 1871. In the *Illustrated London News* of 1862, for example, the Darwinites are described as "reviving the doctrine of Lord Monboddo that men and monkeys are of the same stock".[27] The Free Church of Scotland minister, James Stewart, joining Dr David Livingstone's expedition to the Zambezi River in 1862, noted in his journal on 29th March, during the visit of a group of native tribesmen, "one dandy ... rising to move to another part of the assembly ... presented an appearance which made me think of Lord Monboddo!"[28] However, although Dickens took a keen interest in the subject of evolution, and used it to inform the writing of *Our Mutual Friend* (1865),[29] I have not been able to find further reference to Monboddo anywhere else in his published writings and correspondence. Nor is the Monboddo allusion mentioned in the television dramatization of *Martin Chuzzlewit*, presumably omitted on the grounds of lack of interest to a modern television audience as well as lack of space.[30]

Recently it has been suggested that Dickens was an evolutionist by 1848, more than a decade before the publication of Darwin's *On the Origin of Species*.[31] Although it is moot whether anyone could be an evolutionist before the theory of evolution was enunciated, nonetheless it is argued that Dickens's 1848 review of Robert Hunt's *The Poetry of Science* is the position from which to begin to trace such influences. I suggest that the allusion to the "Monboddo doctrine" in *Martin Chuzzlewit* may indicate that these interests of Dickens in fact date back at least to 1842.

Acknowledgement

Adapted, with minor amendments, from: Larner AJ. Dickens and Monboddo. *The Dickensian* 2004;100(462):36–41.

References

1. A brief article on Dickens's allusion to Monboddo in the first chapter of *Martin Chuzzlewit* has been published: Rosner M. A note on two allusions: *Martin Chuzzlewit*, Chapter 1. *Dickens Studies Newsletter* 1981;12(1):12–13.
2. For Monboddo's life and work, see: Stephen L. (ed.). *Dictionary of National Biography*. London: Smith, Elder & Co., 1886:412–414. Knight W. *Lord Monboddo and some of his contemporaries*. London, 1900. Cloyd EL. *James Burnett Lord Monboddo*. Oxford: Clarendon Press, 1972. Rosner (ref. 1, p.12) erroneously gives Monboddo's date of death as 1770, and gives the title of his work as *Of the Origin and Progress of Learning*. Monboddo was a member of the Canongate Kilwinning Freemason Lodge, where Robert Burns was also introduced; he later wrote an elegy for Eliza Burnett, Monboddo's daughter,

who died aged 24: Chalmers J. Duncan's non-medical clubs and societies. In Chalmers J (ed.). *Andrew Duncan Senior. Physician of the Enlightenment.* Edinburgh: National Museums Scotland, 2010:178–9.

3. Scott W. *Guy Mannering, or The Astrologer.* 1829, II, p.267n.
4. Burnett J, Lord Monboddo. *Of the Origin and Progress of Language.* 1773, pp.270–299, 347.
5. Buffon was a celebrated French naturalist. I am grateful to Professor Malcolm Andrews for pointing out to me that Buffon is mentioned by Dickens in *The Old Curiosity Shop*, chapter 51. Eight volumes of Buffon's *Natural History* (1797–1808) were among Dickens's books at Tavistock House.
6. Tyson E. *Orang-Outang, sive Homo Sylvestris: or, the Anatomy of a Pygmie Compared with that of a Monkey, an Ape and a Man.* London, 1699; republished 1751. For Tyson's account of the chimpanzee, see: Ashley Montague MF. *Edward Tyson, M.D., F.R.S. 1650–1708 and the Rise of Human and Comparative Anatomy in England. A Study in the History of Science.* Philadelphia: Memoirs of the American Philosophical Society, 1943, volume 20. Gould SJ. To show an ape. In: *The Flamingo's Smile.* Harmondsworth: Penguin, 1991:263–280. Larner AJ. Edward Tyson (1650–1708) and *The Anatomy of a Pygmie, 1699. Journal of Medical Biography* 2000;8:78–82. For Tyson's influence on Monboddo, see Ashley Montague, p.290, 409–410. For Rousseau's influence on Monboddo, see: Lovejoy AO. Monboddo and Rousseau. *Modern Philology* 1933;30:275–296. Ashley Montague, p.409n67. The *Philological Essay* was reprinted in: Windle BCA. *A Philological Essay concerning the Pygmies of the Ancients.* London, 1894. See also Ashley Montague, pp.308–345. The skeleton of "Tyson's pygmy" may still be seen in the Natural History Museum, South Kensington, London.
7. Ashley Montague, p.409. Wendy Moore argues that John Hunter (1728–93) discussed the relation of humans and monkeys with James Beattie in 1773, "a full year before Lord Monboddo's shocking assertion": Moore W. *The knife man. Blood, body-snatching and the birth of modern surgery.* London: Bantam Books, 2005:489. As an anatomist, Hunter may have been familiar with Tyson's work, although it has been noted that he was largely uninterested in book learning.
8. Paul Broca's pioneering studies on the neuroanatomical substrates of language were not published until 1861.
9. Brain R. Lord Monboddo: evolutionist and anti-Johnsonian. In: *Some reflections on genius and other essays.* London: Pitman Medical, 1960:101–12.
10. Tillotson K. (ed.). *The Pilgrim Edition of the Letters of Charles Dickens. Volume 4 (1844–46).* Oxford: Clarendon Press, 1977: pp.711–26.
11. Cloyd, p.vii.
12. Garnett D. (ed.). *The novels of Thomas Love Peacock. Volume 1* (2nd edition). London: Hart-Davis, MacGibbon, 1963: pp.91–343, especially chapter VI, pp.127–39. *Of the Origin and Progress of Language* is referred to fourteen times in all, *Antient Metaphysics* twenty-seven. Monboddo is named in the footnote on p.272.

13. House M, Storey G. (eds.). *The Pilgrim Edition of the Letters of Charles Dickens. Volume 1 (1820–39)*. Oxford: Clarendon Press, 1965: p.250n.
14. Brain R. Dickensian diagnoses. *BMJ* 1955;ii:1553–6 (also published in Brain R. *Some reflections on genius and other essays*. London: Pitman Medical, 1960:123–36). Although Lord Brain's interests encompassed both Dickens and Monboddo, he does not seem to have commented on Dickens's allusion to Monboddo which forms the subject of this article.
15. Op. cit., ref. 9.
16. Hill GB, Powell LF. (eds.). *Boswell's Life of Johnson*. Oxford: Clarendon Press, 1950 (henceforward *Life*). Smith-Dampier JL. *Who's who in Boswell?* Oxford: Shakespeare Head Press, 1935: p.67.
17. Martin P. *A life of James Boswell*. London: Weidnefeld & Nicolson, 1999:33.
18. *Life*, V, p.82. Monboddo advised Boswell about potential marriage candidates and discussed Lord Auchinleck's remarriage. Martin, p.253, 254.
19. *Life*, II, p.74. Again indicative of Rousseau's influence on Monboddo. Note that this conversation was prior to the publication of any of Monboddo's works; this may suggest a prior meeting between Johnson and Monboddo, and/or that Monboddo's ideas were already common currency, as perhaps implied by "talked".
20. *Life*, V, p.74, 77–83. Martin, p.306.
21. Johnson S. *A journey to the Western Isles of Scotland*. London, 1775: p.11. Johnson subsequently sent a copy of his book to Monboddo via Boswell; *Life*, III, p.102.
22. *Life*, V, p.46; see also V, p.248.
23. *Life*, IV, p.1 n1; IV, p.273 and n1. Sisman A. *Boswell's presumptuous task. Writing the life of Dr Johnson*. London: Penguin, 2001:114–116.
24. Schlicke P. (ed.). *Oxford reader's companion to Dickens*. Oxford: OUP, 1999:309.
25. Tillotson, pp.724.
26. Wetherill A. Doctor Strong and Doctor Johnson. *Dickensian* 1935;31:59–60. Dr Strong has also been identified with Dickens himself: Welsh A. *From Copyright to Copperfield. The identity of Dickens*. Cambridge: Harvard University Press, 1987: p.116, 119, 121–122, 135, 137.
27. Simpson JA, Weiner ESC. (eds.). *Oxford English Dictionary*. Oxford: Clarendon Press, 1989; IV, p.237.
28. Wallis JPR (ed.). *The Zambesi Journals of James Stewart 1862–1863 with a selection from his correspondence*. London: Chatto & Windus, 1952: p.38 & n.
29. Fulweiler HW. "A dismal swamp": Darwin, design and evolution in *Our Mutual Friend. Nineteenth-Century Literature* 1994;49(1):50–74.
30. Lodge D. Adapting *Martin Chuzzlewit*. In: *The Practice of Writing*. Harmondsworth: Penguin, 1997:230–259.
31. Fielding KJ, Lai SF. Dickens, science, and *The Poetry of Science. Dickensian* 1997;93(1):5–10. See also Collins P. Letter to the editor. *Dickensian* 1997;93(2):136. Fielding KJ, Lai SF. Letter to the editor. *Dickensian*

1997;93(3):205. These debates clearly contradict George Orwell's assertion that Dickens had an "unscientific cast of mind" and that for him "science is uninteresting", at least for biological science. Orwell G. Charles Dickens. In: *The Penguin essays of George Orwell*. Harmondsworth: Penguin, 1991: p.70, 71.

Mrs Elizabeth Inchbald (1753–1821) and Charles Dickens

In his 1848 tour with his amateur theatrical troupe, Dickens "revived an eighteenth-century play entitled *Animal Magnetism*, written at the height of public fascination with Mesmer, and staged several amateur productions with himself in the role of the mesmerist".[1] The use of the term "revived" in this context is unfortunate since, following its first production at Covent Garden in April 1788,[2] *Animal Magnetism* had been performed on several occasions in London, Edinburgh and Dublin in the early years of the nineteenth century. Nevertheless, Dickens's decision to produce this play may occasion little surprise. His interest in mesmerism, or animal magnetism, dating from the late 1830s onwards and developed through his friendships with Dr John Elliotson (1791–1868) and the Reverend Chauncy Hare Townshend (1791–1868), is well attested to, as is the potential influence of mesmerism on his fiction.[3]

Mesmerism was a subject of significant general interest in the 1830s. Basic to the therapeutic system devised by Franz Mesmer (1734–1815) "was the neo-Paracelsian idea of magnetic (or electric) positive and negative forces. These indivisibly dialectical forces of attraction and repulsion … operating though a subtle universal fluid".[4] Mesmerists were apparently able to control these forces by concentration, gaze, or hand movements. As investigations into the nature of electricity and magnetism were central to the academic pursuits of 19th century physics, it is not surprising that the two outstanding scientists of the era, Michael Faraday (1791–1867)[5] and James Clerk Maxwell (1831–1879),[6] both had interactions with mesmerism, if only to confirm that the physical forces they studied had nothing to do with the claims of Mesmer.

In his seminal study of *Dickens and Mesmerism*, Fred Kaplan alludes only briefly and in passing to *Animal Magnetism* and its author, Mrs Inchbald, noting that Dickens had read the play as a boy, citing a letter to John Leach of 1848, and that it was "one of his favorite farces".[7] In his Dickens biography, Michael Slater lists "Elizabeth Inchbald's collection of farces (1806–09)" amongst Dickens's boyhood reading,[8] and Peter Ackroyd suggests that "some of the comic scenes [in *Pickwick Papers*] might have been taken from the farces by Mrs Inchbald".[9] Slater also notes later performances of *Animal Magnetism*, on 5th and 6th January 1857, paired with *The Frozen Deep*.[10] However, little other comment seems to have been made about the connections between Dickens and Mrs Elizabeth Inchbald, suggesting that a brief examination may be worthwhile, the moreso as, at time of writing, the bicentenary of Mrs Inchbald's death (1st August 1821) approaches.

Mrs Inchbald was born Elizabeth Simpson in 1753, near Bury St Edmunds in Suffolk.[11] She seems to have been set on a career on the stage from a young age, despite a stammer, and went to London to pursue her ambitions in 1772, shortly thereafter marrying the actor Joseph Inchbald, who was twice her age. They briefly spent time in France in 1776, which may have afforded her the opportunity to become familiar with the language, a facility of great significance to her eventual career as a writer. She continued to act after Joseph's death in 1779, and had her London debut at Covent Garden in 1780. However, from 1784 onwards her major focus was as a playwright, both translated comedies and farces and her own original works, many of which were produced on the London stage, most being well received. She ceased acting in 1789 in favour of writing, which in addition to her plays included two novels, *A Simple Story* (1791) and *Nature and Art* (1796), and literary criticism, producing prefaces for all 125 plays included in the twenty-five volumes of *The British Theatre*.[12] She died in 1821 and was buried at the church of St Mary Abbots, Kensington.[13]

Elizabeth Inchbald is perhaps best known to readers of 19th century fiction indirectly, through an intertextual appearance in Jane Austen's *Mansfield Park* (1814), chapter XIII, when a staging of the play *Lovers Vows* (1798), freely adapted by Inchbald from *Das Kind der Liebe* by August von Kotzebue, is planned and partially rehearsed but not performed.[14] Inchbald's earlier play, *Animal Magnetism*, was also an adaptation, of *Le Médecin malgré tout le monde* of 1786 by Antoine Jean Bourlin (1752–1828), called Dumaniant, and was well received on its first production in 1788 and revived the following year. She had previously adapted another of Dumaniant's plays, produced as *The Midnight Hour* (1787), with great success.[15] Many of her plays addressed themes of current interest, a fact which undoubtedly contributed to their generally positive reception.

Dickens's production of Inchbald's *Animal Magnetism* encompassed performances at the Haymarket (15th May 1848) followed by Manchester and Birmingham in June and Glasgow in July.[16] The play revolves around a "Doctor" (in fact, a quack) who wishes to learn the art of mesmerism so that he can control and manipulate his much younger ward, Constance, in order to marry her against her wishes. This plan is undermined by a younger lover, whose valet poses as "Doctor Mystery" to teach the Doctor the arts of animal magnetism. Constance and her maid, Lisette, play-act being mesmerised at appropriate moments. The play has garnered some recent critical attention, which notes that the parody accurately echoes Mesmer's own language[17] and satirizes mesmerism as a fraudulent pseudo-science.[18]

Besides his childhood reading, other possible connections between Dickens and Mrs Inchbald may be discerned which might possibly be of relevance to his decision to produce *Animal Magnetism*. In 1833, the *Memoirs of Mrs Inchbald*, edited by James Boaden, had been published by Richard Bentley, not long before Dickens took up the editorship of *Bentley's Miscellany* in 1836. In 1837 Dickens apparently requested a complete set of Bentley's *Standard Novels*,[19] which included (in Volume 26) both of Inchbald's novels, *A Simple Story* and *Nature and Art*.[20] Another stimulus may have been the work of the playwright James Robinson Planché (1796–1880). His play *The Drama at Home, or An Evening with Puff*, produced in London in 1844, featured Charles Mathews, a favourite comic actor of Dickens's youth, in the role of Puff, part of whose dialogue includes the line "You remember *Animal Magnetism*?".[21] If Dickens heard or knew of this, it may have seemed to him an open invitation, a conjunction of his both his childhood reading (Inchbald) and his theatrical inspiration (Mathews). Another Dickens-Inchbald link may have been a shared interest with his acquaintance Leigh Hunt, who quoted from Inchbald's *Nature and Art* in his 1849 work *A Book for a Corner*.[22]

Dickens's choice of producing *Animal Magnetism* may seem an obvious one, and not only because of his known interest in its titular subject matter. The purpose being to raise funds, for the perpetual curatorship of Shakespeare's house, selection of a popular play in the hope of attracting large paying audiences would have been a high priority. In addition, Dickens may have felt some kinship with Elizabeth Inchbald as an actor, perhaps aware that her debut in London was at Covent Garden, the same theatre where he had been scheduled to audition in 1832. It may also be significant that *Animal Magnetism* afforded Dickens the opportunity to appear in the character of "Doctor" (to my knowledge the only role in which Dickens appeared on stage as a doctor). He may have approached this, perhaps subconsciously, as an opportunity to reprise his role as a mesmeric "physician" which he had played for his "patient", Madame Augusta de la Rue, whom he had met during his time in Genoa through her husband, Emile. Dickens mesmerised Madame de la Rue on many occasions during 1844–5. Believing in his powers as a mesmerist, Dickens had undertaken this role with great seriousness.[23] Indeed, a broader argument may be made concerning Dickens in the role of doctor,[24] including his ability, noted by many clinicians, to describe medical conditions, also referred to in his death notice in the *British Medical Journal*. His own experiences with mesmerism may have caused Dickens to relate to some of the action in *Animal Magnetism*. For example, the Doctor's inadvertent mesmerism of the maid, Lisette, as well as the intended target of Constance, was perhaps reminiscent of Dickens's own inadvertent mesmerism of Catherine Dickens on one occasion whilst attempting a long distance mesmerism of

Madame de la Rue,[25] in both instances the mesmeric force acting upon one as well as another.

Whilst *Animal Magnetism* may be seen as no more than a delightful comedy, Dickens's choice might also be seen as problematic, and indeed might in some ways appear counterintuitive. The play does not show mesmerism in a good light, indeed its farcical treatment appears to ridicule the whole notion of mesmerism. More seriously, the Doctor wishes to learn the secrets of the art in order, at least in part, to gain power over his (much younger) ward Constance so that he can marry her against her will. One of the most damning accusations levelled against mesmerism in its London heyday was that it might be put to such unscrupulous ends, male operators taking advantage of mesmerised female subjects. Elliotson himself was subjected, obliquely, to such accusations.[26]

Perhaps it was the case that Dickens had lost interest in mesmerism by 1848 when he first staged *Animal Magnetism*, and so did not much care that it was made a subject of ridicule as long as it afforded a good ensemble piece for his amateur theatricals with the potential to raise charitable funds. However, Kaplan speaks of Dickens's "continued belief in the reality of the phenomenon [of mesmerism] all his life".[27] Moreover, it was three years later that what Slater calls the "only direct literary outcome"[28] of Dickens's mesmeric treatment of Madame de la Rue was published, namely the short story entitled *To be read at dusk*, published in *Heath's Keepsake* for Christmas 1851. The "story of the English bride" was apparently told to him by Elizabeth Gaskell who was certainly furious at its publication.[29] In the part of the short story related by Baptista, a Genoese courier, Clara, the English bride, sees a strange man in a dream before her marriage. This man is then encountered when she travels to Italy, the mysterious Signor Dellombra. Eventually Clara disappears without trace, last seen in a carriage with Dellombra. The presumption seems to be that he has somehow mesmerised Clara ("looking ... fixed upon her out of darkness"), but neither mesmerism nor animal magnetism is mentioned by name.

Further reference to Mrs Inchbald is made in two articles published in *Household Words* in 1853. Although some authors have ascribed these pieces to Dickens,[30] they are in fact by Leigh Hunt.[31] On the subject of Kensington (3rd September; volume VIII, pp.13–17), tight-lacing is blamed for Inchbald's death. It goes on to say of Inchbald (p.15) that "She was a woman of rare endowments - an actress, a dramatist, a novelist - and possessed of virtue so rare, that she would practise painful self-denials in order to afford deeds of charity. Her acting was perhaps of the sensible, rather than the artistical sort; and though some of her plays and farces have still their seasons of reappearance on the stage, she was too much given, as a dramatist, to theatrical and sentimental effects – too melo-dramatic; but her novels are admirable, particularly the *Simple Story*, which has all the elements of duration – invention, passion, and thorough truth to nature in word and deed."

In a subsequent *Household Words* piece (19th November 1853; volume VIII, pp.276–281), entitled Kensington Church, after alluding to Inchbald's grave and its epitaph, the author writes (p.279): "We take the opportunity of observing, in addition to our previous notice of this lady, that although we have spoken but of the latest [*sic*; in fact the first] and profoundest of her two novels, the *Simple Story*; the other, *Nature and Art*, is also full of genius, and would alone have rendered the steps of her pilgrimage in this life worthy the tracing. It is one of the earliest works of fiction in this country that sounded in the ears of the prosperous the great modern note of Justice to All. No reader of the least reflection can forget the impression made on him by the trial of the poor girl, whose crime was owing to the very judge on the bench that sentences her to death."

Dickens evidently enjoyed *Animal Magnetism*, so much so that he directed and performed in several additional private productions, one at Knebworth House in 1850, one at Rockingham Castle in 1851, and four at Tavistock House in 1857. He made one further allusion to Mrs Inchbald, specifically her novel *Nature and Art*, in his memorial piece for Clarkson Stanfield published in *All the Year Round* (1st June 1867).[32]

In conclusion, Mrs Inchbald's plays were known to Dickens from his boyhood and, although any influence on his own writing is speculative, her *Animal Magnetism* provided a vehicle for theatrical entertainment which suited Dickens's requirements as an actor, director, and producer.

Acknowledgement

Adapted with amendments from: Larner AJ. Dickens and Mrs Inchbald: a bicentenary appreciation. *The Dickensian* 2021;117(513):60–66.

References

1. Moore W. *The Mesmerist. The society doctor who held Victorian London spellbound.* London: Weidenfeld and Nicolson, 2017:246. On Dickens's amateur theatricals see Schlicke P. (ed.). *Oxford reader's companion to Dickens.* Oxford: OUP, 1999:12–14.
2. Robertson BP. *Elizabeth Inchbald's reputation: a publishing and reception history.* London and New York: Routledge, 2015:77–83.
3. Kaplan F. *Dickens and Mesmerism. The hidden springs of fiction.* Princeton: Princeton University Press, 1975.
4. Cooter R. Alternative medicine, alternative cosmology. In: Cooter R (ed.).

Studies in the history of alternative medicine. Basingstoke: Macmillan, 1988:63–78 [quote at 66].

5. Moore, 2–3, 73; Cantor G. *Michael Faraday. Sandemanian and scientist. A study of science and religion in the nineteenth century.* Basingstoke: Macmillan, 1991:148.

6. Clegg B. *Professor Maxwell's duplicitous demon. The life and science of James Clerk Maxwell.* London: Icon Books, 2019:53–4.

7. Kaplan, 98.

8. Slater M. *Charles Dickens.* New Haven and London: Yale University Press, 2009:11.

9. Ackroyd P. *Dickens.* London: Minerva, 1990:204.

10. Slater, 417–8. Also Robertson, 81.

11. Jenkins A. *I'll tell you what. The life of Elizabeth Inchbald.* Lexington: University Press of Kentucky, 2003.

12. Robertson, passim, catalogues all these publications and responses to them.

13. Roberston, 22–28, tracked down the memorial tablet, now in the playground of St Mary Abbots primary school. The church has a medical connection, featuring a Healing Window commemorating the eighteenth-century surgeon John Hunter. McHardy G. John Hunter and the "Healing Window" in the church of St Mary Abbots, Kensington, London. *J Med Biogr* 2020:28:96–101.

14. Austen, J. *Mansfield Park* (ed. K Sutherland). London: Penguin Classics, 2003:113–21, 493n1.

15. Roberston, 70–76.

16. Ibid, 81, although Robertson seems to suggest two performances at the Haymarket which is incorrect; see Hanna RC. Selection guide to Dickens's amateur theatricals – Part 1. *The Dickensian* 2011;107:220–7 [at 221–2]. See also Dickens's letters to Julia Fortescue, 12th April 1848 (http://dickensletters.com/letters/julia-fortescue-12–april-1848), and to Charles Evans, 22nd May and 5th June 1848 (http://dickensletters.com/letters/charles-evans-22–may-1848; http://dickensletters.com/letters/charles-evans-5–june-1848).

17. Burwick FL. Inchbald: *Animal Magnetism* and medical quackery. In: Hayden JA (ed.). *The New Science and women's literary discourse. Prefiguring Frankenstein.* New York: Palgrave Macmillan, 2011:165–81.

18. Leach N. Gendering pseudo-science: Inchbald's *Animal Magnetism. Literature Compass* 2014;11:715–23. Leach (722n4) refers to "a [*sic*] performance organized by Charles Dickens in 1857". For a precis of *Animal Magnetism*, see Jenkins, pp.215–20; Burwick, pp.170–7.

19. House M, Storey G. (eds.). *The Pilgrim Edition of the Letters of Charles Dickens. Volume 1 (1820–39).* Oxford: Clarendon Press, 1965: p.250n.

20. Roberston, 129,142.

21. Burwick, 177–8. Slater, 383 notes that in the winter of 1853/4 Dickens produced Planché's *Fortunio and his seven gifted servants.*

22. Roberston, 21.

23. Kaplan, 74–105.

24. Larner AJ. Dickens and neurology. *Brain* 2020:143:1957–61. Many doctors appear in Dickens own works: Waldron Smithers D. *Dickens's doctors.* Oxford: Pergamon Press, 1979.

25. Kaplan, 83.

26. Moore, 200.

27. Kaplan, 234. "Animal magnetism" remained an occasional topic of investigation even amongst orthodox medical practitioners until late in the 19th century, e.g. Charcot's students Charles Féré and Alfred Binet published *Le magnétisme animal* in 1887. See Larner AJ. Charles Féré (1852–1907). *J Neurol* 2011;258:524–5.

28. Slater, 233. This story is not mentioned by Kaplan.

29. Compare Slater, 334 and Uglow J. *Elizabeth Gaskell: a habit of stories.* London: Faber & Faber, 1993:244–5. Mesmerism may possibly have been a subject of interest to Gaskell: Hilton C. Elizabeth Gaskell and mesmerism: an unpublished letter. *Med Hist* 1995;39:219–35. Slater, 233, says of *To be read at dusk* that "Dickens makes the relationship between powerful male mesmerist and female subject explicitly sexual in nature". I confess that, perhaps due a lack of insight, my reading fails to detect this.

30. Roberston, 24 and n123; 31 and n170.

31. I am grateful to Professor MY Andrews and an anonymous reader for correcting my initial misattribution, following Robertson, of these articles.

32. Slater M, Drew J (eds.). *Dickens' Journalism. Volume 4. "The Uncommercial Traveller" and other papers 1859–70.* London: JM Dent, 2000:331,333.

Matthew Baillie (1761–1823)

In the Great Hall of the Royal College of Physicians of Edinburgh (RCPEd), the frieze depicts in carved profiles 15 of the greats of the history of medicine. Amongst the familiar names, such as Avicenna, Boerhaave, Cullen, Galen, Harvey, Hippocrates, Jenner, and Sydenham, one also finds Matthew Baillie (1761–1823), a name perhaps less resonant in the canon of medical history than the others. He never worked in Scotland, let alone Edinburgh, so what is his claim to inclusion in this medical pantheon?

A first-time visitor to the town of Shotts in Lanarkshire, about 30 miles west of Edinburgh and 20 miles east from Glasgow, might consider it an inauspicious location from which to commence a career aspiring to the highest echelons of medicine. Yet it was here on the 27th October 1761 that Matthew Baillie was born, in the manse, the son of the Reverend James Baillie and his wife Dorothea, née Hunter. His mother's maiden name is highly significant in Matthew's biography, since she was the middle sister of William (1718–83) and John Hunter (1728–93), towering figures in the history of medicine (the latter also profiled in the RCPEd Great Hall). Tracing Baillie's biography, he can sometimes appear little more than a bit part player in the biographies of his famous uncles,[1,2] rather than emerging as a figure in his own right. As rather little appears to have been written on Baillie in recent times,[3,4] and as the bicentenary of his death approaches, this seems an opportune moment to evaluate his life and work, mindful as one must be that such an undertaking risks the accusation of "Whiggishness" and that all medical biography is constructed, not least by the subject and his relations.[5]

Early years

Information on Baillie's early years is available in a piece he wrote in 1818 entitled "Some short memoranda of my life", which were published in abridged form in 1896.[6] Some childhood vignettes of Matthew are also available in a memorial by his sister, Joanna (1762–1851), a noted poet and playwright. After basic schooling in Hamilton, he entered the University of Glasgow at the age of 13. His father was appointed Professor of Divinity there in 1775, but his death in 1778 when Matthew was 17 necessitated his uncle, William Hunter, now a leading (and wealthy) figure in London medicine, to step in to pay his fees. After Baillie had distinguished himself in his studies in Glasgow, Hunter facilitated a subsequent move to Balliol College Oxford in April 1779 and obtaining a Snell scholarship there (http://archives.balliol.ox.ac.uk/History/snellexh.asp).

William Hunter's influence determined Baillie's decision to enter the medical profession, his education hitherto having focussed on classical (Latin, Greek) and philosophical studies, science being, in his own words, "very little cultivated at Oxford" at that time. As Hunter was "the relation who had it most in his power to be useful to me with regard to my future prospects, ... this determined me to enter the Medical Profession – I had no strong liking for this Profession ... but I had no dislike to it, and I enter'd upon it willingly".[6] After eighteen months in Oxford, Baillie moved in October 1780 to live with his uncle in London and pursue his studies at the School of Anatomy which William Hunter had founded around 1746 and which he moved to custom built premises in Great Windmill Street in 1767. Baillie first undertook teaching classes there in 1781. He also took classes in chemistry with George Fordyce and in obstetrics with Thomas Denman, whose daughter Sophia became his wife in 1791.

Despite the estrangement of William Hunter from his brother, John, Matthew was able to remain on good terms with both. It was he who summoned John to William's deathbed in 1783, and thereafter ensured that the family estate at Long Calderwood in Lanarkshire which had been bequeathed to him by William should go to his uncle John even though he had not been mentioned in William's will. Baillie subsequently studied under John at St George's Hospital in 1784–5.

Great Windmill Street Anatomy School

Baillie's autobiographical memoranda reported that William Hunter's "manner towards me was never familiar nor warm, but it was mild and kind" and he judged him "probably the best Teacher of Anatomy that ever lived".[6] Nevertheless, William Hunter's will left to Matthew not only the family estate in Scotland but also his entire collection for thirty years, along with £20000 and a half share of the Great Windmill Street Anatomy School, the other half going to William Cruikshank (1745–1800)[7] who had been Hunter's assistant from 1771 and partner in the school since 1774.

The continued popularity of the Great Windmill Street Anatomy School after William Hunter's death was in no small measure a consequence of the excellence of Baillie's teaching. There are no registers available listing the students who attended his lectures there, but some are known, including notable Edinburgh Medical School graduates, such as Andrew Duncan Junior (1773–1832) in 1794, and Peter Mark Roget (1779–1869), later the author of the *Thesaurus*, in 1799.[8] As Edinburgh medical training was far in advance of any other United Kingdom university at this time, the move of these alumni to London to attend Baillie's lectures and dissections may be taken as indicative of the high regard in which such an educational opportunity was held. The polymath Thomas Young (1773–1829), perhaps best remembered for his development of the wave theory of light, also attended Great Windmill Street, in 1793, before he enrolled at Edinburgh University. Baillie was one of those who signed the proposal for Young's election to the Royal Society in 1794, at the age of 21.[9]

The Anatomy School not only provided an income for Baillie but also afforded the opportunity for many dissections which were the basis for his major work, *The Morbid Anatomy of some of the most important parts of the human body*, first published in 1793. In this context, Baillie's close interaction with professional bodysnatchers, as was the case with his uncles, should be noted, although it has been suggested that Baillie was less tainted by this inevitable connection than his uncles.[10] Andrew Duncan Junior notes in a letter of 3rd November 1794 to his father, Andrew Duncan Senior (by then Professor of the Institutes of Medicine at Edinburgh), that "Dr Baillie says there is no managing the resurrection men, one of them called some time ago to see if anything was wanted and atho' several were commissioned, yet nothing has come in".[11]

St George's Hospital

John Hunter's influence could not secure his nephew a physician post at St George's Hospital when he first applied in 1786, but the following year brought the desired appointment. In his autobiographical memoranda Baillie states that "I was not only as attentive as I could be to the Cases of my Patients, but embraced every opportunity of examining the Morbid appearances after death".[6] These studies afforded publications in 1788 and 1789 which facilitated his election to the Fellowship of the Royal Society in 1790, and later the same year he was made a Fellow of the Royal College of Physicians.

Baillie was apparently present at the infamous board meeting at St George's Hospital on 16th October 1793 when his uncle John Hunter collapsed and died. Baillie remained on the hospital staff until 1800, resigning to concentrate his efforts on private medical practice.

The Morbid Anatomy (1793)

It seems highly likely that Baillie would have been familiar with Andrew Duncan Senior's (1744–1828) book *Heads of Lectures upon Pathology*, published in Edinburgh in 1782, as one of the few existing books on pathology published in English. Nevertheless, Baillie was of the opinion that "the Books published hitherto on this subject were too diffuse, and the descriptions of the diseas'd appearances were often indistinct, and very inaccurate."[6] This perception prompted him to compose *The Morbid Anatomy*, based on his immense experience in the Great Windmill Street dissecting room and at St George's. First published in 1793, the book went through several subsequent editions and translations.[12] It was supplemented with engravings, published in fasciculi between 1799–1802 as *A Series of Engravings Accompanied with Explanations which are Intended to Illustrate the Morbid Anatomy of some of the Most Important Parts of the Human Body*. These are based on specimens from Baillie's own collection as well as those of William and John Hunter.[13]

Regarded by some as the first comprehensive text and atlas on morbid anatomy, Baillie's book is perhaps little remembered now, the criticisms of posterity including the absence of microscopical description and of clinico-pathological correlation, although in subsequent editions Baillie did add accounts of symptoms as well as pathological appearances.[14] The *Morbid Anatomy* was probably the first work to illustrate emphysema (or possibly interstitial fibrosis or fibrosing alveolitis), the lungs illustrated perhaps being those of Samuel Johnson (1709–1784), who had been a patient of William Cruikshank,[7] a subject which has been much discussed.[15]

Medical Practice from 1800

In 1799, as his business as a physician began to increase, Baillie "gave up altogether my situation as an Anatomical Teacher" at Great Windmill Street, also in part due to the fact that "my connection with Mr Cruikshank, who had a very odd temper, became more and more unpleasant to me".[6] This increase in clinical practice, which also prompted his resignation from St George's, was in part due to the illness in 1798 of his friend and fellow Scot Dr David Pitcairn (1749–1809), also an Edinburgh alumnus, who recommended his patients to attend Baillie. He also bequeathed Baillie the gold-headed cane, the symbol of physicianly pre-eminence in London, previously held by the likes of John Radcliffe and Richard Mead.[16] Baillie's first appointment to the royal household, to Princess Amelia, came in 1810. Thereafter he was physician extraordinary to the King, George III, and to his grand-daughter Princess Charlotte in 1814. He was in attendance at the latter's lying-in in 1817 which, after a 50–hour labour, resulted in the death of both child and mother, and the subsequent suicide of her accoucheur, Sir Richard Croft, Baillie's brother-in-law.

These were busy years. As his reputation grew, Baillie saw a number of famous patients, including Edward Gibbon, Lord Byron, William Pitt, and

Richard Brinsley Sheridan. Other notable patients may have reached Baillie through connections with his sister, Joanna. As a poet and playwright, she was a long standing friend of the novelist Walter Scott (1771–1832),[10] who requested advice from Matthew Baillie in 1817 for presumed biliary colic.[17] The playwright Elizabeth Inchbald (1753–1821), who consulted Dr Baillie sometime in the second decade of the 19th century,[18] was perhaps also acquainted with Joanna Baillie. She had certainly attended the first night of Joanna's play *De Monfort* and provided a preface for it when it appeared in the multivolume work entitled *The British Theatre* in 1807, opining that it would be "ever rated as a work of genius". It has been argued that the medical careers and interests of her brother and uncles influenced Joanna Baillie, both in terms of career path and subject matter. She dedicated the second volume of her *Plays on the Passions*, published in 1802, to her brother.

Henry Austen, brother of the novelist Jane Austen (1775–1817), was treated by Baillie during an illness in 1801, according to a letter written by his wife Eliza on 29th October: "At length a prescription of Dr Baillie's (who had already tried a variety of medicines to no purpose) removed some of the … symptoms" which had been presumed to indicate "galloping consumption" (tuberculosis).[19] Clery has suggested that Baillie may also have attended Henry Austen during a more serious illness in 1815 when he was being looked after by his sister (Eliza had died in 1813), as a consequence of which Jane, now a published author of three novels (*Sense and Sensibility, Pride and Prejudice, Mansfield Park*) received her invitation to visit the home of Baillie's royal patient, the Prince Regent (later George IV), who reportedly admired her work, and hence gained the dubious privilege of dedicating any future work to him, duly performed with *Emma* (1815), despite her personal distaste for the Prince. It is suggested that Baillie "would have taken an interest in literary ladies" because of his sister's calling.[20]

Baillie is also numbered amongst those general physicians whose practice encompassed home, rather than institutional, care for insane patients from the upper classes,[21] perhaps as a consequence of experience gained in his attendance on King George III. It may have been in this context that Baillie acted as a patron to Alexander Morison (1779–1866), latterly a President of RCPEd (1827–1829), then seeking to establish himself in London.

Character

One indication of Baillie's high standing within the medical profession may be given by the fact that Rene Laennec (1781–1826) sent him a copy of his book on mediate auscultation when it was first published in 1819.[22] Baillie was also the dedicatee of the first edition of John Forbes (1787–1861) translation of

Laennec's book in 1821 (Baillie also provided a testimonial for Forbes in the year before his death).[23] In his translation Forbes noted that Dr Baillie had informed him that he used chest percussion frequently in his practice, and Morison recorded in 1816 Baillie's use of the ausculatory technique (presumably direct rather than mediate) of chest examination. Indeed, Baillie was noted for his "great stress upon the information which he might derive from the external examination of his patient". It is uncertain whether or not an Edinburgh physician of the following generation, Matthew Baillie Gairdner (1808–1888), the first to propose that the second heart sound was caused by closure of the semilunar cardiac valves,[24] was named after his illustrious predecessor.

The encomia of previous centuries often obscure rather than enlighten us as to a clinician's character and clinical method. Despite some errors in his dating of significant events in Baillie's life, Macmichael, writing as the gold-headed cane in 1827, gives information which may have been based on personal observation. He credits Baillie not only with a minute and accurate knowledge of the structure of the human body, as might be anticipated in an anatomist, but also, in consequence, with "the most perfect distinctness and excellent arrangement, in what might be called the art of statement". His utterances were deliberate, easy to follow, and technical terms were avoided. The exertion of common sense was held to be key to successful treatment. However, his manner could be perceived as blunt: "when in the hurry of great business … he was sometimes rather irritable, and betrayed a want of temper in hearing the tiresome details of an unimportant story," an observation to which many clinicians can surely relate.[16]

Final years

In 1806 Baillie purchased an estate at Duntisbourne Abbots near Cirencester in Gloucestershire (https://electricscotland.com/history/other/baillie_matthew.htm is in error with "Dantisbourne"). In the same year his portrait was painted by Thomas Lawrence (1769–1830), the foremost portrait painter in the country (portrait now at RCP London). As per the terms of William Hunter's will, in 1807 Baillie sent his collection to Glasgow University.

Baillie travelled to Scotland in 1809, his first visit there in 26 years: "The Country was much improved, and I met with much to gratify me from the attention of my Countrymen".[6] One such gratification may have been his appointment to an Honorary Fellowship of the RCPEd. This is mentioned in passing in the history of the College,[25] to which more details may now be added. The minutes of the College Quarterly Meeting held on 7th November 1809 record that:

Doctor Spens, Vice President at the request of the President [Dr Charles Stuart], seconded by Dr [Thomas Charles] Hope, moved, that Doctor Mathew [*sic*] Baillie of London should be admitted an Honorary Fellow of the College … which was unanimously agreed to.

A few days later (18th November), Baillie replied, and an excerpt of his letter was read at the Quarterly Meeting of 6th February 1810:

I received the favour of your most obliging letter yesterday and take the earliest opportunity of expressing the deep sense which I feel of the distinguished Honour which has been conferred upon me in being elected an Honorary Fellow of the Royal College of Physicians of Edinburgh. I sincerely wish that I had a better title to this distinction but I hope at least not to forfeit the esteem of the Royal College of Physicians of Edinburgh by any part of my future conduct.

Increasingly Baillie lived in Gloucestershire in his later years, not too distant from his friend Edward Jenner (1749–1823), an erstwhile pupil of his uncle John in London. Baillie died on 23rd September 1823, a few months after Jenner. He was buried in St Peter's Church, Duntisbourne Abbots. More grandly, he also has a bust and inscription in Westminster Abbey, close to that of his erstwhile pupil Thomas Young who died six years later. In a further coincidence, Young's memorial medallion was executed by the same architect, Francis Chantrey, responsible for Baillie's memorial at Duntisbourne Abbots, described as "a plain neo-Greek tablet".[26] Shortly after his death his widow donated the gold-headed cane to the Royal College of Physicians of London,[16] where it remains.

Acknowledgement

Adapted from: Muqit MMK, Larner AJ. Matthew Baillie (1761–1823): from Shotts to Duntisbourne Abbots. *Scott Med J* 2022;67:129–33.

References

1. Moore W. *The knife man. Blood, body-snatching and the birth of modern surgery.* London: Bantam Books; 2005, pp.119,376,383,418,422,460,454–5,460.
2. Bynum WF, Porter R, editors. *William Hunter and the eighteenth-century medical world.* Cambridge: Cambridge University Press; 1985, pp.8,34,40–1,46,118,139,210,228,230,246n116,305.
3. Finkel RI. A memoir of Matthew Baillie. MD thesis, Yale University, 1965. https://ia600600.us.archive.org/25/items/memoirofmatthewb00fink/memoir ofmatthewb00fink.pdf.

4. Crainz F. *The life and works of Matthew Baillie MD, FRS, L&E, FRCP, etc (1761–1823)*. Rome: Peliti Associati; 1995.
5. Nenadic S. Writing medical lives, creating posthumous reputations: Dr Matthew Baillie and his family in the nineteenth century. *Soc Hist Med* 2010; 23: 509–27.
6. Bailey JB. Matthew Baillie. An autobiography, entitled "A short memoir of my life, with a view to furnishing authentic materials". *Practitioner* 1896; 57: 51–65. The memoranda are reproduced in Appendix V of Finkel, pp.120–34. Also in Crainz, pp.7–50, with commentary.
7. McDonald SW. William Cruikshank (1745–1800), anatomist and surgeon, and his illustrious patient, Samuel Johnson. *Clin Anat* 2015; 28: 836–43.
8. Emblen DL. *Peter Mark Roget. The word and the man*. London: Longman; 1970, p.46.
9. Robinson A. *The last man who knew everything. Thomas Young, the anonymous polymath who proved Newton wrong, explained how we see, cured the sick, and deciphered the Rosetta Stone, among other feats of genius*. Oxford: One World; 2006, pp.35,36,38.
10. McMillan D. "Dr" Baillie. In: Cronin R, editor. *1798 The year of the Lyrical Ballads*. London: Palgrave Macmillan; 1998, pp.68–92 [at 71].
11. Chalmers J. Medical jurisprudence and public health. The role of Andrew Duncan Junior. In: Chalmers J, editor. *Andrew Duncan Senior. Physician of the Enlightenment*. Edinburgh: National Museums Scotland; 2010, p.101.
12. Crainz F. The editions and translations of Dr. Matthew Baillie's Morbid Anatomy. *Med History* 1982; 26: 443–52.
13. Spear C, Reilly M, McDonald SW. Matthew Baillie's specimens and engravings. *Clin Anat* 2018; 31: 622–31.
14. Rodin AE. *The influence of Matthew Baillie's Morbid Anatomy: biography, evaluation and reprint*. Springfield, Charles C Thomas; 1973.
15. Sharma OP. Samuel Johnson's lung disease. *J Med Biogr* 1999; 7: 171–4.
16. Macmichael W. *The gold-headed cane*. London: Royal College of Physicians; 1968, pp.152–79.
17. Hutchison R. The medical history of Sir Walter Scott. *Edinb Med J* 1932: 39: 461–85 [at 469].
18. Jenkins A. *I'll tell you what. The life of Elizabeth Inchbald*. Lexington: University Press of Kentucky; 2003, p.494.
19. Le Faye D. *Jane Austen's "Outlandish cousin": the life and letters of Eliza de Feuillide*. London: British Library; 2002, pp.160–1.
20. Clery EJ. *Jane Austen. The banker's sister*. London: Biteback Publishing; 2017, pp.253,257.
21. Scull A, Mackenzie C, Hervey N. *Masters of Bedlam. The transformation of the mad-doctoring trade*. Princeton: Princeton University Press; 1996, pp.137,142.
22. Lefanu WR. Laennec and Matthew Baillie. *Ann R Coll Surg Engl* 1965; 36: 67–8.

23. Agnew RAL. *The life of Sir John Forbes (1787–1861). Royal physician, medical journalist and translator of Laennec – a Victorian polymath* (3rd edition). Shoreham-by-Sea: Bernard Durnford Publishing; 2018, pp.28,36.

24. Nicolson M, Windram J. Matthew Baillie Gairdner, the Royal Medical Society and the problem of the second heart sound. *Proc R Coll Physicians Edinb* 2001; 31: 357–67.

25. Craig WS. *History of the Royal College of Physicians of Edinburgh.* Oxford: Blackwell Scientific Publications, 1976, p.780.

26. Verey D, Brooks, A. *The buildings of England. Gloucestershire I: The Cotswolds.* New Haven and London: Yale University Press, 1999, p.329.

Michael Faraday (1791–1867): "loss of memory" revisited

Michael Faraday (1791–1867) is acknowledged as one of the foremost scientists of the nineteenth century. He is famed for his discoveries of (amongst other things) electromagnetic rotation (1821) and induction (1831) and the laws of electrolysis during a period of over 50 years of experimental work based at the Royal Institution of Great Britain in London. Moreover, through his lectures to the general public, delivered at the Royal Institution, he helped to popularise science, and he also sought to inspire an interest in science in young people through his series of Christmas lectures.

Faraday's life and career have attracted much biographical analysis in the century and a half since his death.[1] It is well attested that in the early 1840s, he suffered some form of illness, a "breakdown" (ref. 2, p.65), which precluded the performance of his experimental work for a period of some 3–4 years and required time away from the Royal Institution to recuperate (ref. 3, p.75). Indeed, an early biographer, John Tyndall, noted that he could no longer engage in society, prompting his description of Faraday as "the great man-child" (cited in ref. 4, p.175). Prominent symptoms of this illness included headaches, dizziness, confusion, and memory difficulties. The nature of this illness has been an occasional subject for comment, some believing that exposure to chemicals (e.g. mercury, aniline) in the course of his experimental work was the cause,[5,6] although the case for such an explanation seems to be inconclusive.

Edward Hare's analysis of Faraday's memory symptoms

In the mid-1970s, the psychiatrist Dr Edward Hare (1917–1996) traced the case notes of Peter Mere Latham (1789–1875), a physician who attended Faraday in November 1839, around the time of what was claimed to be the onset of Faraday's debilitating illness. Using this and the existing sources, Hare made diagnostic formulations concerning the nature of Faraday's illness, focussing in particular on the memory symptoms.[7,8]

In his brief initial report, Hare (ref. 7, p.618) argued that "Faraday's observations on his memory disturbance suggest that it was of the organic type now known as the amnesic syndrome ... which is associated with damage to the hippocampal formation". The transitory attack of vertigo, unsteadiness and strabismus described by Latham in November 1839 was characterised by Hare as a transient ischaemic attack in the territory of the vertebrobasilar arterial system to the brain. Hare suggested that "It is therefore reasonable to suppose that, if Faraday suffered vertebrobasilar attacks, these could account for his loss of memory as well as his bouts of giddiness", and he speculated that carbon monoxide exposure might explain early-onset of atheroma, and hence of vessel narrowing, in the vertebrobasilar system predisposing to these attacks.

In his fuller account, Hare cited many examples of Faraday's memory complaints from his correspondence after 1840, and, basing his formulation on "the present state of medical knowledge" (ref. 8, p.41), reiterated his view of a "transient ischaemic cerebro-vascular attack" to explain the November 1839 episode (ref. 8, p.43). Further, he held that transient ischaemic attacks "could explain Faraday's recurrent symptoms of giddiness, confusion, and headache" (ref. 8, p.44) and now cited the work of Benson et al. (1974) on amnesic stroke secondary to posterior cerebral artery occlusion[9] to justify his conclusion that "the present balance of evidence points to some damage to the memory centres of the brain" (ref. 8, p.45). However, because of Faraday's obsessional traits of character he "became unduly preoccupied with the *belief* – the belief rather than the fact – that his memory was failing" (Hare's emphasis; ref. 8, p.45). Contrary to his earlier paper, Hare did not use the term "amnesic syndrome" in this account.

The purpose of this article is to re-evaluate Faraday's memory symptoms, using the contemporary materials which were available to Hare, but considered in light of changing conceptions of memory disorders and transient ischaemic attacks (TIAs), post-dating Hare's formulation.

Responses to Hare's analysis of Faraday's illness

A number of authors have cited Hare's work on Faraday's "loss of memory". The following does not claim to be an exhaustive survey.

In his biography of Faraday, Geoffrey Cantor (ref. 2, p.282–3) cited Hare's 1976 paper, noting the latter's uncertainty as to whether Faraday's memory problems were due to brain damage. He took the view that Faraday "convinced himself that his memory was substandard" and seemed to favour underlying anxiety as the cause of these symptoms (ref. 2, p.281,283).

Oppenheim, in her work on depression in Victorian England, cited Hare's 1976 paper twice, firstly noting that, at the "start of his prolonged breakdown" in 1839, Faraday "followed Peter Mere Latham's orders and went to Brighton in the hopes of curing an almost incessant headache, accompanied by memory loss" (ref. 10, p.127 and n46). In June 1841, Faraday and his wife undertook a trip to the Swiss Alps, "headaches, giddiness, and loss of memory plaguing him mercilessly" (ref. 10, p.128). Discussing "Faraday's puzzling illness in the 1840s," Oppenheim referred to Hare as "One astute psychiatrist, and historian of psychiatry" and directly quoted his view that, rather than depression, Faraday's symptoms reflected an ""episode of brain damage" late in 1839, specifically "a transient ischaemic cerebro-vascular attack ... in which a part of the brain is transiently deprived of its blood supply"" (ref. 10, p.169 and n76), despite stating in her previous paragraph that "Faraday ... suffered from disabling depression" in the midst of his highly successful career (ref. 10, p.169).

Citing Hare's 1976 paper, Post (ref. 11, p.30) stated that "Faraday had a well-documented transient cerebrovascular ischaemic attack, and, perhaps in relation to this, sustained, many years later, severe memory loss and physical decline". He therefore seemed to accept Hare's diagnostic formulation of the 1839 event.

Citing only the initial (1974) Hare paper, Ohry (ref. 12, p.206) repeated the "TIA ?amnestic syndrome?" formulation. Tweney and Ayala,[13] also citing only the initial (1974) Hare paper, suggested that Faraday's highly developed memory artifacts (viz. his notebooks and records) might have been in part a response to his memory concerns.

All of these authors, with the exception of Cantor, seem to have largely or completely accepted Hare's analysis of Faraday's memory symptoms. Neither Stein[5] nor O'Brien[6] cite Hare's work, perhaps understandably in view of their different conception of the cause of Faraday's memory complaints.

Shortcomings of Hare's analysis

Hare's analysis may be criticised on both historical and neurological grounds. With respect to the former, it is of note that Faraday's memory complaints predate his illness of November 1839, and that his subsequent occupational and social history preclude a diagnosis of an amnesic syndrome.

Hare (ref. 8, p.36) reported that "Faraday's serious complaints about his memory begin in April 1840" and cited many examples of such complaints from Faraday's post 1840 correspondence, although he acknowledged that Faraday "does indeed make several references to his poor memory before his illness of 1839" (ref. 8, p.47). Indeed, Faraday's memory complaints may date from 1812 (letter to Abbott, 12th July 1812) when aged 20 (ref. 8, p.47) or 1822 (letter to Ampère, 26th May 1822) when aged 30 (ref. 13, p.424). Faraday's biographer Pearce Williams was, according to Hare (ref. 8, p.43), of the view that Faraday's memory was always very poor. Faraday's early memory concerns may also be evidenced by his attention to Gregor von Feinagle's system for memory improvement, as noted in his commonplace book in 1816 when aged 25 (ref. 8, p.47; ref. 13, p.429). These activities might be contrasted with Humphry Davy's comment, dated Christmas Eve 1812, that Faraday had given proof of "great zeal power of memory & attention" (ref. 3, p.32, citing *Correspondence* I:17) which undoubtedly aided his first appointment at the Royal Institution in 1813.

Whilst it is certainly true that Faraday's contributions to his diary declined in the period 1840–44, with no entries in 1841 (ref. 2, p.345n69), a number of arguments against a serious loss of memory during this period may be advanced, based on the preservation of some of his social and occupational functions. For example, in March 1840 he discoursed with Grove at the Royal Institution on the correlation of forces (ref. 12, p.205). In October 1840 Faraday became an Elder in the Sandemanian church to which he belonged (ref. 2, p.65) and in 1842 made contributions to services and visited the Sandemanian fellowships in Norfolk and Newcastle (ref. 2, p.67, 68). Despite the paucity of his published work in these years, he nevertheless joined the Chemical Society in January 1842 (ref. 2, p.142). He resumed his work for Trinity House in 1842, and regular research in May 1844 (ref. 8, p.37), making many scientific contributions thereafter, including in 1845 the discovery of diamagnetism. He was able to contribute to the Haswell Colliery Inquiry in October 1844, despite being "at that time afflicted considerably by loss of memory" (ref. 2, p.158). A bibliography of Faraday's lectures and publications is not devoid of material for the years 1840–44, and although 1841 has only two items one of these is a handbill for a course of lectures "adapted to a juvenile auditory" (ref. 14, pp.39–42).

Considering now the neurological perspective, Hare characterised Faraday's symptoms as "loss of memory" which was entirely understandable since Faraday himself used this terminology in some of his letters. To require objective evidence of memory loss or decline would be anachronistic since cognitive testing procedures, including those for memory functions, did not begin to evolve until the late 19th and early 20th centuries.[15] Nevertheless, there are a number of reasons to doubt Faraday suffered "memory loss", let alone an "amnesic syndrome" as understood clinically as a pathology affecting the hippocampal formation or its connections. All Faraday's aforementioned social and occupational activities in the 1840–44 and post 1844 periods would require both the ability to learn new information (anterograde memory) and planning ahead (prospective memory), functions incompatible with a persistent amnesic state. Hare's statement regarding the period before 1839, "I find it impossible to believe that anyone with a pathological degree of memory disturbance could have done these things" (ref. 8, p.47), is surely also applicable to the period after 1839.

A new formulation

What does seem clear from the available evidence is that Faraday consistently made complaints about his memory over an extensive period of time, perhaps dating from his 20s or 30s onwards, and not only during the period 1840–44. Although the latter coincided with a cessation or diminution of scientific activities, this impairment was not persistent as he returned successfully to his work thereafter. In light of this, I venture to suggest that Faraday had a functional cognitive disorder (also sometimes known as "functional neurological disorder, cognitive subtype").

Functional neurological disorders are characterised by inconsistency or incongruence of symptoms. Inconsistency between the presence of subjective memory complaints and the absence of significant objective memory loss is a characteristic feature of functional cognitive disorders (FCD).[16] Individuals with FCD may be able to recall in detail perceived shortcomings of their memory function despite concurrent assertions of memory loss; paradoxically, they are often able to respond eloquently to an inquiry to recount what they have forgotten. Complaints of memory loss should therefore not simply be taken at face value, and are certainly not synonymous with, nor necessarily indicative of, amnesia. Another incongruence often observed in individuals with FCD is the ability to continue working in a demanding occupation without evident complaint from co-workers or managers. It is therefore pertinent to note Hare's report that "even those who knew him [Faraday] well do not seem to have noticed anything really wrong with his memory" and that "between the ages of 50 and 70 his colleagues saw little the matter with him" (ref. 7, p.617; see also ref. 8, p.38).

Current practice aims to establish a positive diagnosis of FCD based on typical clinical features, rather than an exclusionary diagnosis, possibly based on multiple negative investigations for other causes. Certainly Faraday manifested features encompassed in suggested diagnostic criteria for FCD,[17] namely symptoms of impaired cognitive function with evidence of internal inconsistency causing significant distress or impairment in social, occupational, or other important areas of functioning. Moreover, these symptoms are not, I would submit, better explained by another medical or psychiatric disorder.

Why might Faraday have developed FCD? Some possibilities, admittedly somewhat speculative, may be suggested. Pre-existent mood/anxiety problems may predispose to functional neurological disorders (ref. 18, p.170,172). In a brief foray into psychobiography, Cantor (ref. 2, p.283) suggested that "a number of symptoms of which he [Faraday] complained may have been connected with anxiety", including his "loss of memory". Obsessive cognitive styles are also thought to predispose to functional neurological disorders and obsessive traits are common in patients with functional symptoms (ref. 18, p.172,176). Many authors report that Faraday had obsessional traits (e.g. ref. 2, p.283–4,285; ref. 3, p.5,127; ref. 8, p.40,43,45,46).

FCD may reflect dysfunction of metacognition, that is the introspective knowledge or self-awareness of cognitive capabilities, including memory (metamemory), rather than dysfunction of memory per se.[19] Cantor's view that Faraday "convinced himself that his memory was substandard" (ref. 2, p.281) may be pertinent here. Faraday's early interest in a system for memory improvement may be a reflection of this introspection, and his exposure to a child calculating prodigy, sent to him by Davy for investigation, might also have sensitised him to the workings of memory, the moreso as he "failed to gain insight from the boy about how the [mental calculating] tables were constructed" (ref. 13, p.429).

Lest it be thought anachronistic to diagnose a historical figure with a recently described disease category, it is important to emphasize that although the terminology or nosology may be new, the disorder is not: medically unexplained symptoms date to antiquity[20] but their conceptualisation has changed.

As to Hare's suggested mechanism of vertebrobasilar transient ischaemic attacks, concepts about this disorder have subsequently progressed. The classification of vertebrobasilar system TIAs developed by the National Institute of Neurological Disorders and Stroke emphasized the rapid onset of motor dysfunction (weakness, paralysis, or clumsiness) or sensory symptoms (loss of feeling, numbness, or paraesthesia) or loss of vision in one or both homonymous visual fields. The classification noted that whilst loss of balance, vertigo, unsteadiness or disequilibrium, diplopia, dysphagia, or dysarthria were characteristic symptoms, they could not be considered indicative of TIA when occurring in isolation, and that an attack that did not include either motor defect, visual loss, or aphasia should be reviewed carefully before accepting TIA as the diagnosis (ref. 21, pp.653–4). The account of Faraday's acute episode of 1839 does not include unequivocal evidence of motor dysfunction, sensory symptoms, or loss of vision, merely vertigo, unsteadiness and strabismus. Furthermore, TIAs are not expected to present as multiple, recurring, stereotyped episodes. In the rare cases where vertebrobasilar ischaemia causes isolated vertigo this is usually followed within a few days by a stroke.

What of Faraday's other symptoms, in particular the episodic headaches and giddiness? Hare initially dismissed migraine as an explanation (ref. 7, p.618) and subsequently suggested Faraday suffered from "nervous headaches" but "found nothing to suggest these were of a migrainous type" (ref. 8, p.44). However, he does report two episodes of transient loss of vision in the left eye in 1834 (ref. 8, p.45). I think these clinical features would prompt a diagnosis of probable chronic migraine for most neurologists, in which giddiness is often encountered, without necessarily implying the vestibular migraine variant.[22]

Discussion

Any attempt at retrospective diagnosis is, of course, a contentious issue.[23] Muramoto identified ontological and epistemic challenges, as well as ethical issues, when attempting retrospective diagnosis.[24] Faraday's fame, his interest to successive generations, and the many previous attempts at retrodiagnosis, may all be taken as justification for this further attempt.

Prefacing his diagnostic formulation, Hare stated (ref. 8, p.39) that "diseases are continually changing in their manifestations and severity". This sounds like a reference to the ontological argument, questioning whether disease entities persist over time. However, Hare goes on to say that "The symptoms expressed by a sufferer from an illness a century or two ago may be unrecognisable in terms of the symptoms to which the same illness give rise today", which may simply refer to cultural and historical changes in the linguistic expression of (unchanging) disease symptoms. It would seem likely that, human biology being largely transhistorical and transcultural, many disease entities have existed before their clinical description and incorporation into evolving nosologies, rendering invalid the ontological challenge to retrospective diagnosis.

If this be accepted, then the central question therefore becomes the epistemic challenge: how can diagnosis be empirically verified retrospectively? This is seldom possible and certainly not claimed here. Although one can never say never, it seems unlikely that further factual information capable of definitively deciding Faraday's diagnosis will become available. It should be noted that examination of hair samples, should any be available, to search for mercury, as advocated by O'Brien (ref. 6, p.50), would not prove a diagnosis of mercury poisoning, merely confirm exposure.

Muramoto argued that diagnoses are cultural constructs based on hypothesis-making and hypothesis-evaluation, following iterative probabilistic Bayesian reasoning in circumstances of uncertainty, this being the approach used in day-to-day clinical practice.[24] A corollary of this position is that diagnoses are liable to change over time, with new understanding of disease pathogenesis and classification. In consequence, retrospective syndromic diagnosis based on history alone is deemed permissible as an explanatory device, provided that overspecification is avoided. Hence the minimum position stated here, and based on current understanding of memory disorders, is that Faraday's memory symptoms suggest a diagnosis of functional cognitive disorder. Future developments in the understanding and classification of the workings of human memory may render this view obsolete, hence it is offered as a provisional formulation.

In conclusion, a re-evaluation of the historical account of Michael Faraday's memory complaints in the light of current understanding of memory disorders suggests that a diagnosis of functional cognitive disorder, rather than an amnesic syndrome, best explains his symptoms.

Acknowledgement

Adapted from: Larner AJ. Michael Faraday's "loss of memory" revisited. *Journal of the History of the Neurosciences* 2021;30:155–162.

References

1.   Williams LP. Faraday and his biographers. *Bulletin for the History of Chemistry* 1991;11:9–17.
2.   Cantor G. *Michael Faraday. Sandemanian and scientist. A study of science and religion in the nineteenth century.* Basingstoke: Macmillan, 1991.
3.   James FAJL. *Michael Faraday. A very short introduction.* Oxford: Oxford University Press, 2010.
4.   Cantor G. The scientist as hero: public images of Michael Faraday. In: Shortland M, Yeo R (eds.). *Telling lives in science. Essays on scientific biography.* Cambridge: Cambridge University Press, 1996:171–193.
5.   Stein D. *Ada. A life and a legacy.* Cambridge, Mass.: MIT Press, 1985.
6.   O'Brien JF. Faraday's health problems. *Bulletin for the History of Chemistry* 1991;11:47–50.
7.   Hare EH. Michael Faraday's loss of memory. *Proceedings of the Royal Society of Medicine* 1974;67:617–618.
8.   Hare E. Michael Faraday's loss of memory. *Proceedings of the Royal Institution of Great Britain* 1976;49:33–52.
9.   Benson DF, Marsden CD, Meadows JC. The amnesic syndrome of posterior cerebral artery occlusion. *Acta Neurologica Scandinavica* 1974;50:133–145.
10. Oppenheim J. *Shattered nerves. Doctors, patients, and depression in Victorian England.* New York: Oxford University Press, 1991.
11. Post F. Creativity and psychopathology. A study of 291 world-famous men. *British Journal of Psychiatry* 1994;165:22–34.
12. Ohry A. Michael Faraday (1791–1867), science, medicine, literature and his disability. *Progress in Health Sciences* 2011;1:204–207.
13. Tweney RD, Ayala CD. Memory and the construction of scientific meaning: Michael Faraday's use of notebooks and records. *Memory Studies* 2015;8:422–439.
14. Jeffreys AE. *Michael Faraday. A list of his lectures and published writings.* Norwich: Jarrold & Sons, 1960.

15. Eling P. History of neuropsychological assessment. In: Bogousslavsky J, Boller F, Iwata M (eds.). *A history of neuropsychology (Frontiers of Neurology and Neuroscience volume 44)*. Basel: Karger, 2019:164–178.

16. Stone J, Pal S, Blackburn D, Reuber M, Thekkumpurath P, Carson A. Functional (psychogenic) cognitive disorders: a perspective from the neurology clinic. *Journal of Alzheimer's Disease* 2015;48(Suppl1):S5–S17.

17. Ball H, McWhirter L, Ballard C, *et al.* Functional neurological disorder: dementia's blind spot. *Brain* 2020;143:2895–2903.

18. Carson A, Hallett M, Stone J. Assessment of patients with functional neurologic disorders. In: Hallett M, Stone J, Carson A (eds.). *Functional neurologic disorders (Handbook of Clinical Neurology volume 139, 3rd series)*. Amsterdam: Elsevier, 2016:169–188.

19. Larner AJ. Functional cognitive disorders: update on diagnostic status. *Neurodegenerative Disease Management* 2020;10:67–72.

20. Trimble M, Reynolds EH. A brief history of hysteria: From the ancient to the modern. In: Hallett M, Stone J, Carson A (eds.). *Functional neurologic disorders (Handbook of Clinical Neurology volume 139, 3rd series)*. Amsterdam: Elsevier, 2016:3–10.

21. [No authors listed]. Special report from the National Institute of Neurological Disorders and Stroke. Classification of cerebrovascular diseases III. *Stroke* 1990;21:637–676.

22. Li V, McArdle H, Anand Trip S. Vestibular migraine. *BMJ* 2019;365:l4213.

23. Larner AJ. Retrospective diagnosis: pitfalls and purposes. *Journal of Medical Biography* 2019;27:127–128.

24. Muramoto O. Retrospective diagnosis of a famous historical figure: ontological, epistemic, and ethical considerations. *Philosophy, Ethics, and Humanities in Medicine* 2014;9:10.

Samuel Gaskell (1807–1886)

Samuel Gaskell, brother-in-law of the novelist Elizabeth Gaskell (1810–1865), had a distinguished medical career in the 1840s to 1860s in the field of lunacy, what might now be termed mental health. Herein I offer a brief biographical account, and then venture to suggest that Samuel and his work may have had a passing influence on Elizabeth Gaskell's writing.

Biography

Samuel Gaskell (1807–1886) makes only occasional, glancing, appearances in Elizabeth Gaskell's biography: he was best man at the Gaskell's wedding in 1832; an occasional advisor on Marianne Gaskell's health as a child; sometime holiday companion of his elder brother, William, on his walking trips; and a mourner at Elizabeth's funeral.[1] Likewise in the extant correspondence,[2,3] he is only ever briefly mentioned, in letters covering the period 1832 to 1859.

To my knowledge, Samuel has no major biography, but his obituaries in the medical press[4,5] and extant biographical material[6-9] inform us that he was born in Warrington on 10th January 1807, two years William's junior. He had his medical education in Manchester and Edinburgh, but this came about only after a period of some years as apprentice to a publisher and bookseller in Liverpool, William Eyres, Samuel's original wish to study medicine having been thwarted by the family doctor's advice, on account of his poor eyesight apparently caused by an attack of measles. However, the apprenticeship afforded Samuel ready access to medical literature, and seeing his enthusiasm for the subject his employer remitted his apprenticeship.

H.L. Freeman reports that at "the age of 18, he moved to Manchester" and "became apprentice to Mr Robert Thorpe at the Manchester Royal Infirmary. In 1831 he moved to Edinburgh" (ref. 8, pp.89–90). However, John Chapple, whom I am inclined to regard as the most reliable source, reports Samuel was "up in Edinburgh gaining prizes for medicine at the university for two years from 1830" (ref. 9, p.337), based on testimonials from James Syme, a distinguished professor of clinical surgery (he was succeeded by his son-in-law, Joseph Lister, pioneer of antiseptic surgery), and Dr J. Mackintosh, a lecturer in the practice of physic who praised Samuel's service at the Edinburgh Cholera Hospital. Chapple floats the possibility that Elizabeth may have met Samuel in Edinburgh, based on her June 1832 visit at which time her portrait was painted (ref. 9, p.420).

By July 1832, Samuel Gaskell was practicing at the cholera hospital, Swan Street, Ancoats, Manchester, whence he attended Elizabeth and William's marriage in August. Returning to Swan Street, he became embroiled in an unsavoury incident when public accusations amounting to bodysnatching (or "burking", after the events in Edinburgh a few years earlier) were levelled at him and a colleague, charges from which he was eventually exonerated (ref. 9, p.426–8).

The episode is, perhaps unsurprisingly, airbrushed from his obituary in the *Journal of Mental Science*, which reports that once qualified (Member of the Royal College of Surgeons, 1832) Samuel obtained an appointment as Resident Medical Officer to the Cholera Hospital in Stockport.[5] However, whether or not his Stockport days were involved with cholera is uncertain, since he is described as the "House Surgeon at Stockport Infirmary" in an 1845 [*sic*] publication. On 27th September 1844 he presented data to the Statistical Society of the British Association in York on the subject of accidents which he attended as the House Surgeon at Stockport Infirmary, data subsequently published in the *Journal of the Statistical Society of London*.[10] Evidently then, he must have been collecting data during the period 1833–5 (long before the necessity of log books became standard for the purposes of medical training).

Hence, in Edinburgh, Manchester, and possibly Stockport, he had gained experience of cholera, one of the most significant public health issues of the 19th century. He published on the subject of malignant cholera, in a paper dated 22nd February 1834 from Stockport Infirmary.[11] In an 1854 letter (ref, 2, p.305) Elizabeth Gaskell reported Samuel's opinion to be that cholera is not infectious, i.e. does not pass from one person to another, an opinion now known to be erroneous.

The *Journal of Mental Science* obituary then states that in 1834 he was appointed as house apothecary at the Manchester Royal Infirmary and Lunatic Asylum.[5] Presumably this experience engendered or extended his interest in the treatment of the insane, and in 1840 he was appointed medical superintendent of the Lancaster County Asylum following election by the county magistrates. He became an active member of the Association of Medical Officers of Asylums and Hospitals for the Insane, founded in 1841. He gained the Fellowship of the Royal College of Surgeons by election in 1844.

Nineteenth century county asylums were dauting institutions, housing a heterogeneous population of inmates, some suffering from what contemporary commentators called insanity or lunacy (what might now be subsumed under the term psychosis, characterised by hallucinations and delusions sufficient to compromise social and occupational functions) and idiocy (what might now be termed mental deficiency or learning disability), as well as people with epileptic seizures and with cognitive decline resulting from dementing disorders. In addition, forced incarceration of the mentally normal at the behest of their families, for example for pecuniary gain, was not unknown. Institutional abuse of the patients was not uncommon, with poor diet, unclean and sometimes frankly squalid conditions, use of physical restraint and sometimes assault, and little in the way of therapy aside from bleeding and purging. Contrary to the etymology of the word asylum, these were seldom places of refuge, their principal function being custodial.

Samuel Gaskell is credited with ending the system of physical restraint of patients in Lancaster Asylum, one element of the system of "moral treatment" which he promoted, along with the asylum physician, Dr Edward de Vitre (1806–1878). This was part of a revolution in the care of lunatics during this period, which sought not only to abolish restraint but also to encourage recovery from mental illness through the provision of adequate care, diet, and employment, in a therapeutic (i.e. clean) environment with access to exercise and recreation. A detailed study of the Lancaster Asylum records by Walton[12] prompted him to conclude that "[t]he overall impression is of a genuine attempt by the medical officers [Gaskell and de Vitre] to introduce a system of "moral treatment" in the fullest sense, and to change the whole spirit in which the asylum was conducted. There is sufficient evidence to suggest that, up to a point, they succeeded" (p.177). Gaskell is also said to have allocated orphan children to the care of female patients "to develop in the women the great principle of maternal love" (ref. 8, p.90; also ref. 6). His role in the development of mental health services in Lancaster is remembered to this day.[13]

These reforms gained Gaskell notice, particularly that of the Earl of Shaftesbury, which resulted in early 1849 in his appointment as one of the Commissioners in Lunacy, an influential position which he held until 1866. The Lunacy Commission was founded by the Lunacy Acts of 1845 to provide a permanent inspectorate able to visit any asylum or madhouse, public or private, in England and Wales with the power to order changes to patient care if provision was deemed inadequate (a kind of nineteenth century Care Quality Commission, the nearest equivalent organisation in today's health bureaucracy). The thoroughness of Gaskell's inspections was noted, and did not always endear him to proprietors and superintendents of madhouses. He has been described as "possibly the most influential commissioner in the commission's history".[7] His London home was a 2 St James Place.

In June 1851 Gaskell was one of the four Lunacy Commissioners, indeed the nominal head, who inspected Bethlehem or Bethlem Hospital ("Bedlam") in London,[14] the longest standing (founded 1247) and most famous madhouse in the country, which had hitherto been specifically exempted from the Lunacy Acts as a consequence of lobbying by the hospital's influential governors. This exemption was something of a *cause celebre* for the reformers, particularly in light of stories emerging of mistreatment and abuse of patients within Bedlam (perhaps akin to, and recalled by, the final scene of Hogarth's *A Rake's Progress* of 1735).

A highly critical report (Report of Evidence of the Lunacy Commissioners to the Home Secretary on Bethlehem Hospital, contained in the 7th Annual Report of the Lunacy Commissioners) ensued in February 1852 which initiated a gradual process of reform at the hospital. Perhaps surprisingly, the most comprehensive history of Bethlem[15] mentions Gaskell only in passing (and not at all in the index), with the comment on the Lunacy Commissioners that "with Gaskell at their head it was not a group likely to return a favourable verdict" on the hospital. Whatever the procedural shortcomings of the interviewing of concerned individuals, there seems little doubt that Bethlem had a case to answer, and that Gaskell and his colleagues did a service in bringing the hospital's shortcomings to more widespread attention.

Gaskell later published on the provision of mental health services,[16] but a road accident in 1865 forced his early retirement the following year due to "mental infirmity". He died at his home in Walton, Surrey, in 1886. He was described as a "genial and lovable" man,[4] "highly esteemed ... by his colleagues".[5] A Gaskell Medal and Prize was established in 1886 in his memory, administered by the body which later became the Royal College of Psychiatrists.[8,17]

Influence

What relevance, if any, did Samuel Gaskell's career have for Elizabeth Gaskell and her writing? She must have been familiar with insanity and mental deficiency from her own life experience, of family and of parish work in Manchester. For example, "... when I was a girl, there used to be poor crazy women rambling about the country ... they might have been born as idiots ... we called them always "cousin Betty"" (*Morton Hall*, chapter 2; see also *Sylvia's Lovers*, chapter 14, for a further reference to "cousin Betty", a well-known contemporary term for female lunatics).

Elizabeth's Aunt Lumb had married a man with mental illness, a wealthy Yorkshireman from Wakefield named Samuel Lumb. There is evidence, reported by John Chapple (ref. 9, p.88–99), that Samuel Lumb was indeed a patient at the Bootham Asylum in York with a diagnosis of "melancholy" (probably conforming to our category of depression), and later in Leicester, with eventual recovery, but by this time Hannah Lumb had returned to Knutsford. How much Elizabeth knew of her aunt's husband's medical history is, as far as I am aware, unknown.

To my knowledge the insane and mentally deficient, the typical patient clientele of Dr Samuel Gaskell, make few appearances in Elizabeth Gaskell's oeuvre, as the following examples show (this does not claim to be a comprehensive list).

In *Morton Hall* (1853), Alice Carr dies "a poor crazy woman" (chapter 1), which Jenny Uglow (ref. 1, p.473) equates with her being "declared insane". However, in the written account Alice is forcibly bound and abducted by her husband, on the pretence that she is ill ("'It touches her here' continued he, pointing to his head"), on the day of the Puritan preachers' visit to Morton Hall, to be taken to London to see the King's own physician. The tenantry pity Sir John for his mad wife, and thereafter speculate that "she was mad, and shut up in London". It would seem possible to read this as the disposal of a troublesome spouse who is in fact entirely sane (Patsy Stoneman judges her to be so; ref. 18, p.37). The chronology of the story would place this in the later seventeenth century: Sir John is later killed at the Battle of the Boyne, fought in 1690. In passing it should be noted that religious beliefs fall outwith the modern clinical definition of delusion on the ground of cultural sanction.

"Idiots" or "naturals" also occur in Gaskell's works. In *The Well of Pen-Morfa* (1850), Nest Gwynn takes in Mary Williams, variously described as a "half-witted woman", a "poor crazy creature" and an "idiot", who has been beaten and underfed by John Griffiths with whom she has been previously boarded by the parish. Nest receives the same money from the parish but pursues a more caring approach. Following Nest's death, Mary goes to the workhouse.

In *Martha Preston* (also 1850), the eponymous heroine is from a Lakeland Statesmen family. Of note, Gaskell's landlady when staying in Skelwith in Little Langdale near Ambleside was a Mrs Preston, a Stateswoman (ref. 1, pp.231–2, 263–4, 274), and in *Sylvia's Lovers* Bell Robson, née Preston, has a similar background. In *Martha Preston*, Martha's younger brother, Johnnie, at about the age of 16 suffers a raging fever, possibly typhoid, for a period of 20 days, but "as he recovered, his wandering lost senses were not restored" and "stupor remained still upon his poor brain". "Martha knew the truth in her heart, that her brother was an idiot." Martha's intended, Will Hawkshaw, suggests that Johnnie be "shut up in an asylum", the phraseology suggesting the institution has a custodial rather than a therapeutic function, but Martha refuses, knowing the asylum to be a "madhouse", a decision which causes the loss of her marriage prospects.

In *The Half-Brothers* (1859), Gregory (inexplicably Patsy Stoneman calls him Godfrey; ref. 18, p.34), the stepson of one William Preston, is described as "lumpish and loutish, awkward and ungainly", and is labelled "stupid" by his aunt and stepfather. At school he can "never be made to remember his lessons" and the schoolmaster advises he be taken out of school; he proves more successful as a shepherd, and performs a self-sacrificing act to save his half-brother.

Timothy Cooper in *Cousin Phillis* (1863–4) is described as a "half-wit" and makes errors in his labours causing Ebenezer Holman to dismiss him, yet Timothy has the insight to divert carts on Hornby market day so that the sick Phillis is not disturbed by their noise, so he is perhaps not an "idiot" (cf. ref. 1, p.543).

None of these examples provides a very direct or necessary link to Samuel Gaskell and his work, but a connection may perhaps be observed in the revision of *Martha Preston*, which appeared as *Half a life-time ago* in *Household Words* in October 1855 (incidentally the occasion on which Dickens's frustration with Elizabeth prompted his notorious comment about beating her had he been Mr Gaskell). Here, the heroine (no longer eponymous) is Susan Dixon, her brother is Willie, a boy named after his father (names and relationships redolent with personal significance for Elizabeth Gaskell), and her intended is Michael Hurst. As her mother dies, Susan Dixon promises to be a mother to Willie. Later, a feverish illness, possibly typhus fever according to the doctor from Coniston, kills her father and nearly Susan also. On her recovery she is told that "Willie has taken the turn and is doing nicely". However, it becomes apparent that the illness has robbed Willie of the "little wit... he ever possessed", and people fear that he "would end in being a 'natural', as they call an idiot in the Dales". His verbal skills regress, consisting largely of vocalisations, and "he had to have the same care taken of him that a little child of four years old requires". Michael Hurst takes Willie, unbeknown to Susan, to see a Dr Preston, "the first doctor in the county", in Kendal, who is reported by Michael to think that Willie "will get badder from year to year" and advises sending him off, specifically to Lancaster Asylum. Michael, who fears that Willie "may turn into a madman some day", reports that in the asylum "They've ways there both of keeping such people in order and making them happy", but Susan, aware of "stories of the brutal treatment offered to the insane; stories that were, in fact, but too well founded", and of "horrible stories... about madhouses", will not agree, pledging herself to look after her brother, and so her chance of marriage to Michael Hurst is lost.

The reference to Lancaster Asylum in *Half a life-time ago* may, of course, be incidental. There are, to my knowledge, no references in the extant correspondence to *Martha Preston*, and only one to *Half a life-time ago* (ref. 3, p.143), so no particular details of the influences on their composition are available, or likely to be recoverable. Any link is therefore at best conjectural. However, it seems unlikely that Elizabeth Gaskell would not have known that her brother-in-law had worked at Lancaster Asylum for almost a decade (1840–9). The story begins "fifty or fifty-one years ago" which would place it in the first decade of the nineteenth century. This is well before Samuel's medical career and the movement to reform the running of madhouses and the care of the insane. However, as Lancaster Asylum was only opened in 1816, there may be anachronism in the story, albeit that in the period 1816–1840 conditions in that institution were undeniably grim (ref. 12, pp.170–2), and hence all too possibly a subject of "stories of the brutal treatment offered to the insane".

Women taking on the care of fatherless children (*Half a life-time ago*) or those otherwise abandoned (possibly orphaned? – *The Well of Pen-Morfa*) is a feature in some of Elizabeth's stories, a call perhaps to the instinct of maternal love, and hence possibly reminiscent of Samuel Gaskell's innovation in the care of orphans and female asylum patients.

Conclusion

The possible influences of Elizabeth's Holland maternal medical relatives, her uncle Peter (1766–1855) and, perhaps most notably, his son and Elizabeth Gaskell's cousin Henry (1788–1873), later Sir Henry Holland, 1st Baronet, have been previously noted,[19] and there is at least one more clinician in later generations of the Holland family (Charles Thurstan Holland, 1863–1941).[20] It may be the case, based on the account given here, that a clinician from her Gaskell family of in-laws also had a small influence upon Elizabeth Gaskell's work.

Acknowledgement

Adapted from: Larner AJ. Dr Samuel Gaskell (1807–1886): a brief biography, and thoughts on his possible influence on Elizabeth Gaskell's writings. *Gaskell Society Newsletter* 2016;62:11–18.

References

1. Uglow J. *Elizabeth Gaskell. A habit of stories*. London: Faber and Faber (1999 [1993]), 79–80; 105; 109; 448; 455; 616.
2. Chapple JAV, Pollard A (eds). *The letters of Mrs Gaskell*. Manchester: Mandolin (1997 [1966]), 2, 4, 13, 22, 25, 34, 39, 45, 146, 148, 154, 181, 201, 203, 218, 296, 298, 305, 313, 316, 322, 355, 363, 546, 847.
3. Chapple J, Shelston A (eds). *Further letters of Mrs Gaskell*. Manchester: Manchester University Press (2003 [2000]), 113, 117, 283.
4. Anonymous. Samuel Gaskell F.R.C.S. Eng. *British Medical Journal*, 1 (1886), 720.
5. Anonymous. The late Samuel Gaskell, Esq. *Journal of Mental Science*, 32 (1886), 235–6.

6. Anonymous. Gaskell, Samuel (1807–1886). http://livesonline.rcseng.ac.uk/
    biogs/E001972b.htm (last accessed 29/08/2015).
7. Anonymous. Biographies of Medical Lunacy Commissioners 1828–1912.
    http://studymore.org.uk/6biom.htm#M11 (last accessed 29/08/2015).
8. Freeman HL. Samuel Gaskell. In: Elwood WJ, Tuxford AF (eds). *Some
    Manchester doctors. A biographical collection to mark the 150ᵗʰ anniversary of
    the Manchester Medical Society 1834–1984.* Manchester: Manchester Univer-
    sity Press (1984), 89–92.
9. Chapple J. *Elizabeth Gaskell. The early years.* Manchester and New York:
    Manchester University Press (2009 [1997]), 88–99.
10. Gaskell S. Tables of accidents brought to the Stockport Infirmary, and
    attended by the House-Surgeon, in the years 1833, 1834, and 1835. *Journal of
    the Statistical Society of London* 8 (1845), 277–81; http://www.forgotten-
    books.com/readbook/Journal_of_the_Royal_Statistical_Society_1845_v8_1
    000770716 (last accessed 29/08/2015).
11. Gaskell S. An attempt to account for the various methods adopted in the treat-
    ment of malignant cholera. *Edinburgh Medical and Surgical Journal,* 42
    (1834), 75–80.
12. Walton J. The treatment of pauper lunatics in Victorian England: the case of
    Lancaster Asylum, 1816–1870. In: Scull A (ed). *Madhouses, mad-doctors, and
    madmen. The social history of psychiatry in the Victorian era.* Philadelphia:
    University of Pennsylvania Press (1981), 166–97 [esp. 170–83].
13. Fearnley E. Care and confinement: A reflective overview of mental health
    service development in Lancaster and the UK. *Cumbria Partnership Journal
    of Research Practice and Learning,* 4/1 (2014), 56–8 [esp. 57];
    http://wwww.cumbriapartnership.nhs.uk/assets/uploads.cpft-
    journal/CPFT_Journal_4_1_-Fearnley_p56.pdf (last accessed 29/08/2015).
14. Chambers P. *Bedlam. London's hospital for the mad.* Hersham: Ian Allen
    Publishing (2009), 248–9.
15. Andrews J, Briggs A, Porter R, Tucker P, Waddington K (eds). *The history of
    Bethlem.* London: Routledge (1997), 469–73 [Gaskell at 469].
16. Gaskell S. On the want of better provision for the labouring and middle
    classes when attacked or threatened with insanity. *Journal of Mental Science,* 6
    (1860), 321–7; doi: 10.1192/bjp.6.33.321.
17. Tantam D. So you've heard of the Gaskell medal: but who was Gaskell?
    Psychiatric Bulletin, 13 (1989), 186–8.
18. Stoneman P. *Elizabeth Gaskell* (2ⁿᵈ edition). Manchester: Manchester
    University Press (2006).
19. Larner AJ. Headache in the works of Elizabeth Gaskell (1810–1865). *Journal
    of Medical Biography,* 23 (2015), 191–6.
20. Larner AJ. Elizabeth Gaskell and Charles Thurstan Holland – another Liver-
    pool connection. *Gaskell Society Newsletter,* no. 59 (2015), 7–8.

Dickens (1812–1870) and neurology

On Thursday 9th June 1870, the celebrated novelist Charles Dickens died at his home at Gad's Hill Place in Kent at the age of 58 years, a day after suffering a stroke. Perhaps unusually for someone with no clinical qualifications, notices of his death were promptly published in both the *British Medical Journal* (18th June)[1] and *The Lancet* (21st June),[2] the former noting, amongst many other achievements, his facility in the description of medical disorders. Perhaps the most familiar such example of "Dickensian diagnosis" is that of Joe the fat boy, who appears in one of Dickens's earliest works, the *Posthumous Papers of the Pickwick Club* (published 1837, and subsequently known generally as the *Pickwick Papers*): Joe's obesity, ruddy complexion, daytime hypersomnolence, and dropsy later prompted use of the term "Pickwickian syndrome" to describe similar cases, terminology now superseded by "obstructive sleep apnoea-hypopnoea syndrome".

Dickens's interests were very extensive, and these encompassed science as well as literature. An exhibition at the Charles Dickens Museum, located at his former abode in London's Doughty Street, in 2018 was entitled *Charles Dickens: Man of Science*, and was divided into four topics: geology, thermo-dynamics, chemistry, and medicine. Concordant with the breadth of his interests, the latter may be found to include its practitioners and institutions, as well as those suffering illness. Certainly he was familiar with a variety of clinicians, since many "types" appear in his fiction, as later catalogued by another clinician, the radiotherapist Sir David Waldron Smithers.[3] Dickens's own episodes of ill health did occasion some scepticism about doctors.[4] As for institutions, he wrote two articles on workhouse hospitals (Poor Law infirmaries), *A Walk in a Workhouse*, published in his own weekly journal *Household Words* (25th May 1850), and *Wapping Workhouse*, published in his subsequent journal *All the Year Round*, (18th February 1860), as well as a piece on St Luke' Hospital for the insane (*Household Words* 17th January 1852). His interest in and support for Great Ormond Street Hospital is well attested,[5] no doubt related to his care for children, and he also published on the work of the charitable East London Hospital for Children. As for patients, he wrote an article on *The Hospital Patient* as early as 1836 (published in the weekly paper *Carlton Chronicle*, 6th August 1836), the pathos of which might be contrasted with the comedy afforded by the tale in the *Pickwick Papers* told by Sam Weller (chapter XLIV) of the obstinate patient who kills himself to prove that his doctor's proscription of crumpets as unwholesome is wrong. Dickens was also familiar with medical innovations, as evidenced by his insistence, apparently against medical advice, on the use of chloroform to ease his wife's pain during the birth of their eighth child in January 1849.

Unsurprisingly then, Dickens's works have proved of enduring interest for many clinicians, including such distinguished neurologists as Lord Brain (1895–1966) and Macdonald Critchley (1900–1997), both of whom published on Dickens,[6,7] as have John Cosnett (1925–2012), Varun Singh (1948–2019), and David Perkin in more recent times. Another neurological admirer was William Gooddy (1916–2004) who once included a tour of Dickens's London haunts in a Queen Square teaching round. At this sesquicentenary of Dickens's death (2020), this article seeks to explore some possible reasons for this neurological interest, in part through a brief, rather than an exhaustive, catalogue of some of his characters who might be perceived to harbour neurological disorders. I say nothing here of Dickens's own possible neurological problems, since these mostly occurred late in life, post-dating, and hence unlikely to have informed, the majority of his writing.

My own first encounter with Dickens *qua* neurologist may stand as an example. *The Lazy Tour of Two Idle Apprentices* is a facetious account of a trip to the north of England undertaken by Dickens and his friend and co-author Wilkie Collins (1824–1889) in September 1857. In the instalment entitled "Chapter the Fourth" (*Household Words* 24th October 1857), part of the story is set at an inn in Lancaster where Dickens describes:

> A chilled, slow, earthy, fixed old man. A cadaverous man of measured speech. An old man who seemed as unable to wink, as if his eyelids had been nailed to his forehead. An old man whose eyes – two spots of fire – had no more motion that [*sic*] if they had been connected with the back of his skull by screws driven through it, and rivetted and bolted outside, among his grey hair.

> He had come in and shut the door, and he now sat down. He did not bend himself to sit, as other people do, but seemed to sink bolt upright, as if in water, until the chair stopped him.

To a neurologist, trained in the diagnostic skills of pattern recognition, this account may read as indicative of the presence of ophthalmoplegia ("eyes … had no motion"), lid retraction ("eyelids had been nailed to his forehead"), axial dystonia with rigidity ("fixed"; "he did not … bend to sit") and en bloc sitting ("sink bolt upright … until the chair stopped him"), a combination or pattern of clinical features suggesting a possible diagnosis of progressive supranuclear palsy (PSP).[8] This predates the first definitive description of this condition in the neurological literature, by Steele, Richardson, and Olszewski (1964), by more than 100 years.

To be sure, many objections may be raised to retrospective diagnosis of fictional, as for historical, characters, and some may deprecate even the attempt at retrodiagnosis as anachronistic. Nevertheless, such attempts have a venerable history: the anonymous author of the death notice in the *British Medical Journal* opined that Dickens "anticipated Dax, Broca, and Hughlings Jackson, on the connection of right hemiplegia with asphasia [*sic*] (*vide Dombey and Son*, for the last illness of Mrs Skewton)",[1] although this claim is somewhat in error if Marc Dax did indeed describe this phenomenon in 1836 as his son Gustav alleged in 1863 (*Dombey and Son* was published in 1848). Furthermore, neurology and literature may be seen as disciplines that have little, if anything, to do with one another. Is this attempt at retrodiagnosis, then, no more than an amusing parlour game for clinicians insufficiently occupied with other forms of work?

Two major challenges to retrospective diagnosis may be formulated: the ontological and the epistemic.[9] The ontological challenge questions whether disease entities persist over time. Evidently, diseases may come and go (for example, epidemics) even though there is probably little change in human biology over historical time and culture (in other words, it is transhistorical and transcultural), albeit some predispositions or vulnerabilities to disease may vary between times and places. But if it is accepted, as seems likely, that many disease entities did exist before their clinical description and incorporation into evolving nosologies, the central question resolves upon the epistemic challenge: how can diagnosis be empirically verified retrospectively?

This objection, difficult or impossible to address for historical figures, is even more acute for fictional accounts, since literary texts give only a limited view over the reality of the past, the so called "problem of the frame," determined as it is by the author. The text is passive (as Plato notes, in *Phaedrus*, written words cannot answer back when you question them) and therefore permits only a "second hand" form of history taking. Nevertheless, this kind of argument, acknowledging as it does the narrative structure of literary case histories, points up a significant area of overlap between neurology and literature. Medical knowledge, like literature, has a narrative structure, albeit potentially active rather than necessarily passive. Neurologists may understand patient narratives as texts within which particular patterns may be discerned, a process which overlaps with the reading and understanding of literary texts. Hence neurology and literature may be disciplines that, on reflection, have much to do with one another.

Moreover, diagnoses may be seen as cultural constructs, based on hypothesis-making and hypothesis-evaluation, and following iterative probabilistic

Bayesian reasoning in circumstances of uncertainty. This is the approach used in day-to-day clinical practice. A corollary of this position is that diagnoses are liable to change over time, with new understanding of disease pathogenesis and classification. In consequence, retrospective syndromic diagnosis based on history alone may be deemed permissible as an explanatory device, provided that overspecification is avoided.[9]

Clearly, the epistemic challenge cannot be definitively answered for literary diagnoses. Irresolvable differences of diagnostic opinion may therefore occur. For example, Grandfather Smallweed in *Bleak House* (1853), who needs to be carried everywhere and "shaken up" (that is, sat up) at frequent intervals, has been variously diagnosed as having some form of incomplete spinal cord injury (arteriovenous malformation, degeneration, tumour, infection?)[10] or with muscular dystrophy possibly related to progeria![11]

Movement disorders tend to be obvious to external observers, as noted in the possible case of PSP already cited, and hence it is perhaps little surprise that a number of possible instances of such conditions may be detected in the Dickens oeuvre. John Cosnett, a dedicated searcher for medical conditions in Dickens's works, suggested that two characters in *Little Dorrit* (1857) are worthy of note in this context: the description of Jeremiah Flintwinch is highly suggestive of spasmodic torticollis (cervical dystonia), and Mr Pancks manifests features concordant with those of Gilles de la Tourette syndrome:[12]

he ... snorted and sniffed and puffed and blew, like a little labouring steam-engine.

Mr Pancks here made a singular and startling noise, produced by a strong blowing effort in the region of the nose, unattended by any result but that acoustic one.

... Mr Pancks, snorting and blowing in a more and more portentous manner as he became more interested, listened with great attention ...

This account predates the eponymous description by Gilles de la Tourette of 1885. In the same novel, Frederick Dorrit, uncle of the title character, is described as "stooped a good deal", turning round in a "slow, stiff, stooping manner", and speaking with a "weak and quavering voice", features which might suggest parkinsonism. Lord Brain noted that the tremor evinced by Mr Dolls in *Our Mutual Friend* (1865) might simply reflect alcohol withdrawal but might conceivably be essential tremor. In *David Copperfield* (1850), the most autobiographical of Dickens's novels, Uriah Heep's writhings have suggested to some the presence of a generalised dystonia. The sadistic whispering schoolmaster, Mr Creakle, apparently based on William Jones, who owned and ran Wellington House Academy which Dickens attended as a boy, may have a spasmodic dysphonia, and the sleepy waiter at the Golden Cross Inn restless legs syndrome.[13] Cousin Feenix in *Dombey and Son* is described as "meaning to go in a straight line, but turning off sideways by reason of his wilful legs", diagnosed by Lord Brain as an ataxic gait.[6]

Why might Dickens have had a particular facility for description of medical disorders? I would suggest (at least) two reasons. One has already been touched upon, namely his powers of observation. Many references to this faculty may be cited from a lauded biography by Michael Slater (ref. 14; page references in this paragraph relate to this work). Even from an early age a "fascination … with the myriad human life-forms bred or shaped by the city [of London] took hold of him … and found its first expression in his writing." (18) He had "an eye for the grotesque," (32) one aspect of what John Forster, his close friend and early biographer, called the "attraction of repulsion" (18,61; neurological disorders might potentially fall within this category). As early as his Street Sketches of 1834, the "people he presents are … men and women that Dickens himself has actually seen, and heard" (44). His editorial manifesto for the magazine *Bentley's Miscellany* (1836) aims to "set before you the scenes and characters of real life in all their endless diversity" (92). The use of individuals known personally to Dickens as models for particular fictional characters is well attested, such as his own father, John Dickens, as the basis for Wilkins Micawber (*David Copperfield*), and the poet Leigh Hunt (1784–1859) for Harold Skimpole (*Bleak House*). The character of Miss Mowcher, a dwarf hairdresser and manicurist (*David Copperfield*), was based on a Mrs Seymour Hill who recognised herself, both she and her solicitor writing to Dickens, which necessitated a change in the "design of the character" (301,516). Leigh Hunt was also upset by his portrayal. Dickens's commitment to the truth to life of his art as a novelist perhaps underpinned his attempted defence of the demise of Krook (*Bleak House*), by means of spontaneous combustion, in a public argument with George Henry Lewes (1817–1878), a literary critic with some knowledge of physiology.

The second reason for Dickens's ability to describe medical conditions, I would submit, was his interest in theatre. From an early age he was attracted to the theatrical stage, and this became a passion, both for attending and performing in an amateur capacity. Indeed, he considered a career on the stage, only a bad cold, apparently, intervening to prevent a scheduled audition at Covent Garden in early 1832. He later established with various friends a troupe, the Amateurs, who performed various plays, mostly for charitable purposes, with Dickens taking leading roles. The essential theatricality of Dickens's art is well recognised, and he himself once wrote that "every writer of fiction … writes in effect for the stage" (ref. 14, pp.445–6). He was also familiar with medicine, at least in its less orthodox forms, as spectacle, having attended some of the wildly popular public demonstrations of mesmerism given by John Elliotson (1791–1868) at University College Hospital (UCH) in 1838. He evidently became friends with Elliotson, dining with him on occasion (including the night of Elliotson's resignation from UCH), persuading him to examine and find work for an impoverished would-be writer, and taking advice from him on the vexed question of spontaneous combustion. He remained a supporter long after Elliotson's fall from grace, but nevertheless stilll gave an after dinner speech at UCH in April 1864.

Indeed, based on such considerations, one may wonder whether there was something of a clinician, or would-be clinician (even neurologist), in Dickens's make up. His evident observational and descriptive powers put one in mind of Gordon Holmes's words on "what is required of the clinician", namely "In the first place, he must be trained to observe accurately ... In the second place, he must learn to describe observed facts accurately and completely". Moreover, Dickens played the role of "Doctor" in one of the amateur theatricals he staged with his friends, as a mesmerist in Elizabeth Inchbald's (1753–1821) play *Animal Magnetism* dating from the late 1780s, in both 1850 and 1857. He also believed himself to have mesmeric powers, applied to his wife Catherine (initially in March 1842), and on several occasions in 1844–5 to Madame Augusta de la Rue, the wife of an acquaintance first made in Genoa, describing himself on occasion as her "physician".

To my knowledge there is no written evidence that Dickens was aware of the fledgling neurological hospital which opened at Queen Square in 1860, although he was familiar with the location from his London perambulations, as it is mentioned in one of his occasional pieces (*Household Words* 22nd March 1851). However, it is certainly possible, based on his connections with the adjacent Great Ormond Street Hospital and his residence nearby at Tavistock House (later demolished and now the location of the headquarters of the British Medical Association).

In *David Copperfield* there is an account in which some readers have discerned a description of *déjà vu*:

> We have all some experience of a feeling which comes over us occasionally, of what we are saying and doing having been said or done before, in a remote time – of our having been surrounded dim ages ago, by the same faces, objects, and circumstances – of our knowing perfectly what will be said next, as if we suddenly remembered it.

The potential significance of this passage may be heightened by the suggestion, occasionally made, that Dickens himself may have suffered from epilepsy, for example by Matthew Woods (1848–1916), who stated that "Charles Dickens

... had convulsions only in childhood". However, no compelling evidence for this retrospective diagnosis has been forthcoming, and later critics have found nothing in David Copperfield's history to suggest that this experience of "double consciousness" is a result of epilepsy. Moreover, accounts of characters experiencing double consciousness may be found elsewhere in Dickens's works, for example, Oliver Twist, and John Jasper in his final and unfinished novel, *The Mystery of Edwin Drood* (1870). It has been suggested that such accounts might be related to the influence of Dickens's understanding of mesmerism.

Nevertheless, Dickens does write some descriptions suggestive of epileptic seizures.[15] In *Oliver Twist* (1838), Monks is afflicted:

> The man shook his fist, and gnashed his teeth, as he uttered these words incoherently, and advancing towards Oliver as if with the intention of aiming a blow at him, fell violently on the ground, writhing and foaming in a fit.

Monks also has other attacks:

> He remained silent for a few moments, and then removing his hands suddenly from his face, showed ... that it was much distorted, and nearly blank.

Oliver believes the first of these events to be the "fearful struggles of the madman", perhaps reflecting an authorial conflation of epilepsy with mental illness so typical of 19th century conceptions of the disease. Of possible note is the fact that these descriptions were written around the time (1838) that Dickens witnessed the mesmeric demonstrations which Elliotson was using to investigate, amongst other things, their potential role as a treatment for epilepsy. Other Dickensian characters afflicted with seizures include Guster (*Bleak House*), Bradley Headstone (*Our Mutual Friend*), and possibly John Jasper (*The Mystery of Edwin Drood*) in the context of taking opium for pain relief. Dickens was also aware of the risk of sudden unexpected death in epilepsy, various characters expiring this way, for example Josiah Bounderby dies "of a fit in the Coketown street" in *Hard Times* (1854).

Many other neurological disorders have been discerned by clinicians reading Dickens's works: recourse to the medical literature discloses publications on sleep disorders,[16] learning disabilities,[17] and physical disabilities.[18] In the latter category, the most celebrated case of attempted rehabilitation is that of Tiny Tim Cratchit in *A Christmas Carol* (1843). He uses a little crutch and his limbs are supported by an "iron frame". In *Nicholas Nickleby* (1838), some of the boys exiled to Dotheboys Hall are described as "children with the countenances of old men, deformities with irons upon their limbs". These examples may fall within the "child as innocent victim" trope so frequently used by Dickens,[18] and may be a forerunner of the literary examples of temporary childhood paralysis as formative experience dating from the late 19th and early 20th century.[19,20] In *Our Mutual Friend* (1865), Miss Jenny Wren, real name Fanny Cleaver, who works as a dolls' dressmaker, often complains that her back is so bad and her legs are so queer, and requires a little crutch-stick to aid her steps, which is shown by Marcus Stone, one of Dickens's original illustrators (in Book 4, Chapter 9 of Dickens's last completed novel).

Limb prostheses are also reported by Dickens. Noah Claypole, the charity boy who goads *Oliver Twist* (1838) to violent remonstrance whilst working for Mr Sowerberry the undertaker, is reported to be the offspring of a "drunken soldier, discharged with a wooden leg". In *Our Mutual Friend*, Silas Wegg has lost a leg, as a consequence of an unspecified "accident", by means of a "hospital amputation". Little more than a stump, this wooden leg proves a significant hindrance to Wegg when he attempts to climb the dust heaps in search of Mr Boffin's buried treasure. Marcus Stone's illustrations (Book 3, Chapters 7 and 14) show Wegg to be missing his left leg. *Our Mutual Friend* also features a "gruff and glum old pensioner" with two wooden legs, a resident of Greenwich Hospital for disabled seamen. Captain Cuttle, in *Dombey and Son* (1848), has "a hook instead of a hand attached to his right wrist" which conveniently doubles as a toasting fork and is illustrated being thus used by "Phiz" (Hablot K Browne, another of Dickens's original illustrators). Curiously, two other of Phiz's illustrations of Captain Cuttle clearly show the hook on his left hand.

Chairbound characters in Dickens's novels have also attracted attention,[21] examples including Mrs Skewton in *Dombey and Son*, whose chair becomes a wheelchair, and Mrs Clennam in *Little Dorrit* (1858). Unlike the accounts of childhood disability, these adults are often portrayed as having a wilful suppression of mobility or self-inflicted paralysis, reflecting their malevolent inner characters.[18] On a more positive note is the account of a wheeled chair used by Mr Omer in *David Copperfield* (1850) to address his failing mobility, and which he describes as an easy chair on wheels which "runs as light as a feather, and tracks as true as a mail-coach".

George Orwell opined in his 1939 essay on Dickens that he was of an "unscientific cast of mind" and had "little intellectual curiosity," observations perhaps related to an absence of any education in science. Furthermore, whereas "he can describe an *appearance*, Dickens does not often describe a *process*", leading to his characterisation as a caricaturist, and hence "except in a roundabout way, one cannot *learn* very much from Dickens" (Orwell's italics). Any insights Dickens might have had into the workings of the brain are unknown. His attendance at Elliotson's demonstrations seems more likely to reflect the lure of fashionable spectacle rather than any particular interest in the workings of the brain per se. However, Dickens certainly was fascinated by imagination and its role in his creativity, and memory, particularly of his childhood, was critical to many of his novels. It has been suggested that a passage in *Little Dorrit* was instrumental in prompting Sherrington's characterisation of the brain as an "enchanted loom".[22] Moreover, in the Postscript of *Our Mutual Friend*, Dickens refers to himself as "the story-weaver at his loom".

Hence, Macdonald Critchley's statement that "Both as a stylist, and as a recorder of the *comédie humaine*, Charles Dickens is still insufficiently acclaimed"[7] may still hold currency. It seems likely that Dickens may continue to be read with interest and profit by neurologists (and non-neurologists) for many years to come.

Acknowledgement

Adapted and extended from: Larner AJ. Dickens and neurology. *Brain* 2020;143:1957–61.

References

1. Anon. Charles Dickens. *Br Med J* 1870;i:636.
2. Anon. Charles Dickens. *Lancet* 1870;i:882.
3. Smithers DW. *Dickens's doctors*. Oxford: Pergamon Press, 1979.
4. Hunting P. Charles Dickens (1812–1870): 'The longer I live the more I doubt the doctors'. *J Med Biogr* 2012;20:182–3.
5. Kosky J. *Mutual friends. Charles Dickens and Great Ormond Street Children's Hospital*. New York: St Martin's Press, 1989.
6. Brain R. *Some reflections on genius and other essays*. London: Pitman Medical, 1960:123–36.
7. Critchley M. *The divine banquet of the brain and other essays*. New York: Raven Press, 1979:136–40.
8. Larner AJ. Did Charles Dickens describe progressive supranuclear palsy in 1857? *Mov Disord* 2002;17:832–3.
9. Muramoto O. Retrospective diagnosis of a famous historical figure: ontological, epistemic, and ethical considerations. *Philos Ethics Humanit Med* 2014;9:10.
10. Ohry A. "Shake me up, Judy!": on Dickens, medicine and spinal cord disorders. *Ortop Traumatol Rehabil* 2012;14:483–91.
11. Singh V. Reflections: neurology and the humanities. Description of a family with progeria by Charles Dickens. *Neurology* 2010;75:571.
12. Cosnett JE. Dickens, dystonia and dyskinesia. *J Neurol Neurosurg Psychiatry* 1991;54:184.

13. Garcia Ruiz PJ, Gulliksen LL. Movement disorders in David Copperfield. *Neurologia* 1999;14:359–60.
14. Slater M. *Charles Dickens*. New Haven and London: Yale University Press, 2009.
15. Larner AJ. Charles Dickens (1812–1870) and epilepsy. *Epilepsy Behav* 2012;24:422–5.
16. Cosnett J. Charles Dickens and sleep disorders. *Dickensian* 1997;93(3):200–4.
17. Grove T. Barnaby Rudge: a case study in autism. *Dickensian* 1987;83:139–48.
18. Wainapel SF. Dickens and disability. *Disabil Rehabil* 1996;18:629–32.
19. Keith L. *Take up thy bed and walk: death, disability and cure in classic fiction for girls*. London: Routledge, 2001.
20. Larner AJ. Some literary accounts of possible childhood paraplegia and neurorehabilitation. *Dev Neurorehabil* 2009;12:248–52.
21. Lesser MJ. Dickens and the chairbound. *Dickensian* 1977;73(1):25–32.
22. O'Brien J, Bracewell RM. A Dickensian origin for Sherrington's enchanted loom? *J R Coll Physicians Edinb* 2015;45:236–7.

William Carpenter (1813–1885): a scientific influence on Elizabeth Gaskell?

In his article on Charles Darwin and Mrs Gaskell,[1] Gordon Chancellor mentions in passing his fascination with "Elizabeth's friendship with the leading Unitarian physiologist and marine biologist William Benjamin Carpenter". Having a similar interest, I venture to share some preliminary findings in the hope that they might be of interest.

Son of the Unitarian preacher Lant Carpenter (1780–1840), William Benjamin Carpenter was born in Exeter in 1813. He studied in Bristol, London, and Edinburgh, where he undertook microscopical research on the nervous system of invertebrates. This work led to his election as a fellow of the Royal Society in 1844 and also to appointment as Fullerian Professor of Physiology at the Royal Institution in London (Michael Faraday was also at the Royal Institution at this time). For many years he was registrar of the University of London. Carpenter was a prolific author, writing textbooks on human and animal physiology (he was cited frequently by John Hughlings Jackson[2]), and in later life on mental physiology (1875) and Mesmerism (1877). Despite his principal interest being marine zoology, probably his most noted publication was the 1850 essay entitled *The use and abuse of alcoholic liquors in health and disease* in which he attempted to show that "occasional moderate use, so far from promoting the health and vigour of the human frame, ... is, on the contrary, under all circumstances, rather injurious than beneficial". He remained a member of the Unitarian church throughout his life.

A few references to William Carpenter appear in the published Gaskell correspondence. He evidently stayed with the Gaskells at Plymouth Grove from Thursday 27th March 1851, this visit anticipated in Elizabeth's letters to her daughter Marianne of 10th and 17th March (Letters 91a, 91b).[3] On Friday 28th March (Letter 92) she tells Marianne that "Dr Carpenter is staying here; he lectures on Fridays & Mondays; and between Mondays and Fridays he goes to Hale to lecture there. He is going to Warrington for next Sunday".[4]

These lectures were, according to William Axon, on the subject of "Microscopic Research" and commenced on March 28th in the Royal Manchester Institution.[5] Although Carpenter's lectures are noted in Uglow's biography,[6] it is not clear whether or not Elizabeth attended these. Andrew Mangham states that "Elizabeth attended one lecture on Microscopical Research"[7] but I can find nothing specifically to that effect in his cited source.[8]

An invitation "to tea on Friday Evening next" addressed to Mrs Susanna Schunck from Elizabeth, dated 2nd April 1851, states that "Dr Wm Carpenter will be staying with us".[9] It may be that Dr Samuel Gaskell, by this time working as one of the Lunacy Commissioners based in London,[10] was also present at this gathering, since in Elizabeth's letter to Marianne of the previous Friday (28th March) she says "Uncle Sam is coming on Friday",[11] just before the mention that Dr Carpenter is staying with them. On 17th April 1851 Elizabeth excuses herself to Marianne for not writing because, amongst other things, "Dr Carpenter was here" (Letter 94).[12]

Aside from this visit, there are only glancing references to Carpenter in the correspondence. Marianne apparently visited the family in London in November 1851 (Letter 107), and Elizabeth "left Mrs Hensleigh Wedgwood's card with mine at the Carpenter's" in July 1855 (Letter 259).[13] William's sister, Mary Carpenter (1807–1877), a noted educational reformer based in Bristol, was the addressee of one letter from Elizabeth (Letter 138).[14] Their father, Lant Carpenter, was well known in Unitarian circles for his educational work in Exeter and Bristol and was also, like his son, active in the affairs of the British Association for the Advancement of Science.[15]

So what might Elizabeth have learned from Dr Carpenter, either during his visit to her home in 1851 or, possibly, from reading his books? Jill Matus, discussing *North and South*, has observed that "the narrator draws consistently on the language of dream and trance" and that "[t]his focus puts Gaskell in the company of mid-century mental physiologists such as William Carpenter, a Unitarian and one of Gaskell's acquaintances".[16] Carpenter's work specifically referred to is the fifth edition of the *Principles of Human Physiology* published in 1855, wherein he used the term "unconscious cerebration" to indicate that much human cognitive function operates outside awareness (an idea which is now a commonplace). In this context, it would be interesting to know if any of Carpenter's books was available in the Portico library and, if so, borrowed by William Gaskell.

In the absence of definite evidence, any other possible influence of Carpenter on Elizabeth and her work must needs be speculative, but I venture to suggest two possible ways. Concerning the perils of alcohol, as described in Carpenter's 1850 book, these were of course already familiar to Elizabeth as portrayed in the character of Esther in *Mary Barton* (1848), but may have contributed to the description of Edward Wilkins in *A dark night's work* (1863) as he gradually sinks deeper into alcohol misuse to the horror of his daughter and the chagrin of his intended son-in-law. Through her friendship with Charlotte Brontë, Elizabeth was evidently aware of Branwell Brontë's intemperance, eventually leading to alcohol addiction.[17]

As regards Carpenter's visit of 1851 it might be surmised that, since the subject of his lectures was "Microscopic Research",[5] this topic might have been discussed at Plymouth Grove. Carpenter's entry in the *Oxford Dictionary of National Biography* states that he was "a leading popularizer of the microscope" and in 1856 he published a book entitled *The microscope and its revelations*. The prevailing view is that Elizabeth deliberately modelled the career of Roger Hamley in *Wives and Daughters* (1866) on that of Charles Darwin,[18–20] based no doubt on her letter (550) to George Smith of May 1864 outlining the novel, suggesting that Roger has "a large offer to go around the world (like Charles Darwin) as naturalist".[21] Nevertheless I suggest that Carpenter and his work may have contributed to the portrayal of Roger (e.g. "That evening he adjusted his microscope …"),[22] albeit many years after his visit to the Gaskells.

Acknowledgement

Adapted and extended from: Larner AJ. *Gaskell Society Newsletter* 2023; 75: 10–14.

References

1. Chancellor G. Mr Darwin and Mrs Gaskell – a tale of two storytellers. *Gaskell Society Newsletter* 2022; 74: 17–22 [at 19].
2. Greenblatt SH. *John Hughlings Jackson. Clinical neurology, evolution, and Victorian brain science*. Oxford: Oxford University Press, 2022.
3. Chapple JAV, Pollard A (eds). *The letters of Mrs Gaskell*. Manchester: Mandolin (1997 [1966]), 830–2 [at 831], 832–4 [at 833].
4. Ibid., 146–7 [at 146].
5. Axon WEA (ed.). *The annals of Manchester: a chronological record from the earliest times to the end of 1885*. Manchester: John Heywood (1886), 256.
6. Uglow J. *Elizabeth Gaskell. A habit of stories*. London: Faber and Faber (1999 [1993]), 270.
7. Mangham A. *The science of starving in Victorian literature, medicine, and political economy*. Oxford: Oxford University Press (2020), 116.
8. Henson L. The "Condition-of-England" debate and the "Natural History of Man": an important scientific context for the social-problem fiction of Elizabeth Gaskell. *Gaskell Society Journal* 2002; 30–47 [at 30].
9. Chapple J, Shelston A (eds). *Further letters of Mrs Gaskell*. Manchester: Manchester University Press (2003 [2000]), 55.
10. Larner AJ. Dr Samuel Gaskell (1808–1886): a brief biography, and thoughts on his possible influence on Elizabeth Gaskell's writings. *Gaskell Society Newsletter* 2016; 62: 11–18.
11. Chapple and Pollard, 146–7 [at 146].
12. Ibid., 149–51 [at 149].
13. Ibid., 169–70 [at 170] and 363–5 [at 364].

14. Ibid., 206–7.
15, Chapple J. *Elizabeth Gaskell. The early years.* Manchester: Manchester University Press (2009 [1997]), 140, 142, 242.
16. Matus JL. *Mary Barton* and *North and South.* In: Matus JL (ed). *The Cambridge Companion to Elizabeth Gaskell.* Cambridge, Cambridge University Press (2007), 27–45 [at 37, 40, 41].
17. Easson A (ed). *Elizabeth Gaskell. The life of Charlotte Brontë.* Oxford: Oxford World's Classics (2009 [1857]), 226–7, 237.
18. Morris P (ed). *Elizabeth Gaskell. Wives and Daughters.* London: Penguin Classics (2003 [1866]), xxv, xxxii.
19. Hughes LK. *Cousin Phillis, Wives and Daughters,* and modernity. In: Matus JL (ed). *The Cambridge Companion to Elizabeth Gaskell.* Cambridge, Cambridge University Press (2007), 90–107 [at 98].
20. Henry N. Elizabeth Gaskell and social transformation. In: Matus JL (ed). *The Cambridge Companion to Elizabeth Gaskell.* Cambridge, Cambridge University Press (2007), 148–63 [at 162].
21. Chapple and Pollard, 731–2 [at 732].
22. Morris, 120.

William Alexander (1844–1919): epilepsy care in Liverpool in the late 19th century

William Alexander (1844–1919) is a name sometimes cited in histories of Liverpool medicine and surgery,[1] but he is probably unfamiliar to most. Over 25 years ago, John Ross described him as a "forgotten pioneer"[2] and this analysis, to my way of thinking, still prevails. He is a figure of interest to gynaecologists, in particular for his operation to correct the retroflexed uterus (sometimes known as Alexander's operation[3,4]) first described in 1881, and to neurologists for his interests in epilepsy. The focus on epilepsy, the topic of this article, was to have social as well as clinical consequences, the former far more significant than the latter. The founding of the Maghull Home for Epileptics, sometimes known as the Epileptic Colony or Epileptic Institution, set a precedent for the care of individuals with epileptic seizures which was subsequently emulated elsewhere.

Epilepsy care in the middle of the 19th century

Some insights into how epilepsy was "managed" in the middle years of the 19th century may be found in accounts written by Charles Dickens (1812–1870).[5] In *A Walk in a Workhouse*, published in his journal *Household Words* in May 1850, he reports:

> In another room, a kind of purgatory or place of transition, six or eight noisy mad-women were gathered together, under the superintendence of one sane attendant. Among them was a girl of two or three and twenty, very prettily dressed, of most respectable appearance, and good manners, who had been brought in from the house where she had lived as domestic servant (having, I suppose, no friends), on account of being subject to epileptic fits, and requiring to be removed under the influence of a very bad one. She was by no means of the same stuff, or the same breeding, or the same experience, or the same state of mind, as those by whom she was surrounded; and she pathetically complained that the daily association and the nightly noise made her worse, and was driving her mad – which was perfectly evident.

A further account, *Wapping Workhouse*, dating from some 10 years later and published in the journal *All the Year Round*, also mentions epilepsy, and suggests little improvement in the care received:

... everybody ... in the room had fits, except the wardswoman: an elderly, able-bodied pauperess ... biding her time for catching or holding some-body. This civil personage ... said, "They has 'em continiwal [sic], sir. They drops without no more notice than if they was coach-horses dropped from the moon, sir. And, when one drops, another drops, and sometimes there'll be as many as four or five on 'em at once, dear me, a rollin' and a tearin', bless you!

The truly dire consequences for epileptics in an age without effective medical treatment, and in which the distinctions between epilepsy and mental subnor-mality, and indeed criminality, were largely elided, is all too evident in these accounts.

Bromides, the first partially effective medication for epilepsy, came into general use in the 1850s and 1860s, in part based on the comments of Sir Charles Locock (a gynaecologist) and the studies of the physician Samuel Wilks,[6] but it is unlikely that these remedies were widely used outside of specialist hospitals such as the National Hospital for the Paralysed and Epilep-tic at Queen Square in London, founded in 1860. Arsenic, borax, and belladonna were also part of the therapeutic armamentarium, and chloroform was used on occasion for recurrent seizures (status epilepticus).

Biography

To my knowledge there is no dedicated biography of William Alexander. The available secondary sources[2,7-9] note that he was born in Holestone, Antrim, Northern Ireland, and following his graduation at the Royal (Queens) Univer-sity of Ireland in Belfast in 1870 he travelled to Liverpool. He was appointed to the full-time post of Resident Medical Officer at the Brownlow Hill Work-house in May 1872.[10] In 1875, he set up in general practice in Rodney Street and two years later, 1877, became a fellow of the Royal College of Surgeons (FRCS).[11] As recorded in his obituary, he won the 1881 Jacksonian Prize on "The pathology and surgical treatment of diseases of the hip-joint" and the 1883 Sir Astley Cooper Prize for a paper on "The pathology and pathological relation of chronic rheumatoid arthritis".

In 1883 he became Honorary Medical Officer to the Liverpool Central Relief and Charity Organisation Society, a philanthropic body which sought to help the poor of the city. Appointed to the committee, he came into contact with influential people including the Secretary, Mr Henry Cox. These contacts were to have important consequences in the following years for the manage-ment of patients with epilepsy.

Alexander was Surgeon to the Royal Southern Hospital from 1889 to 1910, and Visiting Surgeon to the Liverpool Workhouse Infirmary at Brownlow Hill.[12]

Macalister's history of the Royal Southern features Alexander several times.[13] He reports that Alexander pointed out the design flaw of the mortuary and the post-mortem room being immediately below the operating theatre at the hospital, an issue subsequently resolved by repurposing these areas. He describes Alexander as a "diehard so far as antiseptics were concerned", although he combined them with modern aseptic surgery. Alexander's student years coincided with Lister's first publications on antisepsis, so although no direct link between Lister and Alexander is evident Lister's practices must nevertheless have made a significant impact on him; he published on the topic as late as 1886 (Alexander W. Antiseptics. *Liverpool Med Chirurg J* 1886;10:58–68). Macalister reports that Alexander maintained a general practice until comparatively late in his career, and that the "gynaecological work in the Hospital was carried out by ... William Alexander between ... 1888 and 1910 as a branch of general surgery". As for epilepsy, "At a very early period he concluded that the routine use of potassium bromide in epilepsy was inadvisable and often harmful and he limited its employment considerably". There is no mention by Macalister of Alexander's work at Maghull (vide infra). He does report Alexander supporting the toast at the Farewell Dinner for Dr William Carter[14] on 27 January 1908. Macalister reproduces Alexander's portrait by F.T. Copnall.[15]

Shepherd's history of the LMI[16] mentions Alexander occasionally, all in the context of general surgery, although one note refers to a presentation on "puerperal convulsions" (subject of a paper published in the *Lancet* in 1911: Alexander W. Puerperal convulsions, or eclampsia, at the Liverpool Workhouse Hospital. *Lancet* 1911;177:217–20). Alexander was elected a member of the LMI in 1872 and served on the committee several times and was vice-president in 1886–7. Certainly he was a frequent contributor to the *Liverpool Medical-Chirurgical Journal*.

As a surgeon he was, perhaps unsurprisingly, interested in experimental surgical approaches to epilepsy (as for gynaecology), such as trephination and removal of the superior cervical sympathetic ganglia. He published on ligation of the vertebral arteries as a possible treatment,[17] methods which do not feature in canonical histories of epilepsy surgery.

Although Alexander was contemporary in his practice in Liverpool with Francis Imlach (1851–1920), and despite his interest in gynaecological surgery, there is no evidence that he ever undertook this approach to try to treat epilepsy, as Imlach had done.[18] In his 1882 report of the round ligament surgery, Alexander mentions a patient, Elizabeth D, whose "menstrual period ... [was] marked by the occurrence of epileptic fits" but the seizures were unaffected by the operation.[19] According to Rivlin,[20] Alexander was subsequently one of the panel of clinicians who sat in judgment on Imlach and his work, with unfavourable outcome for the latter.

Alexander's epilepsy interests resulted in a monograph, *The treatment of epilepsy*, published in 1889,[21] which makes it clear that by this time he had abandoned vertebral artery ligation in favour of sympathectomy and trephination. Despite Macalister's comments, the use of bromides features in a number of the cases reported by Alexander.

Epilepsy in Liverpool

There is no reason to believe that the circumstances for individuals with epilepsy in Liverpool were substantially different in any way from those reported by Dickens in London. Although Richard Caton had, whilst working in Liverpool in 1875, first recorded the electrical activity of the brain, an observation which was to prove the forerunner of the electroencephalograph (EEG) which transformed the investigation of epilepsy in the 20th century, this advance had absolutely no contemporary clinical impact.[22,23] In the era of "Squalid Liverpool", the title of a series of articles and a pamphlet published in 1883,[24] options for epileptics were limited. Inability to work because of seizures condemned many to the workhouse. It is said by Barclay[7] that Alexander had many epileptic patients at Brownlow Hill Workhouse.

William Alexander and Henry Cox, working together in the Central Relief and Charity Organisation Society committee, saw the need for provision for people with chronic epilepsy.[7] Using the model of the Bethel Epileptic Colony founded in 1867 at Bielefeld, Westphalia, in Germany,[25] which had previously been visited by other committee members, Alexander and Cox initiated a plan to open a home for people with epilepsy near Liverpool. Alexander reports that:

> In the early part of the year (1888) I was consulted as to the desirability of establishing a hospital for epilepsy in Liverpool, by a philanthropic gentleman, who saw the great difficulties in the treatment of the disease, that both doctors and patients laboured under.

> I immediately objected to a hospital for such cases, ... but proposed a home in the country, where work, treatment, education, and all good influences could be brought to bear ...[26]

With the support of the Society, they looked for a country house to rent, and found the Manor House in Maghull to be available and suitable. Of possible note, even before this time, Alexander reports on epilepsy patients being sent to Maghull to a convalescent home.[27]

Alexander himself visited Bielefeld in June 1888 to develop his ideas about the nature of the planned institution, a visit described at some length in his book, *The treatment of epilepsy*, along with a briefer account of the founding of the Maghull Home for Epileptics.[28]

The first patient was admitted on 28 December 1888. Dr Alexander was the Acting Honorary Medical Consulting Officer, to whom applications for admission were to be addressed (at 100 Bedford Street South) using a proforma.[29] However, the Local Honorary Medical Officer with responsibility for day-to-day treatment of the patients was Dr JF Gordon, a general practitioner in Maghull.[30] Places were quickly taken up at the Home, funded by either private or public means, and early reports indicated patients were by and large healthy and happy. It may well be that their quality of life at the Home was far better than would have been the case living in the community or obliged by want of other resources to enter the workhouse. One of Alexander's later publications contains several photographs of colony residents in their occupations and recreations.[31]

It should be pointed out that the Maghull Homes for Epilepsy was entirely distinct from the Moss Side Red Cross Hospital, sometimes known as the Moss Side Military Hospital or Maghull Hospital,[32] situated about a mile away. Although the Poor Law authorities of Liverpool originally intended this site to be developed as an epilepsy colony, part of the expansion of the system in the early years of the 20th century, the onset of the First World War brought about a change of plan, the institution becoming a military establishment. Here treatments for soldiers who had sustained shell shock were pioneered, by WHR Rivers (1864–1922)[33] amongst others, along with the training of medical officers in psychiatry.[34,35] Moss Side Hospital later (1989) became incorporated as part of Ashworth Hospital.

Epileptic Colonies

> Near my sister's house was an Epileptic Colony which helped to support itself by its own farm, which owned several hundred acres and was inhabited by some four hundred men, women and children. There was a school for the children, playing fields, gardens, pigs and a herd of fine Ayrshires. The men and women were kept apart, but moved about freely in the district in pairs or parties. None might go alone outside the grounds.[36]

This description is by the author Margiad Evans (*nom de plume* of Peggy Whistler, 1909–1958), herself destined to develop epilepsy in 1950, shortly after this visit.[37] As one of Margiad's biographies indicates that she was visiting her sister, Nancy, in Chalfont St Peter in Buckinghamshire at this time,[38] the colony described is identifiable as Chalfont,[39] but the account might also serve for the similar institution in Maghull.[7] Certainly Alexander's vision for

Maghull was to "maintain a home-life away from the homes of the patients", but that "all must be employed in some way or other",[40] what we might now characterise as "ergotherapy".

Consequences

The precedence of the Maghull epileptic colony, claimed by the committee in a pamphlet published in 1898–9 to commemorate the first ten years of its existence,[41] has been widely acknowledged subsequently. For example, in 1913, McDougall and Allington Plant wrote that:

> The Colony plan of bettering the lot of epileptics was begun in England some twenty-five years ago by the instituting of the Home for Epileptics at Maghull near Liverpool.[42]

Almost 100 years later, modern scholarship does not appear to demur from this judgment. Alexander's advice was apparently sought by the founders of the Chalfont colony, both at its foundation and some years later (1910), regarding his opinions on the contested issue as to whether or not a resident medical officer was necessary in such institutions: "As Alexander put in reply to questions – the Centre was 'under the control of ladies because we think that epileptics are better controlled by ladies, better controlled by persuasion than by force, and ladies exercise persuasion better than men'".[43]

In one of his late publications, Alexander asked (rhetorically, no doubt):

> What have we gained by the "home" or "colony" system of treating epileptics? Are the results worth the trouble and expense? Has the system come to stay, or is it only an ephemeral fad?

Unsurprisingly his responses were positive, concluding:

> There is no doubt that an epileptic colony is the best atmosphere for an epileptic as far as health, life, and happiness is concerned.[44]

Neither Alexander nor Epileptic Colonies/Homes feature in Temkin's seminal history of epilepsy,[45] but in his celebrated textbook on epilepsy published in 1960 William Lennox noted that "a home for epileptics was established at Mughall [sic] near Liverpool in 1888".[46]

In her book examining representations of epilepsy, Jeanette Stirling entitles a whole chapter "The colonies" although the discussion ranges much more widely.[47] Maghull is mentioned in passing only three times (and Alexander not at all),[48] the main emphasis being on Chalfont, apparently because of its association with the National Society of the Employment of Epileptics (NSEE), its founding body. This seems to ignore the fact that, despite its name, the NSEE had no national profile for many decades, all its efforts being focused initially on Chalfont.[39] Moreover, the claim that the NSEE "turned outwards for inspiration" as evidenced by the fact that "one of its founders – Miss Burdon-Sanderson – had notes on the Bielefeld epileptic colony in Germany"[49] is hardly convincing: Alexander, on behalf of Maghull, had been there before.

The epileptic colony model was also exported to America and Australia.[47] The Ohio Hospital for Epileptics opened in 1893,[50] and the Craig Colony located at Sonyea in New York State ("the flagship of the American colony system"[51]) in 1896. What influence, if any, the institution at Maghull had on these developments remains to be determined, but certainly Alexander was aware of the Craig Colony.[52]

Commentary

Alexander died after a few days' illness on 9 March 1919,[53] at Heswall, and was buried there. His *BMJ* obituary stated that "he was unostentatious in manner, his opinions were lucidly expressed, and in speech he was never redundant".[8] Macalister described him as a "tower of clinical experience", of strong physical make-up, and of a kindly nature and very sympathetic to the sufferings of his patients.[54] Perhaps surprisingly, then, his name does not feature amongst the obituaries of members of the LMI in the Annual Report for 1919, or 1920. Indeed, his name disappears from the listing of LMI members published in the Annual Reports after 1912, without explanation.

Maghull Homes built a Special Care Home in the mid-1970s which was named Alexander Home in his memory, opened by the then prime minister, Harold Wilson. This building was later demolished.

To adjudge now, as we may, the enterprise of "epilepsy colonies" as segregating, isolating, excluding, marginalising, custodial, and stigmatising is to indulge in (what EP Thompson called) the condescension of posterity. In Victorian society epilepsy was stigmatised, and the colony environment may well have been far more accepting of individuals with this disorder, albeit catering for only a small minority of all those with epilepsy (numbers at Maghull were never more than around 400). Alexander's belief that "an epileptic colony is the best atmosphere for an epileptic as far as health, life, and happiness is concerned" may have been true at that time (no written testimony from a colonist which might corroborate or contradict this view is known to survive). Indeed, Lannon sees colonies as supporting innovative care and as a response to the repression of social and eugenic laws of the times.[55]

Liverpool clinicians have maintained an interest in epilepsy over the years, including Robert Hughes's (1911–1991) in his 1961 book on electroencephalography (wherein he is listed, amongst other appointments, as "Honorary Neurologist, Maghull Epileptic Colony"),[56] and Kenneth Slatter (1921–2013).[57,58] In recent years, Liverpool has developed a significant reputation in epilepsy research, based on the work in clinical trials of anti-epileptic drugs coordinated at the Walton Centre for Neurology and Neurosurgery, initially by Professor David Chadwick and subsequently by Professor Tony Marson. It should not be forgotten that, long before these developments, contributions to epilepsy care were being pioneered in Liverpool by William Alexander and his colleagues. Certainly Alexander's career endorses the view that the developing specialty of gynaecology in this period was a "protean" and "enormous field of activity".[59]

Bibliography of Alexander's publications

NB: It is not claimed that this listing is comprehensive, since a systematic search of all relevant journals has not been attempted. Alexander's many contributions to case presentations and discussions at LMI meetings as recorded in the *Liverpool Medical-Chirurgical Journal* (at least 45 by my reckoning) are not included here, only substantive papers.

1872:
Alexander W. An enlarged heart. *Lancet*, 100:585.

1873:
Alexander W. Liverpool Workhouse Hospital. Acute inflammation of the spleen; abscess; peritonitis; death. *Lancet*, 102:264.

1876:
Alexander W, Hamilton AMS. Progressive muscular atrophy. *Lancet*, 107:10–1 and 44–6.

1877:
Alexander W, Bare J. A case of a new form of pseudo-paraplegia, ending in true paralysis. Caries of dorsal vertebrae; death; autopsy. *Lancet*, 109:903–5.
Alexander W. Liverpool Workhouse Hospital. Case of depressed fracture of skull in which temporary relief followed the use of the trephine; abscess of brain. *Lancet*, 110:426–7.

1878:
Alexander W. The mortality of lying-in hospitals. *Lancet*, 111:145.
Alexander W. Notes of two cases of disease of the bladder relieved by somewhat novel operative methods of treatment. *Lancet*, 112:209–10.

1879:
Alexander W. Liverpool Workhouse Hospital. A case of oesophagotomy. *Lancet*, 113:155–6.
Alexander W. Liverpool Workhouse Hospital. Four cases of amputation through the hip joint; remarks. *Lancet*, 114:544–5.

1881:
Alexander W. Case of cancer uteri treated with Chian turpentine. *Liverpool Med. Chirurg. J.*, 1:83–5.
Alexander W. Ovariotomy at Liverpool workhouse. *Med. Times Gaz.*, 2:63–5.
Alexander W. An attempt to cure epilepsy by ligature of the carotid or vertebral arteries; with reports of some cases in which ligature of one or both of these vessels was performed. *Med. Times Gaz.*, 2:598–600.
Alexander W. Gonorrhoea followed by abdominal tumour: contents removed by aspirator; recovery. *Lancet*, 117:538–9.
Alexander W. On some rare forms of disease, accompanied by lesions of trophic nerves or trophic centres, and illustrative of trophic changes. *Lancet*, 117:986–7 and 1023–4.

1882:
Alexander W. The radical cure of hernia. *Liverpool Med. Chirurg. J.*, 2:124–34.
Alexander W. The treatment of epilepsy by ligature of the vertebral arteries. *Brain*, 5:170–87.
Alexander W. Observations on the effect of ligature of the vertebral arteries in certain diseases of the spinal cord. *Liverpool Med. Chirurg. J.*, 3:232–42.
Alexander W. On the cure of epilepsy by ligature of the vertebral arteries. *Med. Times Gaz.*, 1:250–2.
Alexander W. A new method of treating inveterate and troublesome displacements of the uterus. *Med. Times Gaz.*, 1:327–8.

1883:
Alexander W. A new method of treating displacement of the uterus. *Liverpool Med. Chirurg. J.*, 4:113–24.
Alexander W. The treatment of parturition and of the puerperal state in hospital practice. *Med. Times Gaz.*, 1:381–2, 470–1, 524–5.
Alexander W. Prolonged suspension of vitality through the subcutaneous injection of morphia and atropine. *Med. Times Gaz.*, 1:582–3.

1884:

Alexander W. Interesting cases of bladder disease. *Liverpool Med. Chirurg. J.*, 6:245–57.

Alexander W. *The treatment of backward displacements of the uterus, and of prolapsus uteri by the new method of shortening the round ligaments.* London, J&A Churchill.

Alexander W. Curious cases of aneurism. *Med. Times Gaz.*, 1:246–8.

Alexander W. On some cases of trephining. *Med. Times Gaz.*, 2:145–7.

1885:

Alexander W. On excision of the hip. *Liverpool Med. Chirurg. J.*, 9:289–303.

Alexander W. Case of bifacial paralysis (Patient). *Liverpool Med. Chirurg. J.*, 9:467–9.

Alexander W. The cure of some uterine displacements by shortening the round ligaments. *Ann. Surg.*, 1:426–39.

1886:

Alexander W. Antiseptics. *Liverpool Med. Chirurg. J.*, 10:58–68.

1887:

Alexander W. Report on the hygienic treatment of "struma" at the Liverpool Workhouse, being the first part of a report on recent practical advancements in the treatment of struma. *Liverpool Med. Chirurg. J.*, 12:44–55.

Alexander W. Removal of advanced cancerous disease of the rectum by a new method. *Liverpool Med. Chirurg. J.*, 13:235–45.

Alexander W. On some points in the pathology and treatment of caries of the vertebrae. *Liverpool Med. Chirurg. J.*, 13:361–82.

Alexander W. Purulent encephalitis with obscure symptoms occurring in a pregnant woman at full term; child saved by abdominal section (Porro's operation). *Lancet*, 129:169–70.

1888:

Alexander W. Second part of a report on recent practical advancements in the treatment of struma. *Liverpool Med. Chirurg. J.*, 14:127–44.

Alexander W. The "Sea-Side" treatment of scrofula: the third part of a report on recent practical advancements in the treatment of struma. *Liverpool Med. Chirurg. J.*, 15:373–86.

1889:

Alexander W. Report on some rare diseases that have recently come under the writer's observation. *Liverpool Med. Chirurg. J.*, 17:281–300.

Alexander W. *The treatment of epilepsy.* Edinburgh and London, Young J. Pentland.

1890:
Alexander W. Report on recent advances in the surgery of the intestinal tract. *Liverpool Med. Chirurg. J.,* 18:183–95.
Alexander W. Interesting gynaecological cases. *Liverpool Med. Chirurg. J.,* 19:357–68.

1891:
Alexander W. Cancer of the tongue: its treatment and results. *Liverpool Med. Chirurg. J.,* 20:99–108.

1892:
Alexander W. Papers on practical surgery; or, the experience of twenty years of operative work. *Liverpool Med. Chirurg. J.,* 22:49–72.
Alexander W. Papers on practical surgery; or, the experience of twenty years of operative work. *Liverpool Med. Chirurg. J.,* 23:393–428.
Alexander W. Two cases of intestinal surgery. *Liverpool Med. Chirurg. J.,* 23:498–502.

1893:
Alexander W. Papers on practical surgery; or, the experience of twenty years of operative work. *Liverpool Med. Chirurg. J.,* 24:159–214.
Carter W, Alexander W. Two cases of post-diphtheritic paralysis with contractures. *Liverpool Med. Chirurg. J.,* 24:229–31.
Alexander W. On some points in the treatment of epilepsy. *Liverpool Med. Chirurg. J.,* 25:271–86.
Alexander W, Humphreys R. The report of the select committee on midwives' registration. *Lancet,* 142:717–8 and 839–41.

1894:
Alexander W. Papers on practical surgery; or, the experience of twenty years of operative work. *Liverpool Med. Chirurg. J.,* 26:157–203.
Alexander W. Puerperal fever. *Liverpool Med. Chirurg. J.,* 27:354–67.

1896:
Alexander W. On some successful cases of intestinal surgery. *Liverpool Med. Chirurg. J.,* 30:116–35.

1897:
Alexander W. Practical gynaecology. *Liverpool Med. Chirurg. J.*, 32:123–44.
Alexander W. Practical gynaecology. *Liverpool Med. Chirurg. J.*, 33:317–29.
Alexander W. Report of the lying-in wards of the Liverpool Workhouse hospital for the year 1895 and 1896; or, workhouse midwives, their training and practice. *Lancet*, 149:545–6.
Alexander W. Ophthalmia in Liverpool. *Lancet*, 149:1435 and 1571–2.
Alexander W. Another method of ameliorating by operation otherwise incurable incontinence of urine. *Lancet*, 150:16–7.

1898:
Alexander W. Practical gynaecology. *Liverpool Med. Chirurg. J.*, 34:1–21.
Alexander W. The treatment of deserted infants. *Liverpool Med. Chirurg. J.*, 35:313–29.
Alexander W. Practical gynaecology. *Liverpool Med. Chirurg. J.*, 35:444–68.
Alexander W. An object-lesson on the necessity for the education, registration, and control of midwives. *Lancet*, 151:1636–7.
Alexander W. Royal Southern Hospital, Liverpool. A case of acute intestinal obstruction; latent hernia; laparotomy; reduction of hernia from within; drainage; recovery. *Lancet*, 152:553.

1899:
Alexander W. Practical gynaecology. *Liverpool Med. Chirurg. J.*, 36:120–44.

1900:
Alexander W. Ophthalmia amongst the poor of Liverpool: its prevalence, prevention and cure. *Liverpool Med. Chirurg. J.*, 39:275–90.
Alexander W. Liverpool Workhouse Hospital. Trephining and drainage in an apparently moribund case of status epilepticus; recovery. *Lancet*, 156:877–8.
Alexander W. Liverpool Workhouse Hospital. A case of presentation of the head, cord, and foot; contracted pelvis; caesarean section; recovery. *Lancet*, 156:1201–2.

1902:
Alexander W. Obstruction of bowels. *Liverpool Med. Chirurg. J.*, 43:314–7.
Alexander W. The education of epileptics. *Lancet*, 159:805–7.

1903:
Alexander W. Liverpool Workhouse Hospital. A case of rupture of the right kidney into fragments; operation; recovery. *Lancet*, 162:1234.

1904:

Alexander W. A peculiar case of carcinoma mammae. *Liverpool Med. Chirurg. J.*, 45:73–7.

1905:

Alexander W. Scientific and clinical reports on epilepsy. *Liverpool Med. Chirurg. J.*, 46:136–65.
Alexander W. Scientific and clinical reports on epilepsy. *Liverpool Med. Chirurg. J.*, 47:419–46.

1907:

Alexander W. Scientific and clinical reports on epilepsy. *Liverpool Med. Chirurg. J.*, 51:167–78.
Alexander W. Scientific and clinical reports on epilepsy. *Liverpool Med. Chirurg. J.*, 52:98–112.
Alexander W. Liverpool Workhouse Hospital. Rupture of the spleen; splenectomy; recovery. *Lancet*, 169:90–1.
Alexander W. Aseptic and septic midwifery at the Liverpool Workhouse Hospital. *Lancet*, 169:940–3.

1908:

Alexander W. Scientific and clinical reports on epilepsy. *Liverpool Med. Chirurg. J.*, 53:99–111.

1909:

Alexander W. Aphasia succeeded by Jacksonian epilepsy; operation; recovery. *Lancet*, 173:1750.

1910:

Alexander W. A note on a case of post-peritoneal haematocele complicating a large uterine fibroid; operation; cure. *Lancet*, 175:643.
Alexander W. Maternity cases in the Liverpool Workhouse during 1907, 1908, and 1909. *Lancet*, 175:1405–6.
Alexander W. The freedom of the feeble-minded in the Liverpool Workhouse and some of its results. *Lancet*, 175:1783–4.

1911:

Alexander W. Puerperal convulsions, or eclampsia, at the Liverpool Workhouse Hospital. *Lancet*, 177:217–20.
Alexander W. The surgical treatment of some forms of epilepsy. *Lancet*, 178:932–8.

1913:
Alexander W. Necessity of a better classification of epileptics. *Lancet*, 181:263–5.

Acknowledgements

Thanks to Sue Curbishley and Adrienne Mayers for accessing relevant books at LMI Library; and to Maggie O'Neill at Parkhaven Trust for information on the Alexander Home. Adapted and extended from: Larner AJ. William Alexander (1844–1919): epilepsy care in Liverpool in the late 19th century. *Medical Historian* 2019;29:15–32.

References

1. Larner AJ. A brief bibliography of papers related to the history of medicine in Liverpool and Merseyside. *Medical Historian* 2015;25:35–51.
2. Ross JA. William Alexander, a forgotten Liverpool pioneer. *Medical Historian* 1992;5:27–29.
3. Longo LD. A new method of treating inveterate and troublesome displacements of the uterus: William Alexander. *Am J Obstet Gynecol* 1976;15:1043.
4. http://www.whonamedit.com/doctor.cfm/156.html (accessed 21/02/18).
5. Larner AJ. Charles Dickens (1812–1870) and epilepsy. *Epilepsy Behav* 2012;24: 422–5.
6. Eadie M. Sir Charles Locock and potassium bromide. *J R Coll Physicians Edinb* 2012;42:274–9.
7. Barclay J. *"The first epileptic home in England". A centenary history of the Maghull Homes 1888–1988.* Glasgow: Heatherbank Press, 1990, pp.18–20.
8. Anonymous. Obituary. William Alexander, M.D., F.R.C.S. *Br Med J* 1919;1:302.
9. Larner AJ. William Alexander (1844–1919): contributions to gynaecology and neurology. *Ulster Med J* 2018;87:184–7.
10. Alexander W. Papers on practical surgery; or, the experience of twenty years of operative work. *Liverpool Med Chirurg J* 1892;22:49–72. This fact attested to at p.49.
11. *Plarr's Lives of the Fellows online*, https://livesonline.rcseng.ac.uk/biogs/E000665b.htm (accessed 21/02/18), which is based largely on ref. 8. Barclay, op. cit., ref. 7, p.19, states "In 1878, Dr Alexander obtained higher surgical qualifications (F.R.C.S.) in London."; this dating, possibly a typographical error, is incorrect.
12. King CD. The Liverpool Brownlow Hill institution. In: Hillam C, Bone JM (eds.). *The Poor Law and after: workhouse hospitals and public welfare* (*Medical Historian* special issue). Liverpool: Liverpool Medical History Society, 1999, pp.23–37.

13. Macalister CJ. *The origin and history of the Liverpool Royal Southern Hospital with personal reminiscences.* Liverpool: WB Jones & Co. Ltd., 1936, pp.31–2, 33, 57, 73, 129, 139–40. At p.139, Macalister gives "1833" as the date of Alexander's Sir Astley Cooper Prize, evidently a typographical error.

14. Sykes AH. Dr. William Carter – a medical life in Victorian Liverpool. *Medical Historian* 2009–2010;21:49–61. Alexander is not mentioned by Sykes.

15. Reproduced in ref. 9. Current whereabouts of this portrait are unknown to me. Copnall (1870–1949) is also responsible for the portrait of Charles Thurstan Holland located in the Gallery at LMI. Larner AJ. Charles Thurstan Holland: a genealogical note. *Medical Historian* 2015;25:31–3, erroneously calls the artist "Copthall" [at 31].

16. Shepherd JA. *A history of the Liverpool Medical Institution.* Liverpool: Liverpool Medical Institution, 1979, pp.157, 159, 163.

17. Alexander W. The treatment of epilepsy by ligature of the vertebral arteries. *Brain* 1882;5:170–87. Barclay, op. cit., ref. 7, p.19, states that "Dr Alexander's first major article on surgery in epilepsy appeared in 1883 in Brain, the neurological journal"; this dating, possibly a typographical error, is incorrect; the same dating error is also found in the list of publications in ref. 11. Alexander also published on the surgery of epilepsy in the *Medical Times and Gazette* in 1881 and 1882 (Alexander W. An attempt to cure epilepsy by ligature of the carotid or vertebral arteries; with reports of some cases in which ligature of one or both of these vessels was performed. *Med Times Gaz* 1881;2:598–600; Alexander W. On the cure of epilepsy by ligature of the vertebral arteries. *Med Times Gaz* 1882;1:250–2).

18. Imlach F. A case of hystero-epilepsy of twenty years' duration, treated by removal of the uterine appendages. *BMJ* 1888;1:740.

19. Alexander W, A new method of treating inveterate and troublesome displacements of the uterus. *Med Times Gaz* 1882;1:327–8.

20. Rivlin JJ. Francis Imlach (1851–1920) and the Liverpool medical establishment. In: Hillam C, Bone JM (eds.). *Wives and whores in Victorian Liverpool. Varieties in attitude towards medical care for women. Papers delivered at a meeting of the Society 4 April 1998* (*Medical Historian* special issue). Liverpool: Liverpool Medical History Society, 1999, pp.42–50.

21. Alexander W. *The treatment of epilepsy.* Edinburgh and London: Young J. Pentland, 1889. The copy in LMI has a handwritten note on the flyleaf, which I read as "With the authors compliments". Sadly this is unsigned and undated so it is not clear whether this is in Alexander's hand, although this seems likely to be the case. Review of the book appears in *Liverpool Med Chirurg J* 1889;17:320–5.

22. Caton R. The Electric Currents of the Brain. *Br Med J* 1875;ii:278.

23. Sykes AH. Dr Richard Caton (1842–1926): Medicine, education and civic affairs in Liverpool. *Medical Historian* 2010–2011;22:11–27.

24. Sykes AH. "*Squalid Liverpool*" revisited. *Medical Historian* 2011–2012;23:53–6.

25. Grewe P, Bien CG. 150th anniversary of the Bethel epilepsy center in

Germany: an important milestone in the evolution of epilepsy care. *Seizure* 2017;53:110–3.

26. Op. cit., ref. 21, pp.161–2.
27. Ibid., p.39, 54, 63, 67, 71, 90, 95. He also mentions an epileptic home or institution in Dingle, p.78, 200.
28. Ibid., Bielefeld, pp.163–77; Maghull, pp.177–81.
29. Ibid., p.178–9.
30. Rowlands JK. *"Fifty years a surgeon in this parish." The history of the Westway Medical Centre Practice and other Maghull general practices.* Maghull, 1998, pp.22–3.
31. Alexander W. Scientific and clinical reports on epilepsy. *Liverpool Med Chirurg J* 1905;46:136–65; occupations at p.137, 139, 141, 143, 147, 151, 153; recreations at p.155, 157, 159.
32. Larner, op. cit., ref. 1, p 38, erroneously elides these completely separate institutions.
33. Young A. W.H.R. Rivers and the war neuroses. *J Hist Behav Sci* 1999;35: 359–78.
34. Lane J. *A social history of medicine. Health, healing and disease in England, 1750–1950.* London: Routledge, 2001, p.181.
35. Jones E. Shell shock at Maghull and the Maudsley: models of psychological medicine in the UK. *J Hist Med Allied Sci* 2010;65:368–95.
36. Evans M. *A ray of darkness.* London: John Calder, 1978 [1952], pp.34–5.
37. Larner AJ. "'A ray of darkness'": Margiad Evans's account of her epilepsy (1952). *Clin Med* 2009;9:193–4; Larner AJ. Margiad Evans (1909–1958): a history of epilepsy in a creative writer. *Epilepsy Behav* 2009;16:596–8; Larner AJ. A "herstory" of epilepsy in a creative writer: the case of Margiad Evans. In: Bohata K, Gramich K (eds.). *Rediscovering Margiad Evans: marginality, gender and illness.* Cardiff: University of Wales Press, 2013, pp.129–41.
38. Lloyd-Morgan C. *Margiad Evans.* Bridgend: Seren Press, 1998, p.114.
39. Barclay J. *A caring community. A centenary history of the National Society for Epilepsy and the Chalfont Centre, 1892–1992.* London: National Society for Epilepsy, 1992.
40. Op. cit., ref. 21, p.177, 180.
41. Anonymous. *The first epileptic home in England; an account of the ten years' pioneer work in the treatment of epileptics in homes or colonies in England.* Liverpool: D Marples, 1899.
42. McDougall A, Allington Plant W. Schools for epileptics and the education of epileptic children in England. *Epilepsia* 1913;A4:358–61 [at p.358].
43. Shorvon S, Shepherd L. *The beginning of the end of the falling sickness. Epilepsy and its treatment in London 1860–1910.* London: Institute of Neurology, 2012, p.44, 64. Barclay, op. cit., ref. 39, pp.74–6, does not mention Alexander in her account of this debate at Chalfont.
44. Alexander W. Scientific and clinical reports on epilepsy. *Liverpool Med Chirurg J* 1907;51:167–78 [at pp.170, 176].

45. Temkin O. *The falling sickness. A history of epilepsy from the Greeks to the beginnings of modern neurology* (2nd edition). Baltimore and London: Johns Hopkins Press, 1971.

46. Lennox WG, Lennox MA, *Epilepsy and related disorders* (2 volumes). London: J&A Churchill; 1960, p.1042.

47. Stirling J. *Representing epilepsy. Myth and matter.* Liverpool: Liverpool University Press, 2010, pp.131–77.

48. Ibid., p.151, 152, 157.

49. Ibid., p.152. Stirling is in error in giving the location of the NSEE colony as "Chalfont St Peters".

50. Kissiov D, Dewall T, Hermann B. The Ohio Hospital for Epileptics – the first "epilepsy colony" in America. *Epilepsia* 2013;54:1524–34.

51. Op. cit., ref. 47, p.158.

52. Alexander W. Scientific and clinical reports on epilepsy. *Liverpool Med Chirurg J* 1905;47: 419–46 [at p.429n]; Alexander W. Scientific and clinical reports on epilepsy. *Liverpool Med Chirurg J* 1907;52:98–112 [at p.100].

53. Hence just over a month after the death of William Barnett Warrington (2nd February 1919), another pioneer of clinical neurology in late 19th and early 20th century Liverpool; see Bracewell RM, Larner AJ. William Barnett Warrington (1869–1919): neurology in Liverpool around the turn of the 20th century. *Medical Historian* 2018;28:51–61; Bracewell RM, Larner AJ. William Barnett Warrington (1869–1919). *Eur Neurol* 2019;81:323–6. A picture of Alexander's grave appears in ref. 9.

54. Op. cit., ref. 13, p.140.

55. Lannon SL. Free standing. Social control and the sane epileptic, 1850–1950. *Arch Neurol* 2002;59:1031–6. She also quotes from Margiad Evans, at p.1034.

56. Hughes RR. *An introduction to clinical electro-encephalography.* Bristol: John Wright, 1961.

57. Slatter KH. Alpha rhythms and mental imagery. *Electroencephalogr Clin Neurophysiol* 1960;12:851–9.

58. Slatter KH. Some clinical and EEG findings in patients with migraine. *Brain* 1968;91:85–98.

59. Weisz G. *Divide and conquer: a comparative history of medical specialization.* New York: Oxford University Press, 2006, p.205.

Sir William Gowers (1845–1915): his comments on cognitive dysfunction

2015 marked the 100th anniversary of the death of Sir William Gowers, one of the towering figures of clinical neurology in the late 19th and early 20th centuries, who has rightly entered the pantheon of neurological greats.[1,2] A splendid recent biography has provided many insights into his life and career.[3]

Gowers' neurological contributions are manifold. Most, if not all, neurologists will be familiar with Gowers' sign or manoeuvre observed in patients with proximal lower limb and trunk weakness as they attempt to rise from the ground, a sign also known as "climbing up oneself" or, in North America, as the "butt-first manoeuver", most typically seen in boys with Duchenne muscular dystrophy, a disorder which Gowers knew as pseudohypertrophic muscular paralysis and on which he wrote a monograph. Those familiar with the anatomy of the spinal cord will know of Gowers' tract (ventral or anterior spinocerebellar tract).

Gowers was a fecund and, unlike Hughlings Jackson, lucid writer, author of many publications, both papers (more than 300) and books (see Box), which culminated in the *Manual of Diseases of the Nervous System*. This book has been variously described as "the greatest single-author comprehensive text-book of clinical neurology ever published" (Ref 3, p.250) and as the "Bible of Neurology",[4] and is perhaps Gowers' most enduring monument. Its two volumes first appeared in 1886 ("Diseases of the nerves and spinal cord") and 1888 ("Diseases of the brain and cranial nerves. General and functional diseases of the nervous system"), with a second edition in 1892 (Volume 1) and 1893 (Volume 2). A third edition of volume 1 appeared in 1899, co-authored with Dr James Taylor, but although preparations for a third edition of volume 2 were made this was never published. Parts of a manuscript marked with Gowers' proposed corrections survive in the Queen Square archives (Ref 3, p.149), with new information particularly relating to nystagmus and myasthenia.[4]

Gowers' neurological interests were very broad, but perhaps particularly related to epilepsy,[5] syphilis (especially tabes and locomotor ataxy), movement disorders, including "paralysis agitans" (Parkinson's disease) and "scrivener's palsy" (writer's cramp), and migraine. The student of cognitive neurology is disappointed to learn from his biographers that "from a survey of all Gowers' publications one gains the impression that he was not particularly interested in higher cerebral function" (Ref 3, p.167), presumably because many of the conditions afflicting these faculties were at that time seen by "alienists" (psychiatrists) rather than by neurologists. That said, he evidently took an interest in his own powers of recollection, which were said to be remarkable (Ref 3, p.238), although perhaps not unexpectedly tailed off in his later years.[6]

Prompted by the biographical suggestion of lack of interest in cognitive neurology, I visited the Liverpool Medical Institution which holds copies of all the editions of the *Manual of Diseases of the Nervous System* (see www.lmi.org.uk and follow the link to Online Library Catalogue). I have examined these volumes, in particular the second edition of volume 2 of 1893, in order to try to gain some appreciation of Gowers' knowledge of and approach to what we might now define as cognitive disorders (unless otherwise stated, all subsequent page citations are to the 1893 edition of the *Manual*, volume 2, although I wish to emphasize that, since I have not read all the 1050 pages of text in the LMI copy, this does not purport to be a comprehensive account).

A brief perusal is initially discouraging: for example, there is no index entry for "dementia", although it is evident that this word was certainly part of Gowers' clinical vocabulary since he does use it on occasion (e.g. pp.107, 648, 983). Much of what we call "dementia" is probably subsumed in his categories of "mental failure" and "insanity". It is clear that Gowers was familiar with many of the symptoms of cognitive dysfunction, and many of the disorders causing such problems.

Cognitive symptoms

Amnesia

In describing "Mental symptoms" (98), Gowers noted that "mental functions of the brain are frequently disturbed in organic disease", and that "Simple mental failure is indicated first and chiefly by *defect of memory*, 'amnesia' in the widest sense of the word" (Gowers' italics; 107). Hence, "The diseases of the brain that affect memory are extremely numerous", including "various degenerative processes, which are for the most part classed as forms of insanity, e.g. senile dementia and general paralysis of the insane" (107). Under the heading of "Mental failure", the index includes references to epilepsy, chorea, and tumour, amongst others (1060).

Aphasia

It has been acknowledged that the *Manual* contains a very good account of aphasia (Ref 3, p.167). Gowers noted of cerebral defects of speech that "The subject abounds in difficulty" (111). Amongst the most important writings on the subject, Gowers cited Broca (111n), Wernicke (109n), and Hughlings Jackson (109n, "in many places, but especially in 'Brain' vols. i and ii").

Gowers drew a clear distinction between motor aphasia (116–119) in which the "patient is able to understand whatever is said to him" despite impaired speech output, and sensory aphasia (119–122) in which "heard words are not understood". He seems to have used the term "word deafness" interchangeably with "sensory aphasia". The defects of writing (agraphia) and reading (alexia) accompanying these two forms of aphasia are also described.

As regards the causation of aphasia, "The region of the cortex in which the speech-centres are situated is supplied by the middle cerebral artery ..., and obstruction of this is the most frequent cause of aphasia" (124). Transient aphasia in the context of right-sided convulsions and of migraine is also noted (124).

"Agnosia"

As far as I can see, Gowers does not use the word "agnosia", coined by Sigmund Freud in 1891, but he was clearly aware of what we would now regard as agnosic phenomena, which 19th century neurologists had called "imperception" or "asymbolia".

He described "word-blindness" as an isolated loss of the power of comprehending visual word-symbols, after Kussmaul, with an inability to read even simple words (122). He noted that such patients could write spontaneously or from dictation but could not copy (123) and that there may be an associated hemianopia (124). Hence this corresponds with what we might now call pure alexia, alexia without agraphia, or pure word blindness. Gowers thought this resulted from a lesion in the lower and hinder part of the left parietal lobe including the angular gyrus. He also characterised word-blindness as a partial form of "mind-blindness", after Munk, that being impaired power to recognise the nature of seen objects, including words, although they could be "recognised at once when some other sense is employed" (23). Gowers' possible role in defining the pathological substrate of one of Hughlings Jackson's patients with agnosia has been described (Ref 3, p.167).

Cognitive disorders

Senile amnesia, Senile dementia

Gowers reported, in a section headed "Senile atrophy" (581–582), that "In old age the brain wastes, like many other organs ... The amount of fluid in the ventricles and on the surface is increased in proportion to the lessened bulk of the brain ... this wasting of the brain is commonly attended by no symptoms. Senile mental failure is often ascribed to it, but ... caution should be observed in attributing to it any mental change that may co-exist". He recognised "senile dementia" as a condition, and a temporal gradient in "senile amnesia", in which "... the events of early life may be vividly remembered, and those of later years be lost" (107).

Paralysis agitans

In his descriptions of what we would now call Parkinson's disease, Gowers noted that the "intellect may be unaffected throughout", as per James Parkinson's original 1817 description of the disease, but noted that "in the later stages of the disease ... mental weakness and loss of memory" are occasionally present and that these might also occur early in the disease course (648). "If tremor is inconspicuous, they add considerably to the misleading aspect of the case. Very rarely they are accompanied by a tendency to delusions, and occasionally they amount to actual dementia" (648). One wonders in retrospect if Gowers is describing here what we might now call dementia with Lewy bodies (DLB).[7] (Other possible cases of DLB may have been described prior to the delineation of diagnostic criteria, suggested examples including the philosopher Immanuel Kant[8] and the writer Mervyn Peake.[9])

Hereditary chorea, Huntington's chorea

Gowers noted that George Huntington's original 1872 description of this disorder mentioned "mental failure" as one aspect of the disease (624). Gowers' own focus was principally on the chorea, but he did note that "Mental changes are generally associated, especially mental weakness, and hence many of the cases have been reported from asylums" (625).

Epilepsy

In the section on "Mental disturbance in Epileptics" (747–749), Gowers noted that the "interparoxysmal mental state of epileptics ... often presents grave deterioration ... In its slightest degree there is merely defective memory, especially for recent acquisitions. In greater degree the intellect suffers generally ... " (748). Furthermore, "The mental state is not, in all cases, entirely the result of the attacks of epilepsy. In some it is, in part at least, the expression of a cerebral imperfection, of which the epilepsy is another manifestation. In such instances mental defect may exist before the occurrence of the first fit" (748). Certainly there is some modern evidence corroborating this formulation.

The possible adverse cognitive effects of medication, specifically bromides, of which Gowers was an enthusiastic prescriber,[5] are noted: "... patients may become ... forgetful ... The effect is often ascribed to the remedy used, especially if this is bromide" (749).

Disseminated or insular sclerosis

In disseminated or insular sclerosis (multiple sclerosis), Gowers noted that "slight mental change is common; considerable alteration is very rare. ... There may be failure of memory, but especially frequent is an undue complacency and contentment" (552).

Alcohol

Describing the effects of "Chronic alcoholism", Gowers noted that "persistent mental changes" such as "failure of memory" might occur (981). "Chronic alcoholism may aid in the production of many forms of definite insanity, but the only variety that can be certainly ascribed to this cause, acting alone, is chronic dementia – failure of memory, commonly progressive for a time" (983). He noted a resemblance to general paralysis of the insane but "differing in the non-progressive character of the disorder if alcohol is given up". He makes no reference, as far as I can see, to the alcohol-related amnesic syndrome described by Korsakoff in 1887, or the earlier work of Robert Lawson which had appeared in the inaugural volume of *Brain* in 1878.[10]

Syphilis

Although Gowers' major interest related to tabes and locomotor ataxy, he was aware that this might co-exist with general paralysis of the insane and noted that "syphilis predisposes to both" (1892 edition of *Manual*, volume 1, p.417).

Discussion

Evidently, from a brief perusal of some parts of his *Manual*, Gowers was familiar with the symptoms of cognitive dysfunction and with disorders of the nervous system causing such dysfunction. This reflects his astute clinical skills. His comments on cognitive impairment in Parkinson's disease may be prescient, and certainly the cognitive impairments he noted in multiple sclerosis and epilepsy were relatively little studied until recent times. Lacking specific tools to assess cognitive function, the development of which was in its infancy, he could not really take these clinical observations much further.

It is intriguing to wonder what new information relevant to cognitive disorders might have been contained in the 3rd edition of volume 2 of the *Manual*. "Brain degenerations" is apparently one of the surviving sections of the proposed third edition of volume 2, with Gowers' handwritten revisions, although Eadie et al. state that in this section "deletions were trivial" (Ref 4, p.3180). It would be fascinating to know if this section mentioned the seminal publications of Arnold Pick on focal lobar degenerations of 1892 and 1906 (Gowers had learnt German), and likewise those of Alois Alzheimer of 1907 and 1911, although it was not until 1912 that the first publication on "Alzheimer's disease" in English appeared, by Solomon Carter Fuller,[11] by which time Gowers had ceased to publish .

Acknowledgement

Adapted from: Larner AJ. Sir William Gowers (1845–1915): a centenary celebration, with an examination of his comments on cognitive dysfunction. *Adv Clin Neurosci Rehabil* 2015;15(1):16–17.

References

1. Tyler KL. William Richard Gowers (1845–1915). *J Neurol* 2003;250:1012–1013.
2. Rose FC. *History of British neurology.* London: Imperial College Press, 2012:130–137.
3. Scott A, Eadie M, Lees A. *William Richard Gowers 1845–1915. Exploring the Victorian brain: a biography.* Oxford: Oxford University Press, 2012.
4. Eadie MJ, Scott AE, Lees AJ, Woodward M. William Gowers: the never completed third edition of the "Bible of Neurology". *Brain* 2012;135:3178–3188.
5. Shorvon S, Shepherd L. *The beginning of the end of the falling sickness. Epilepsy and its treatment in London 1860–1910.* London, 2012:30–32.
6. Sacks O. Gowers' memory. *Neurology* 1996;46:1467–1469.
7. Larner AJ. Was dementia with Lewy bodies described by Sir William Gowers (1845–1915) in the nineteenth century? *Prog Neurol Psychiatry* 2015;19(2):10.
8. Miranda M, Slachevsky A, Garcia-Borrequero D. Did Immanuel Kant have dementia with Lewy bodies and REM behaviour disorder? *Sleep Med* 2010;11:586–588.
9. Sahlas DJ. Dementia with Lewy bodies and the neurobehavioral decline of Mervyn Peake. *Arch Neurol* 2003;60:889–892.
10. Larner AJ, Gardner-Thorpe C. Robert Lawson (?1846–1896). *J Neurol* 2012;259:792–793.
11. Larner AJ. Solomon Carter Fuller (1872–1953) and the early history of Alzheimer's disease. *Adv Clin Neurosci Rehabil* 2013;12(6):21–22.

Major books published by Sir William Gowers

A Manual and Atlas of Medical Ophthalmoscopy

Pseudo-hypertrophic Muscular Paralysis

The Diagnosis of Diseases of the Spinal Cord

Manual of Diseases of the Nervous System

Syphilis of the Nervous System

Epilepsy and Other Chronic Convulsive Disorders

The Border-land of Epilepsy: Faints, Vagal Attacks, Vertigo, Migraine, Sleep Symptoms and their Treatment

Medical practitioners and practice on Livingstone's Zambesi expedition, 1858–1864

Between 1853 and 1856, Dr David Livingstone (1813–1873) made the first of his major African journeys, from the west coast (in modern-day Angola) to the east (Mozambique).[1,2] During this transcontinental journey he became increasingly aware of the African slave trade, and he became convinced that the Portuguese, nominally the colonial masters of much of this territory, colluded in the traffic in human lives.[3] Livingstone determined that the solution to the problem of slavery would be to introduce British civilization, commerce and Christianity into the interior of Africa.

On furlough in Britain between 1856 to 1858, he canvassed support for this idea, gaining the sponsorship of the British government for an expedition to the Zambesi river. At a meeting in the Senate House of the University of Cambridge in December 1857, Livingstone called on the young men of the University to assist in completing his work in Africa,[4] a consequence of which was the foundation of a University Mission to Central Africa and, subsequently, the sending of Christian missionaries to Africa. Livingstone and the Expedition party embraked on the SS Pearl at Liverpool in March 1858, beginning a journey which was to last for almost six years.[5–9]

Health problems dogged members of both the Expedition and the subsequent Mission, principally the "African fever", a condition which had claimed the lives of many Europeans on previous expeditions in tropical Africa. Difficult and dangerous as it is to extrapolate from 19th century disease categories to our own, this was most probably in large part due to malaria; the Expedition took place in areas now known to be high risk for malaria. Livingstone's favoured remedy for attacks of African fever, developed during his previous travels, was a combination of quinine and purgatives. To four grains of quinine were added resin of jalap eight grains, calomel eight grains, and rhubarb four grains, the whole mixed well together, made into pills with spirit of cardamoms and given when required in a dose of ten to twenty grains. Following the discharge of bile, quinine was given until the ears were ringing ("cinchonism"). This mixture apparently relieved headaches and pain within four to six hours, and Livingstone reported it to be "successful in every case". Among the members of the Expedition it became known colloquially as the "Zambesi rouser". However, Livingstone found no prophylactic role for quinine: "It is decidedly curative but questionably prophylactic, if we deduct the effect on the imagination". For Livingstone the best preventative against fever was "plenty of exercise and abundance of good food".[10]

Dr Charles Meller (1836–1869)

Further medical observations from the Zambesi expedition were later reported in the British medical press by Dr Charles James Meller.[11] He joined Livingstone in February 1861, almost three years after the expedition had first reached Africa. He published two papers, the first in the *British Medical Journal* in October 1862. Meller characterized fever as "asthenic and remittent", whereas Livingstone's previous report described the fever to be "sthenic and intermittent", thus implying that the course of the fever was more chronic, if less severe acutely. However, Meller did endorse the regime of quinine and purgatives (the "Livingstone specific") but he quotes four grains of quinine, eight grains of resin of jalap, four grains of calomel, and ten grains of rhubarb, with quinine then given every two to three hourly in a dose of five to ten grains until deafness was produced, the greater the deafness the speedier the restoration of the patient.[12] The difference in regime does suggest a lack of uniformity in prescribing practice. Meller stated that with this treatment headaches associated with the fever might persist for three to seven days, hence he was less optimistic about its efficacy than Livingstone. It seems likely that Livingstone underplayed the medical hazards of Africa, not wishing to discourage in any way immigration and colonisation. Meller agreed with Livingstone that quinine had no role as a prophylactic.[12] Meller thought that African fever resulted from exposure to miasmata arising from decomposing vegetable matter. The miasmatic theory of malaria transmission was a common belief in the mid-19th century. It was almost forty years later that the mosquito vector transmission of malaria was demonstrated by Ronald Ross.[13]

Meller's second paper based on observations made on the Zambesi expedition was published in the *Lancet* in October 1864, with Meller tilted as "surgeon-naturalist in medical charge".[14] There are a number of case reports, including details of Meller's own febrile illness which necessitated his return to the Cape for recuperation, from April to October 1862 (it seems likely his first paper was written and sent during this period). The case of Richard Wilson, a stoker on the expedition, is presented: during a severe attack of fever his urine was noted to darken progressively, from deep green to brown to almost black, after which he became jaundiced, dull and listless. Subsequent readers have identified this account as almost certainly one of blackwater fever, a complication of falciparum malaria due to massive intravascular haemolysis, sometimes precipitated by quinine, although Wilson had not had quinine before the changes in urinary colour. This report has been acknowledged as one of the earliest descriptions of blackwater fever in Africa, although it is not mentioned in the extensive monograph on the subject by Stephens published in 1937.[15]

It was well known that Europeans in Africa were more susceptible to fever than the indigenous peoples. Travelling with Livingstone's party were a number of Johanna men, natives of the Comoros Islands off the coast of East Africa, "hybrids of Arab and Negro" as Meller described them. Meller's *Lancet* paper reports a quantitative analysis of fever incidence among the Europeans and the Johanna men, performed during April 1863. It was found that the Europeans spent 20% of their time on the sick list and were four times more likely to be struck by fever than the Johanna men. Natives of the river (Zambesimen) "had almost perfect immunity". For this work, Meller has been credited with having performed "the first disease survey in Central Africa, on malaria".[16]

Meller's papers seem at first sight, to be pioneering contributions to the developing field of "tropical medicine". However, with the advent of further information, the analysis may be carried further, and suggests that matters are not in fact so straightforward.

Dr John Kirk (1832–1922)

When Livingstone first conceived the Zambesi expedition, he was keen to have the services of a botanist to study the indigenous flora in the hope that plants suitable for commercial development might be discovered. On the recommendation of Sir William Hooker, the Director of Kew Gardens, London, Livingstone appointed Dr John Kirk, a medical graduate of Edinburgh University and a keen botanist with some overseas experience of collecting plants, to the post of "Economic Botanist and Medical Officer" to the Expedition. It was Kirk who, at Livingstone's behest, equipped the expedition with the necessary medical supplies, obtained from Apothecaries Hall, London, in February 1858, and Kirk who travelled to Liverpool in early March 1858 to embark on the SS Pearl. He had signed up for three years, but in the event served for almost the whole duration of the Zambesi expedition, much of the time as *de facto* second-in-command to Livingstone. Kirk and Livingstone, trekking alone, became the first Europeans to reach Lake Nyassa (Lake Malawi) in September 1859. Livingstone wrote in his *Narrative* of the expediton[5] that Kirk:

> collected above 1000 species of plants, specimens of most of the valuable woods, of the different native manufactures, of the articles of food, and of the different kinds of cotton from every spot we visited, and a great variety

of birds and insects; besides making meteorological observations, and affording, as our instructions required, medical assistance to the natives in every case where he could be of any use.[17]

Kirk kept a daily journal of his work and experiences throughout his time in Africa. Livingstone hoped Kirk would use this as the basis for his own account of the Expedition, focusing on botanical and medical issues not covered in his own *Narrative*. However, this did not come about, and it was not until 1965, one hundred years later, that Kirk's journals entered the public domain,[18] although their contents had been made use of in earlier biographical works.[19,20] The journals' account of the expedition is often harrowing: it describes the hard labour of hauling the paddle steamer over shallows where its draught was too deep for the river, of cutting wood for its voracious and inefficient boiler; the mischievous behaviour of certain members of the Expedition; problems with the indigenous population; the ill-health and death of friends; the failure to realise the stated aims of the Expedition.

The journal bears out Livingstone's statement in his *Lancet* paper of 1861 that, for the treatment of African fever, "Dr Kirk ... entertain[s] the same opinion of the value of our pills as I do".[10] Initially Kirk envisaged diarrhoea as a mechanism for getting rid of malaria, but after a couple of years in Africa he was advocating quinine and magnesia or even quinine alone for slight febrile attacks, and reserving "active purgatives" for more severe attacks. Kirk also observed the inefficacy of unbleached quinine, which was impure, as opposed to pure quinine, in the treatment of fever.

Expedition policy regarding quinine prophylaxis is clarified by Kirk's journal. On the outward journey, Kirk records: "Today we began the quinine (2 grains in half glassful of wine) to each man. We shall continue this daily." However, two months later, once in Africa, we read: "Quinine again recommended. It has been intermitted for about 12 days." Arrival at a marshy location again prompted the precautionary use of quinine. With this piecemeal approach to prophylaxis it is perhaps not surprising that it proved ineffective. Moreover, the dosages of quininie used were too low by modern standards.

It is clear from Kirk's journal that Dr Meller's arrival in Africa in February 1861 came as a complete surprise to Kirk; evidently Livingstone had not informed him of his plans. Despite this difficult start, Kirk tried hard to get on with the newcomer but occasional comments in the journal suggest that he was not entirely enamoured of him.

A comparison of the medical information contained in Kirk's posthumously published journal and Meller's publications makes for interesting reading, since there are significant areas of overlap. As in Meller's 1864 *Lancet* paper,

Kirk's journal for 7–8 February 1863 also relates the story of Wilson, the stoker with blackwater fever, and also of Macleod, a blacksmith, who was similarly afflicted (8–10 February 1863). In addition to the clinical features, Kirk gives an account of the findings in the urinary sediment:

> when boiled, it almost solidified with a coagulum which was rendered more dense by nitric acid. Heated with nitric acid, it became bright green. Through the microscope nothing could be seen save a very few epithelium scales and mucus corpuscles, not a blood disc full or collapsed. The colour is most certainly due to bile; the mucus, a pus corpuscle, may come from anywhere ... But whence comes the albumen in such quantities [?].

The circumstantial details provide added verisimilitude to what may be regarded as a remarkable piece of medical science, considering the prevailing working conditions.

Kirk's journal contains the results of an epidemiological analysis of fever in Europeans and Johanna men which he undertook between April to July 1862, hence several months before Meller undertook his, briefer, analysis (in April 1863). Kirk notes that of 23 Europeans, 532 days were lost sick and off duty, whereas six Johanna men lost only 29 days. Hence there was more than four times as much sickness amongst the Europeans, who spent one-fifth of their time on the sick list, four-fifths of this due to fever. These results are almost identical to those subsequently found by Meller.

On the basis of the existing documentary evidence, I am not able to advance any explanation for the similarities in the work of Kirk and Meller. They may have seen the same patients, together or independently, but certainly the epidemiological surveys could not have been collaborative work, since for the whole period that Kirk was collecting data Meller was recuperating at the Cape, and Kirk doubted that he would return to the Expedition. Certainly the availability of the journal indicates that the credits given by posterity to Meller for his publications are at least equally merited by Kirk.

Epilogue: Kirk and Meller after the Zambesi expedition

Why did Kirk not write up his journal for publication, as Livingstone had hoped? I suspect that, by the time he was able to leave, he was fed up: with Livingstone, the struggle of exploration, arguments with other Expedition members, the loss of his collections and of friends. He needed to recuperate from his own ill health. He may have preferred to put the Zambesi behind him and look to the future, and indeed new opportunities were opening up.

He returned to Africa as Vice-Consul in Zanzibar in 1866. In his Zambesi journal he had written that it was a "duty of humanity" to reduce the slave trade. In 1873, as Consul-General, he was able to conclude an anti-slavery treaty with the Sultan of Zanzibar, thus in the year of Livingstone's death partially achieving one of the aims of the Zambesi expedition.[21]

Following the death of Richard Thornton, the geologist to the Expedition, Meller asked to leave Africa. Livingstone accused him of "mortal funk on poor Thornton's death" and balked at the request, pointing out to Meller his agreement to serve for three years and that his sick leave at the Cape could not count. It was thus not until July 1863 that Meller was allowed to leave. Bad feeling persisted: amongst other things Meller labelled Livingstone's proposed *Narrative* as a "composition of untruth". In June 1865, he took up an appointment as HM Vice-Consul in Madagascar. Conacher reports that he became director of the Pamplemousses Gardens in Mauritius, with a brief to find new sugar cane varieties. He died and is buried in New South Wales, Australia.[22]

Acknowledgement

Adapted and updated from: Larner AJ. Medical aspects of Dr Livingstone's Zambesi expedition, 1858–1864. *Medical Historian (Journal of the Liverpool Medical History Society)* 2002–2003;13:5–11; and Larner AJ. Charles Meller and John Kirk: medical practitioners and practice on Livingstone's Zambesi expedition, 1858–64. *J Med Biogr* 2002;10:129–134.

References

1. Livingstone D. *Missionary travels and researches in South Africa; including a sketch of sixteen years' residence in the interior of Africa, etc.* London: John Murray, 1857.
2. Schapera I (ed.). *Livingstone's African journal 1853–1856*. London: Chatto & Windus, 1963 (2 volumes).
3. Newitt MDD. The Portuguese on the Zambezi: an historical interpretation of the Prazo system. *J Afr Hist* 1969;10:67–85.
4. Monk W (ed). *Dr Livingstone's Cambridge Lectures together with a prefatory letter by the Rev. Professor Sedgwick* (2nd edition). Cambridge: Deighton Bell, 1860.
5. Livingstone D, Livingstone C. *Narrative of an expedition to the Zambesi and its tributaries: and the discovery of the lakes Shirwa and Nyassa 1858–1864*. London: John Murray, 1865.
6. Wallis JPR (ed.). *The Zambesi Expedition of David Livingstone 1858–1863*. London: Chatto & Windus, 1956 (2 volumes).
7. Shepperson G (ed.). *Livingstone and the Rovuma*. Edinburgh: Edinburgh University Press, 1965.
8. Martelli G. *Livingstone's river: a history of the Zambezi expedition 1858–1864*. London: Chatto & Windus, 1970.

9. Dritsas L. *Zambesi: David Livingstone and expeditionary science in Africa.* London: IB Tauris, 2010.
10. Livingstone D. On fever in the Zambesi. *Lancet* 1861;ii:184–186.
11. Larner AJ. Charles Meller and the medicine of the tropics in the mid-nineteenth century: pioneer or plagiarist? *St Mary's Gazette* 1998;104(2):47–49.
12. Meller CJ. Fever of the South-East coast of Africa. *BMJ* 1862;2:437–440.
13. Cook GC, Webb AJ. Perceptions of malaria transmission before Ross' discovery of 1897. *Postgrad Med J* 2000;76:738–740.
14. Meller CJ. On the fever of the East Central Africa. Encountered by Livingstone's Zambesi expedition. *Lancet* 1864;ii:459–461.
15. Stephens JWW. *Blackwater fever: a historical survey and summary of observations made over a century.* London: University of Liverpool/Hodder & Stoughton, 1937.
16. King MS, King E. *The story of medicine and disease in Malawi. The 130 years since Livingstone.* Blantyre: Montfort Press, n.d. [but after 1992]:12.
17. Foskett R (ed.). *The Zambesi Doctors: David Livingstone's letters to John Kirk, 1858–1872.* Edinburgh: Edinburgh University Press, 1964.
18. Foskett R (ed.). *The Zambesi journal and letters of Dr John Kirk, 1858–63.* Edinburgh: Oliver & Boyd, 1965.
19. Coupland R. *Kirk on the Zambesi: a chapter of African history.* Oxford, Clarendon Press, 1928.
20. Chadwick O. *Mackenzie's Grave.* London: Hodder & Stoughton, 1959.
21. Liebowitz D. *The physician and the slave trade. John Kirk, the Livingstone expeditions, and the crusade against slavery in East Africa.* New York: WH Freeman, 1999.
22. Conacher ID. Last resting places of the Zambezi Expedition (1858–1864) doctors. *J Med Biogr* 2018;26:68–69.

Richard Wolfgang Semon (1859–1918)

The name of Semon may be familiar to some neurologists because of (Sir) Felix Semon (1849–1921), a significant pioneer in the field of otolaryngology who held an appointment at the National Hospital for the Paralysed and Epileptic at Queen Square in London between 1887 and 1909. In an 1881 publication he described the paralysis of extensor before flexor muscles in lesions of the anterior horn cells, later known as Semon's law (or the Rosenbach-Semon law) [10], although its status as a "law" may be contested.

Felix's younger brother, Richard Wolfgang Semon (1859–1918), may be less well remembered in neurological circles, but his contributions to the study of memory in the early twentieth century, though initially largely neglected, have recently been noted increasingly and indeed may possibly be more significant in the history of neurobiology than his brother's contributions. At this time surrounding the centenary of the translation of his key works into English, it is apposite to review Richard Semon's life and career.

Born in Berlin, he obtained a doctorate in zoology at the University of Jena (1883) and then a medical qualification (1886) after studying in Heidelberg but he never practiced medicine. His interests in evolutionary biology, prompted in part by his mentor Ernst Haeckel (1834–1919), led to an associate professorship in Jena (1891). From 1891–3 Semon undertook a zoological expedition to Australasia, the collections from which led to the identification of many new species [7]. Semon's name is commemorated in the Linnean binomial taxonomy by a species of green-blooded skinks and a family of parasitic spiny-headed worms discovered on this expedition.

He moved from Jena to Munich in 1897, following an affair with Maria Krehl, the wife of one of the professors in Jena. It was in Munich, as a private scholar (*Privatgelehrter*), that his work on memory developed. Because of his circumstances, this work was entirely theoretical, for although relevant literature was considered Semon undertook no empirical studies.

In his 1904 work *Die Mneme*, which attempted to link the mechanisms of heredity and memory, Semon introduced the concept of the engram: "the enduring though primarily latent modification of the irritable substance produced by a stimulus". The process giving rise to new engrams he termed "engraphy", hence stimuli acted engraphically to create engrams. He clearly envisaged engrams as physical changes in the state of the brain although did not speculate on the precise nature of such changes. Semon introduced a further term, ecphory, to describe memory retrieval: "the influences which awaken the mnemic trace or engram out of its latent state into one of mani-fested activity". *Die Mneme* proved controversial, principally because of Semon's apparent commitment to the neo-Lamarckian position of inheritance of acquired characteristics in his understanding of heredity. Consequently *Die Mneme* was generally not well received.

Semon's second book, *Die mnemischen empfindungen*, published in 1909, was devoted entirely to memory, particularly retrieval phenomena, including the idea that "each ecphory of an engram-complex produces not only a mnemic sensation ... but through this creates a new engram". Unlike *Die Mneme*, *Die mnemischen empfindungen* was largely ignored. This lack of recognition hurt Semon, as is evident from his correspondence with August Forel (1848–1931), an ardent supporter of his work. This disappointment was compounded by the death of his wife Maria from cancer and Germany's defeat in World War 1, both in 1918, all of which may have been triggers for Semon's suicide later that year.

It was not until after his death that Semon's books were translated into English, as *The mneme* (1921) [8] and *Mnemic psychology* (1923) [9], but again little attention seems to have been paid to them. Donald Hebb was apparently unaware of Semon's notion of the engram when developing his ideas about modifiable synapses as the substrate of memory in the 1940s, and Karl Lashley's publication which popularised the term engram (1960) did not reference Semon's work [3]. Although Semon was still known in the German speaking world [6], it was not until the 1970s that his work was "rediscovered" by the Anglophone world, principally due to the work of Daniel Schacter [4,5].

Although published in its current form in 2001, Schacter's biography of Semon [4] was based on his research dating from the late 1970s and early 1980s. In the interim, there has been increased neurobiological interest in the notion of the engram, the only one of Semon's neologisms to have persisted and which has been largely equated with the notion of "memory traces". Contemporary research seeking for "hippocampal memory engrams" and for "motor engrams encoding motor experience" may be found in the literature. Indeed, as a consequence of his apparent anticipations, for example of pattern completion and multiple trace theory, Semon has been accounted one of the "heroes of the engram" [2], a status which may serve to justify Semon's belief that recognition of his contributions would have to await future generations.

Be that as it may, overlooking any anachronism in reinterpreting Semon's work in the light of current ideas, and whatever recent empirical studies may discover, Semon's core idea of the engram remains vulnerable to conceptual attack. Semon's introduction of the engram is mentioned in the second (but not the first) edition of Bennett & Hacker's *Philosophical Foundations of Neuroscience*, although misdated to 1921 rather than 1904 [1], as part of their discussion of the conceptual incoherence of memory traces being encoded or stored in the brain. The etymology of the term "engraphy" (understood as the making of an engram) implies something being written down, or engraved, on or in the brain. However, it makes no sense to say that what one remembers, the ability to recollect, is dependent upon something written down (or stored, or encoded) in the brain. Certainly one may not be able to remember without certain neural configurations or synaptic connections within the brain, and future empirical studies may further define with increasing precision what these neural configurations or synaptic connections may be, but they will not identify an engram because conceptually this idea makes no sense.

Acknowledgment

Adapted from: Larner AJ, Leff AP, Nachev PC. Richard Wolfgang Semon (1859–1918). *J Neurol* 2022;269:2822–2823.

References

1. Bennett MR, Hacker PMS (2022) Philosophical foundations of neuroscience (2nd edition). Oxford: Blackwell, p.173
2. Josselyn SA, Köhler S, Frankland PW (2017) Heroes of the engram. J Neurosci 37:4647–4657
3. Lashley K (1960) In search of the engram. In: Beach FA, Hebb DO, Morgan CT, Nissen HW (eds). The neuropsychology of Lashley. New York: McGraw-Hill
4. Schacter DL (2001) Forgotten ideas, neglected pioneers: Richard Semon and the story of memory. Philadelphia: Psychology Press
5. Schacter DL, Eich JE, Tulving E (1978) Richard Semon's theory of memory. J Verbal Learning Verbal Behav 17:721–743
6. Schatzmann J (1968) Richard Semon (1859–1918) und seine Mnemetheorie. Zurich: Juris-Verlag
7. Semon R (1899) In the Australian Bush, and on the Coast of the Coral Sea: being the Experiences and Observations of a Naturalist in Australia, New Guinea, and the Moluccas. London: Macmillan
8. Semon R (1921) The Mneme. London: George Allen & Unwin
9. Semon R (1923) Mnemic psychology. London: George Allen & Unwin
10. Shorvon S, Compston A (2018) Queen Square. A history of the National Hospital and its Institute of Neurology. Cambridge: Cambridge University Press, p.370–371

William Barnett Warrington (1869–1919)

Time spent thumbing through old copies of the *Liverpool Medical-Chirurgical Journal*, for example those available in the Library of the Liverpool Medical Institution (LMI), reveals that certain names, some of them well known in the history of Liverpool medicine and surgery,[1] occur frequently. Other names, although occurring with similar frequency, may be less familiar. One such is William Barnett Warrington (1869–1919). Although he has been noted in a history of British physiologists,[2] only recently has there been any acknowledgement of his contributions to neurology,[3,4] although his published works encompass not only neurology but also extend more broadly to general medicine.

Biography

Most of the readily available biographical detail about William Warrington comes from his *BMJ* obituary[5] and his (brief) entry in *Munks Roll*.[6] He was born in Liverpool, on 11th May 1869, the son of John T Warrington, JP, and Margaret Warrington. As Liverpool had no University at the time, he was obliged to study medicine elsewhere, at Owens College, Manchester, and at the Rotunda Hospital, Dublin. In Manchester, he was one of the earliest students (number 12) to be admitted to the Hulme Hall of Residence.[7] He took the Manchester MB ChB degrees in 1891 and the London MB in 1893. His house appointments included one as house physician at Manchester Royal Infirmary, whence his earliest publication, dated 1892, and at the National Hospital for the Paralysed and Epileptic (later the National Hospital for Nervous Diseases, and later still the National Hospital for Neurology and Neurosurgery) at Queen Square in London in 1894. He then spent some time studying in Leipzig.

Returning to Liverpool, he worked in the laboratory of Charles Scott Sherrington (1857–1952), then the Holt Professor of Physiology. Thereafter he undertook medical practice in Liverpool, initially with an honorary appointment to the Stanley Hospital, then as honorary physician at the Northern Hospital and as demonstrator in pathology at University College Liverpool (later lecturer in clinical medicine and neuropathology, University of Liverpool). He eventually became assistant physician to the Liverpool Royal Infirmary.

The *BMJ* obituary states that he gained the MRCP in 1905 and his FRCP ten years later (hence 1915). However, this appears to be incorrect since he is listed as "MD MRCP" in all his *Brain* papers published from 1898 onwards, and as FRCP at least from a *Lancet* paper of 1905, a date corroborated by *Munks Roll*. He lived in Rodney Street (variously listed as number 69, 35, and 63 in *LMI Reports* between 1896 and 1918), handily placed for visits to the LMI of which he was an active member from 1896 onwards. He was a great supporter of the meetings which served as a focal point for clinicians from the several general hospitals in the city and roundabout. Shepherd's history of the LMI notes that he served as Librarian (1907–8) and as Vice-President (1913–14).[8]

During the Great War he served as a captain in the Royal Army Medical Corps. In the aftermath of the conflict he fell victim to influenza complicated by pneumonia, dying on Sunday 2nd February 1919. He is recorded as "Captain William B Warrington" on the wall plaque in the foyer of the LMI "In Arduis Fidelis 1914–1919", a gift of Thelwell Thomas, LMI President 1918–1919, commemorating those who "gave their lives for their country" (Victor Horsley's name appears on the same memorial). Warrington is also commemorated on the War memorial at Anfield Cemetery,[9] and also at the University of Manchester War Memorial located on the John Owens' building in Oxford Road, Manchester.

Physiology

How Warrington came to have the opportunity to work with Sherrington is uncertain, but his Queen Square credentials are unlikely to have been immaterial. Sherrington spent the years 1895–1913 in Liverpool as Holt Professor of Physiology, the midpoint of which (1904) saw him deliver the Silliman Memorial Lectures at Yale which were to become his seminal work, *The integrative action of the nervous system* (1906). However, this is a period in Sherrington's life about which relatively little is written, or perhaps known, in contrast to his subsequent years as Waynflete Professor of Physiology in Oxford. Lord Henry Cohen's Sherrington Lectures (1958),[10] Ragnar Granit's *Appraisal* (1966),[11] and Eccles and Gibson's biography (1979),[12] devote no more than a few pages to Sherrington's Liverpool years, although Granit (p.84) acknowledges that this was a "period of intense creation and study". Some possible remnants of teaching materials used by Sherrington in Liverpool, as well as in Oxford, have recently been described.[13]

Neither Granit nor Eccles and Gibson, as far as has been seen, mention William Warrington. Granit[11] states that "[g]uest workers came and stayed on to experiment under Sherrington's guidance" (p.88) but although he "was a teacher of many young men" they are often "difficult to trace unless they were actual co-workers" (p.97). This is perhaps a little disingenuous, since we hear much of Harvey Cushing, who stayed for about a month, but nothing of Warrington who was around for perhaps 5 years. In his list of Sherrington's pupils, Lord Cohen[10] lists Warrington first, before Cushing (p.13).

Warrington does get a solitary mention in *The integrative action of the nervous system* (1906): in Lecture IX, on "The physiological position and dominance of the brain", in a section entitled "Richness of the extero-ceptive field in receptors; comparative poverty of the intero-ceptive", Sherrington writes: "The afferent nerve fibres in the sympathetic system as judged by their number are comparatively few; Warrington's recent observations show this conclusively",[14] with a reference to a paper co-authored by Warrington in 1904.[15]

Hence it is difficult to envisage clearly the working relationship of Sherrington and Warrington. O'Connor[2] merely states that "Warrington's connexion with physiology *apparently* came through Sherrington" (my italics). Derek Denny-Brown (1901–1981), in his account of the "Sherrington School" of physiology, notes Warrington amongst the "many others [who] published work from his laboratory under his guidance" (p.543), a group which he distinguishes from Sherrington's collaborators.[16]

Certain it is that Warrington single authored four papers in the *Journal of Physiology* between 1898 and 1904 on the subject of structural alterations in nerve cells following various nerve lesions. In all but the second of these he expressed his obligation and thanks to Professor Sherrington. This work in experimental physiology was also shared with members of the LMI, both in publications and demonstrations, for example when Warrington "showed sections of the spinal cord" (see *Liverpool Med Chirurg J* 1900;20:332, not 433 as given in the Journal index).

The three later *J Phys* papers (1899, 1900, 1904) are all designated as coming from the Thompson Yates Laboratories in Liverpool. This facility was opened in 1898 and was the location for research in both physiology, under Sherrington, and pathology and bacteriology, including tropical medicine, under Professor Rubert Boyce (1863–1911). The laboratories issued a house journal, the *Thompson Yates Laboratories Report*, from 1898 to 1903, edited by Boyce and Sherrington "with the co-operation of" (amongst others) Warrington, who is listed under both "Pathology and Bacteriology" and "Neurology". From 1905, following the opening of further purpose-built laboratory space, the journal became the *Thompson Yates and Johnston Laboratories Report*, again edited by Boyce and Sherrington "assisted by" (amongst others) Warrington. The exact form of the co-operation and assistance provided by Warrington is not clear.

In the copies of these journals available in the University of Liverpool

Library Special Collections and the Liverpool School of Tropical Medicine, Warrington only appears in Volume II, dated 1898–9. This includes (pages 79–89) a co-authored paper on a case of "myelopathic albuminosuria", probably myeloma, which was later also published elsewhere. In the report of the "Department of Histology" (page 91) it is stated that Mr EE Laslett "investigated, in conjunction with Dr W.B. Warrington, the pathological anatomy of a spinal case of much neurological interest" subsequently published in *Brain*.[17] There is also a report (pages 119–121) from "The Pathological Diagnosis Society of Liverpool" written by Warrington as the "Director". The purpose of the society was to put the facilities of a clinical laboratory at the disposal of local medical practitioners, to which end instructions were given about the submission of samples for diagnosis of tuberculosis, diphtheria, and typhoid, as well as tissues for tumour analysis. Nothing further is heard of either Warrington or this society in subsequent editions of the journal.

Medicine in general; neurology in particular

By the end of the nineteenth century, neurology in the United Kingdom had evolved as a discipline to the point where a very small number of physicians devoted all of their working time to neurological problems, and at least one hospital, the National Hospital for the Paralysed and Epileptic in Queen Square, London, was dedicated to the care of neurological patients (although the clinicians there preferred to call themselves physicians rather than neurologists). However, outside the metropolis, neurology remained largely a component of general medicine, with certain practitioners taking an interest in neurological disorders as one part of their more general work as physicians. One such clinician was William Barnett Warrington.

Warrington was clearly an indefatigable writer, publishing many articles, not only in high profile international journals such as the *Lancet* and *Brain*, but also in local publications such as the *Liverpool Medical-Chirurgical Journal* (the LMI house publication) and the *Medical Chronicle. A monthly record of the progress of the medical sciences*, a publication based at Owens College in Manchester. These included case reports and series, reviews on topical issues and of the works and publications of others, as well as lectures. Although most of his presentations were undertaken in Liverpool, there are also published lectures originally presented to medical societies in Southport (1907, "Some observations on the more common nervous diseases"), Wigan (1908, "Some acute cerebral diseases"; published in 1910), and Birkenhead (1913, "A review of some recent work in neurology"). In addition to substantive papers, Warrington's comments on papers presented by others were often recorded in transactions of the meetings, and he also gave demonstrations of pathology (e.g. an axillary sarcoma, and specimens illustrating vascular disease of the brain; *Liverpool Med Chirurg J* 1902;22:404 and 1903;23:412, respectively).

Warrington collaborated with other notable figures in Liverpool medicine, for example the orthopaedic surgeon (Sir) Robert Jones with whom he reported cases of Charcot-Marie-Tooth disease (1901) and paralyses of the brachial plexus (1906); the neuropathologist Alfred W. Campbell[18] who looked at the pathology of Warrington's case of African sleeping sickness (*Liverpool Med Chirurg J* 1903;23:162) and whose report to the LMI on "The pathology of progressive muscular atrophy" Warrington commented on (*Liverpool Med Chirurg J* 1903;23:407–8); the surgeon Keith Monsarrat[19] with whom he reported cases of cerebellar pathology (1902)[3] and of paraplegia (1908); and the radiologist Charles Thurstan Holland[20] who provided some of the x-ray images for Warrington's 1910 paper "On the relationship of injury to certain conditions of the spine and spinal cord and their differential diagnosis".

To the clinician of today, the breadth of Warrington's publications is staggering, including renal and hepatic disease, endocrinology (diabetes mellitus and insipidus, thyroid disease), infectious diseases (mostly syphilis, but also comments on typhoid), and metabolic disease ("myelopathic albuminosuria", or multiple myeloma). However, his publications are mostly related to disorders of the nervous system, perhaps particularly the peripheral nervous system but also cerebral disorders including aspects of psychology.

Despite this astonishing productivity, Warrington is almost entirely unknown in neurological circles today, perhaps because he made no obviously seminal contribution to the discipline. With the benefit of hindsight, it may be conjectured that he narrowly missed eponymous fame with descriptions of cases of what later came to be known as Guillain-Barré syndrome (GBS) following a paper published by these authors (and Strohl) in 1916. Reports by Warrington published in 1903 and 1914 in the *Liverpool Medical-Chirurgical Journal* presented a patient who developed proximal limb weakness which steadily progressed upwards segment by segment, with onset two weeks after a febrile illness. Four days after symptom onset the patient could not lift his legs from the bed, the shoulder girdle muscles were affected and the tendon reflexes were lost, but the paralysed muscles "acted strongly to faradism". The clinical phenotype is thus suggestive of GBS (accepting the difficulties of retrospective diagnosis), and predates the eponymous account by some years.[21,22] However, lumbar puncture was not reported in this patient, and hence no information is available concerning the typical dissociation between raised protein and normal cell count seen in the cerebrospinal fluid (CSF) in GBS patients, as reported in the eponymous authors' description. This is disappointing, not least because Warrington was certainly familiar with lumbar puncture and CSF analysis, topics on which he had published; the *Liverpool Medical-Chirurgical Journal* in 1904 (24:398) reported that "Dr Warrington showed stained preparations of the cerebrospinal fluid obtained by lumbar puncture in cases of different varieties of meningitis", and he was one of the discussants of the value of CSF analysis in meningitis in the *BMJ* (1905;2:1017–8).

Another potentially significant neurological description may be found in Warrington's 1903 paper "On some uncommon forms of neuritis of the upper limb with an unusual etiology" published in the *Lancet*. This paper may contain an early description of the condition now called neuralgic amyotrophy or brachial neuritis (see Case 2), and predates by more than 50 years the eponymous description by Parsonage and Turner in the same journal.[23]

During the Great War, Warrington served as a captain in the Royal Army Medical Corps. His war experience led to a paper in 1916 on "musculo-spiral" (i.e. radial) nerve injuries, but tragically this proved to be (as far as we have been able to ascertain) his last publication, since in the aftermath of the conflict he fell victim to influenza complicated by pneumonia.[5]

Commentary

Warrington was not a neurologist as we understand the term today, since he did not devote all his clinical time to disorders of the nervous system – very few physicians did so at this time. The effective absence of competition meant that he had the opportunity of the prepared mind to work in virgin territory. Although a significant contribution to neurology had already been made in Liverpool by Richard Caton who had recorded brain electrical activity, the forerunner of the EEG, in laboratory animals in 1875, this was largely unacknowledged. Certainly the experimental work of Sherrington stimulated interest in clinical disorders of the nervous system.

Warrington's *BMJ* obituary noted that "As a physician Dr Warrington was in the front rank in all that related to nervous disease".[5] Certainly his publications attest to the truth of this statement. His career illustrates that general physicians with an interest in neurology could make noteworthy contributions prior to greater specialisation (this did not begin in Liverpool, as in other regional centres, until the 1970s). William Warrington deserves to be better remembered as a significant contributor to the early history of neurology as a clinical discipline.

Bibliography of Warrington's publications

NB: It is not claimed that this listing is comprehensive, since a systematic search of all relevant journals has not been attempted. This listing does not include comments made by Warrington at meetings and which were published in reports of those meetings, mostly at the LMI but also at BMA Annual Meetings, mostly appearing in the *Lancet* but also in the *BMJ* and the *Liverpool Medical-Chirurgical Journal.*

1892:
Warrington WB. Two cases of Erb's juvenile paralysis. *Med. Chronicle*, Oct 1891–March 1892;15:299–301.

1896:
Warrington WB. A note on Nissl's stain for nerve cells. *Med. Chronicle*, April 1896–Sept 1896;5(New series):402–5.

1898:
Laslett EE, Warrington WB. The morbid anatomy of a case of lead paralysis. Condition of the nerves, muscles, muscle spindles and spinal cord. *Brain*, 21:224–31.
Warrington WB. On the structural alterations observed in nerve cells. *J. Physiol.*, 23:112–29. [Comment in *Med. Chronicle*, Oct 1899–March 1900;2(SeriesIII):98–100.]

1899:
Laslett EE, Warrington WB. Observations on the ascending tracts in the spinal cord of the human subject. *Brain*, 22:586–92. [See also *Liverpool Med. Chirurg. J.*, 19:401–2 and 1900;20:318, latter not mentioned in the Journal index.]
Warrington WB. Further observations on the structural alterations observed in nerve cells. *J. Physiol.*, 24:464–78. [Comment in *Med. Chronicle*, Oct 1899–March 1900;2(SeriesIII):98–100.]
Bradshaw TR, Warrington WB. The morbid anatomy and pathology of Dr. Bradshaw's case of myelopathic albuminosuria. *Med. Chir. Trans.*, 82:251–68. [Also *Liverpool Med. Chirurg. J.*, 1900;20:147–9 and 1902;22:329–30.]

1900:
Warrington WB, Dutton JE. Observations on the course of the optic fibres in a case of unilateral optic atrophy. *Brain*, 23:642–56. [Also *Liverpool Med. Chirurg. J.*, 1901;21:210–24.]
Warrington WB. Further observations on the structural alterations in the cells

of the spinal cord following various nerve lesions: Part III. *J. Physiol.*, 25: 462–7.

1901:
Raw N, Barendt FH, Warrington WB. Epidemic arsenical poisoning amongst beer drinkers. *BMJ*, 1:10–12.
Warrington WB, Jones R. A family of three cases of the peroneal type of muscular atrophy (Charcot-Marie-Tooth-Hofmann). *Lancet*, 158:1574–7. [Also *Liverpool Med. Chirurg. J.*, 1901;21:403–5, as "A family of three cases of peritoneal [*sic*] type of muscular atrophy."]

1902:
Warrington WB. Two cases. *Liverpool Med. Chirurg. J.*, 22:92–9.
Warrington WB. Lumbar puncture and its value, especially in cases of meningitis. *Liverpool Med. Chirurg. J.*, 22:409–15.
Warrington WB, Monsarrat K. A case of arrested development of the cerebellum and its peduncles with spina bifida and other developmental peculiarities in the cord. *Brain*, 25:444–78. [Also Monsarrat K, Warrington WB. Case of arrested development of the cerebellum and its peduncles, with spina bifida and other developmental peculiarities in the cord. *Liverpool Med. Chirurg. J.*, 1902;22:434–6; also available at LMI as a pamphlet.]

1903:
Warrington WB. On some uncommon forms of neuritis of the upper limb with an unusual etiology. *Lancet*, 2:878–81. [Also "Author's abstract" in *Med. Chronicle*, Oct 1903–March 1904;39:176–8.].
Warrington WB. The pathology of sleeping sickness. *Liverpool Med. Chirurg. J.*, 23:159–63.
Warrington WB. Two cases. *Liverpool Med. Chirurg. J.*, 23:261–8.
Warrington WB. Some recent work on the condition of the deep reflexes and other symptoms in transverse lesions of the cord. A critical review. *Med. Chronicle*, Oct 1902–March 1903;37:101–19.
Warrington WB. Two cases of Brown-Séquard's paralysis. *Med. Chronicle*, April 1903–Sept 1903;38:29–40.

1904:
Warrington WB, Griffith F. On the cells of the spinal ganglia and on the relationship of their histological structure to the axonal distribution. *Brain*, 27:297–326.
Warrington WB. Note on the ultimate fate of ventral cornual cells after section of a number of posterior roots. *J. Physiol.*, 30:503–6. [Comment in *Med. Chronicle*, April 1904–Sept 1904;40:66–7.]

Warrington WB. Two cerebral cases. *Liverpool Med. Chirurg. J.*, 24:227–32.

Warrington WB. A review on some recent work on the diagnosis and treatment of cerebral tumour. *Med. Chronicle*, April 1904–Sept 1904;40:17–25.

Warrington WB. Myasthenia gravis with ophthalmoplegia: with some observations on ocular palsies. *Med. Chronicle*, April 1904–Sept 1904;40:319–24.

1905:

Warrington WB. A case of tumour of the cauda equina removed by operation, with remarks on the diagnosis and nature of lesions in that situation. *Lancet*, 2:749–53.

Warrington WB. Plantar reflexes. *Liverpool Med. Chirurg. J.*, 25:104–10.

Warrington WB. On compression paraplegia, and an account of a case in which a tumour was removed from the cauda equina. *Liverpool Med. Chirurg. J.*, 25:176–93.

Warrington WB. On the present position of the problem of localisation of the great-brain – the frontal lobe. *Med. Chronicle*, Oct 1904–March 1905;41:379–84.

Warrington WB. Cerebellar tumour. *Med. Chronicle*, April 1905–Sept 1905;42:144–7.

Warrington WB. Review of some recent clinical papers on cerebellar tumours. *Med. Chronicle*, April 1905–Sept 1905;42:151–7.

Warrington WB. Neurology. *Med. Chronicle*, April 1905–Sept 1905;42:161–4.

1906:

Warrington WB, Jones R. Some observations on paralyses of the brachial plexus. *Lancet*, 2:1644–9. [Also available at LMI as a pamphlet.]

Warrington WB. Some cases of chronic rigidity of the spine. *Liverpool Med. Chirurg. J.*, 26:140–2.

Warrington WB. Recent works on psychology. *Med. Chronicle*, Oct 1905–March 1906;43:24–9.

Warrington WB. Some cases of chronic rigidity of the spine. *Med. Chronicle*, Oct 1905–March 1906;43:343–53.

1907:

Warrington WB. Some observations on the more common nervous diseases. *Liverpool Med. Chirurg. J.*, 27:49–61.

1908:

Warrington WB, Monsarrat KW. A case of paraplegia due to an intramedullary lesion and treated with some success by the removal of a local accumulation of fluid. *Lancet*, 1:94–6.

Warrington WB. A clinical lecture on granular kidney. *Lancet*, 2:517–20.

Warrington WB. Two clinical studies of cases of enlargement of the spleen. *Liverpool Med. Chirurg. J.*, 28:74–84.

Warrington WB. Introduction to a discussion at the Liverpool Medical Institution on exophthalmic goitre. *Liverpool Med. Chirurg. J.*, 28:311–25.

Warrington WB. The treatment by diet of a severe case of diabetes mellitus and a note on three cases of diabetes insipidus. *Med. Chronicle*, Oct 1907–March 1908;47:1–7.

Warrington WB. Some recent works on nephritis. *Med. Chronicle*, April 1908–Sept 1908;48:82–93.

1909:

Warrington WB. Visceral syphilis. *Liverpool Med. Chirurg. J.*, 29:87–100.

Warrington WB. Note on natural history and diagnosis of cirrhosis of the liver with reference to the value of the Talma-Drummond-Morison operation. *Liverpool Med. Chirurg. J.*, 29:282–95.

1910:

Warrington WB, Murray RW. On the failure of nerve anastomosis in infantile palsy. *Lancet*, 1:912–4.

Murray RW, Warrington WB. On the failure of nerve anastomosis in infantile palsy. *Lancet*, 2:1168.

Warrington WB. Note on tuberculous meningitis, with especial reference to the invasion of symptoms when the disease occurs in adults. *Lancet*, 2:1754–5.

Warrington WB. Some results of treatment in the severer forms of diabetes mellitus. *Liverpool Med. Chirurg. J.*, 30:77–86.

Warrington WB. Some acute cerebral diseases. *Med. Chronicle*, Oct 1909–March 1910;51:150–65.

Warrington WB. On the relationship of injury to certain conditions of the spine and spinal cord and their differential diagnosis. *Med. Chronicle*, April 1910–Sept 1910;52:215–42.

1911:

Warrington WB. Neurasthenia. *Med. Chronicle*, Oct 1910–March 1911;53:137–172. [Journal contents and index erroneously gives first page as 143.]

Warrington WB. Neurasthenia. *Med. Chronicle*, Oct 1910–March 1911;53:203–15.

Warrington WB. The after later effects of head injuries. *Med. Chronicle*, Oct 1910–March 1911;53:273–302.

Warrington WB. Traumatic myelitis. *Med. Chronicle*, Oct 1910–March 1911;53:350–7.

Warrington WB. Injury as an etiological factor in the causation of organic nervous disease. I. General considerations. *Med. Chronicle*, April 1911–Sept 1911;54:1–5.

Warrington WB. Injury as an etiological factor in the causation of some well-defined nervous diseases. *Med. Chronicle*, April 1911–Sept 1911;54:121–41.

Warrington WB. The effects of injury on the nervous system. [Also available at LMI as a pamphlet.]

Warrington WB. A case of lymphadenoma terminating in paraplegia. *Liverpool Med. Chirurg. J.*, 31:53–57.

Warrington WB. II. Carcinoma of the stomach. *Liverpool Med. Chirurg. J.*, 31:559–62.

1912:

Warrington WB. The treatment of syphilis of the nervous system and of the parasyphilitic diseases. *Liverpool Med. Chirurg. J.*, 32:79–87.

Warrington WB. Remarks on syphilitic pseudo-tabes, with the record of a case. *Q. J. Med.*, 5:371–6. [Comment in *Med. Chronicle*, April 1912–Sept 1912;56:170.]

1913:

Warrington WB. A review of some recent work in neurology. Being some account of the sensory representation within the nervous system, and of Freud's views on abnormal psychology. *Liverpool Med. Chirurg. J.*, 33:69–88.

1914:

Warrington WB. Acute generalised infective paralyses in adults. *Liverpool Med. Chirurg. J.*, 34:67–76.

1916:

Warrington WB, Nelson P. War injuries to the musculo-spiral nerve. *Liverpool Med. Chirurg. J.*, 36:51–70.

Acknowledgements

Adapted from: Bracewell RM, Larner AJ. William Barnett Warrington (1869–1919): neurology in Liverpool around the turn of the 20th century. *Medical Historian (Journal of the Liverpool Medical History Society)* 2018;28:51–61; and Bracewell RM, Larner AJ. William Barnett Warrington (1869–1919). *European Neurology* 2019;81:323–326.

References

1. Larner AJ. A brief bibliography of papers related to the history of medicine in Liverpool and Merseyside. *Medical Historian* 2015;25:35–51.
2. O'Connor WJ. *British physiologists 1885–1914: a biographical dictionary.* Manchester and New York: Manchester University Press, 1991:369.
3. Compston A. Editorial. *Brain* 2010;133:643–644.
4. Bracewell RM, Larner AJ. William Barnett Warrington (1869–1919). *J Neurol* 2015;262:1794–1795.
5. Anonymous. Obituary. William Barnett Warrington, M.D.Lond., F.R.C.P. *BMJ* 1919;1:203.
6. http://munksroll.rcplondon.ac.uk/Biography/Details/4636   (accessed 26/09/17).
7. Hern J. *Chairs that stand empty. The men behind the names on the Hulme Hall First World War Memorial.* Matador: Kibworth Beauchamp, 2017:14,133–135.
8. Shepherd JA. *A history of the Liverpool Medical Institution.* Liverpool: Liverpool Medical Institution, 1979:205, 207, 224.
9. https://www.cwgc.org/find/find-war-dead/results/?cemetery=LIVER-POOL+(ANFIELD)+CEMETERY&csort=surname&tab=wardead&casualty pagenumber=45 (accessed 13/01/18).
10. Cohen of Birkenhead, Lord. *Sherrington. Physiologist, philosopher and poet.* Liverpool: Liverpool University Press, 1958.
11. Granit R. *Charles Scott Sherrington. An appraisal.* London: Nelson, 1966.
12. Eccles JC, Gibson WC. *Sherrington. His life and thought.* Heidelberg: Springer International, 1979.
13. Molnar Z, Brown RE. Insights into the life and work of Sir Charles Sherrington. *Nat Rev Neurosci* 2010;11:429–436.
14. Sherrington CS. *The integrative action of the nervous system.* London, Constable [1906] 1915:318, 402.
15. Warrington WB, Griffith F. On the cells of the spinal ganglia and on the relationship of their histological structure to the axonal distribution. *Brain* 1904;27:297–326.
16. Denny-Brown D. The Sherrington School of physiology. *J Neurophysiol* 1957;20:543–548.
17. Laslett EE, Warrington WB. Observations on the ascending tracts in the spinal cord of the human subject. *Brain* 1899;22:586–592.
18. Macmillan M. Alfred Walter Campbell's Rainhill days. *Medical Historian* 2011–2012;23:29–52.
19. Carmichael J. In the beginning was Monsarrat – medicine in war-time Liverpool. *Medical Historian* 2010–2011;22:35–44.
20. Larner AJ. Charles Thurstan Holland: a genealogical note. *Medical Historian* 2015;25:31–33.
21. Larner AJ. GBS100: some literary and historical accounts. In: Willison HJ, Goodfellow JA (eds.). *GBS100: Celebrating a century of progress in Guillain-*

Barré syndrome. Peripheral Nerve Society, 2016:20–27 [at 26].

22. Ziso B, Larner A. William Warrington (1869–1919): GBS before G, B, and S? *Eur J Neurol* 2016;23Suppl1:868 (abstract 32236).

23. Turner JW, Parsonage MJ. Neuralgic amyotrophy (paralytic brachial neuritis); with special reference to prognosis. *Lancet* 1957;2:209–212.

Semiology

Dolichocephaly and brachycephaly

When a schoolboy, aged perhaps 12 or 13, a friend and I took great delight in discovering new and unusual words (e.g. mnemonic, id). We were particularly pleased when he discovered "dolichocephalic" whilst reading Sherlock Holmes (it was many years later before I read the Holmes canon). The passage in question comes from chapter 1 of Arthur Conan Doyle's *The Hound of the Baskervilles* (1902), in which a medical man, Dr James Mortimer MRCS, notes:

> "You interest me very much, Mr Holmes. I had hardly expected so dolicho-cephalic a skull or such well-marked supraorbital development. ... A cast of your skull, sir, until the original is available, would be an ornament to any anthropological museum."

This report may possibly shape (no pun intended) individual perceptions of the physiognomy of Sherlock Holmes.[1]

Head size and shape is generally of little interest to neurologists dealing with adult patients, whilst paediatric neurologists may be more aware of these features in the context of dysmorphology syndromes, developmental problems, and hydrocephalus.[2] Large head size has been reported to be a feature of normal pressure hydrocephalus, the authors suggesting that this condition may be a consequence of congenital hydrocephalus which becomes symptomatic in later life.[3,4]

Heads longer (dolichocephaly) or shorter (brachycephaly) than expected, rather than normal (mesaticephalic or mesocephalic), may be defined using a cephalic or cranial index: the ratio of the maximum width of the head (biparietal diameter) multiplied by 100 and divided by maximum head length (occipitofrontal diameter). Once a staple of human physical anthropology, and by association inferences for unjustified assumptions about intelligence, often referred to race, the cephalic index is now of most interest to dog breeders, boxer dogs being typically brachycephalic, whippets and greyhounds dolicho-cephalic.

A few other literary references to dolichocephaly and brachycephaly have come to my attention over the years. Most significant is Aldous Huxley's (1894–1963) novel *Brave New World* (1932). In this dystopia, people are genetically engineered into five classes, Alpha through Epsilon, each further subdivided as Plus or Minus, with Alpha Double-Plus individuals at the apex of society, with declining intellectual and physical capacity going down the scale to the regular or semi-moron Epsilons. An Alpha Minus who is a "mine of irrelevant information and unasked-for good advice" is described as brachycephalic, as are noseless black Deltas working in a factory and a golden-haired Beta-Plus female, whereas the "menial staff of the Park Lane Hospital for the Dying" consist of Deltas including "seventy-eight dark dolichocephalic male twins". Head shape does not, therefore, seem to be particularly engineered in direct association with class or intelligence, although no data are vouchsafed on head shape in the Alpha Double-Plus class.[5]

Is it possible that Aldous learned the terminology from his grandfather, the biologist Thomas Henry Huxley (1825–1895)? In his biography of THH, Adrian Desmond notes that after the publication of *Evidence as to Man's Place in Nature* in 1863 the argument between Huxley (as Darwin's bulldog) and his opponents in the "ape-brain debate", particularly the comparative anatomist Richard Owen (1804–1892), became heated. This spilled over into popular culture, and in a broadsheet Huxley was caricatured as yelling that Owen was a "lying Orthognathous Brachycephalic Bimanous Pithecus".[6]

A final example: the Anglo-Welsh poet RS Thomas (1913–2000) uses the terminology in his poem *Brochure*, dating from 1964, in which he describes the Welsh as:

The people with dark hair,
Small in the thigh,
A large proportion
Dolichocephalic.

References

1. Larner AJ. Sherlock Holmes as "an exact embodiment of somebody or other". *The Sherlock Holmes Journal* 2017;33:60–61.
2. Gatrad AR, Solanki GA, Sheikh A. Baby with an abnormal head. *BMJ* 2014;348:f7609.
3. Graff-Radford NR, Godersky JC. Symptomatic congenital hydrocephalus in the elderly simulating normal pressure hydrocephalus. *Neurology* 1989;39:1596–1600.
4. Krefft TA, Graff-Radford NR, Lucas JA, Mortimer JA. Normal pressure hydrocephalus and large head size. *Alzheimer Dis Assoc Disord* 2004;18:35–37.
5. Huxley A. *Brave New World.* London: Granada [1932] 1983:87,130,137,168.
6. Desmond A. *Huxley. The devil's disciple.* London: Michael Joseph, 1994:316.
7. Brown T, Walford Davies J (eds.). *R.S. Thomas Uncollected Poems.* Tarset: Bloodaxe Books, 2013:54.

Echo phenomena

A number of echo phenomena are described in the neurological literature,[1] some of which are briefly considered here.

Echophenomena/Imitation behaviour

Much acquired human social behaviour is imitative in origin, both adaptive and maladaptive, but in neurological practice the term "imitation behaviour" is reserved for the reproduction by the patient of the examiner's words or gestures without preliminary instruction to do so ("naive imitation behaviour") or even despite explicit instruction not to do so ("obstinate imitation behaviour").[2] The term echophenomena has sometimes been used interchangeably with imitation behaviour.

To be labelled as such, the behaviours must be consistent and, as implied in the "obstinate" terminology, have a compulsive quality to them. Echophenomena may be accompanied by frontal release signs and utilization behaviour (another reflection of environmental dependency), and are usually attributed to frontal lobe dysfunction, though have been associated on occasion with either basal ganglia or thalamic lesions, and exceptionally with parietal lesions.

Kahlbaum's 1874 description of catatonia included the symptoms of echophenomena, and echolalia and echopraxia feature amongst the symptoms listed in the criteria for catatonia in *DSM-5*. Obstinate imitation behaviour has been reported to distinguish frontotemporal dementia from Alzheimer's disease,[3] but I think this is likely to be a specific (few false positives) but not very sensitive (many false negatives) sign.

Echolalia

Echolalia is the involuntary repetition of an interviewer's speech utterances (as opposed to the voluntary mickey-taking which characterises an irritating game typical of childhood, but sometimes indulged in by adults). As well as frontal lobe lesions, catatonia, and dementia syndromes, echolalia may also be encountered in children with autism, in Tourette syndrome,[4] and rarely as an ictal phenomenon, possibly with a left supplementary motor area origin.[5]

Echolalia may also occur in certain aphasia syndromes, for example in transcortical sensory aphasia, a fluent aphasia with well-preserved repetition skills. The aphasia of Alzheimer's disease has sometimes been likened to transcortical sensory aphasia, and a "mixed transcortical aphasia" with echolalia has been reported in Creutzfeldt-Jakob disease.

In contrast, "effortful echolalia" has been reported in left medial frontal lobe infarction including the supplementary motor area, with a non-fluent output typical of transcortical motor aphasia.[6]

In "dynamic aphasia" speech output is characterised by a difficulty in initiation, with the phenomenon of "incorporational echolalia" when the patient uses the examiner's question to help to form an answer. This has sometimes been conceptualised as a form of transcortical motor aphasia, and may sometimes be seen in progressive supranuclear palsy.

Echopraxia

Charcot used the term "echokinesis" to describe involuntary imitation of a movement in the context of what came to be known as Gilles de la Tourette syndrome.[7] However, the involuntary repetition of an interviewer's movements or gestures is now generally known as echopraxia. As with echolalia, echopraxia may be seen in frontal lobe disorders, catatonia, Tourette syndrome,[4] and rarely as an ictal phenomenon.[5] A mechanism for echopraxia in schizophrenia has been postulated which invokes activity in mirror neurones providing representation to the inferior frontal gyrus and motor cortex which becomes an executed movement due to decreased inhibition and/or increased arousal.[8]

Echolocation

An entirely separate echophenomenon is echolocation.

Visiting the Liverpool Asylum for the Blind in 1805, the American chemist Benjamin Silliman (1779–1864) reported:

> "How ... can we account for the acuteness of hearing which enabled a particular blind man, by means of the echo produced by his whistling, to decide when he was approaching any object of some magnitude ...".[9]

Echolocation is the comparison of outgoing sound pulses with the returning echoes in order to navigate or hunt. Though echolocation is most familiar (and studied) in bats and dolphins,[10] some blind individuals have developed the ability to use self-generated sounds, such as tongue clicks or finger snaps, as a form of sensory substitution to perceive the environment (YouTube has some informative videos). Sighted individuals can also be trained to do this.

A possible answer to Silliman's question has been provided by a functional magnetic resonance (MR) imaging study of two blind echolocators which found that calcarine ("visual") but not auditory cortex was activated when the subjects listened to recordings of echolocation clicks and echoes, suggesting a possible role for cross-modal brain plasticity in the development of this faculty of compensatory enhancement.[11] It would be interesting to learn if this was also the case in sighted individuals trained to echolocate.

Acknowledgement

Adapted from: Larner AJ. Neurological signs: echo phenomena. *Adv Clin Neurosci Rehabil* 2015;15(3):16.

References

1. Larner AJ. *A dictionary of neurological signs* (4th edition). London: Springer, 2016:109–110.
2. Lhermitte F, Pillon B, Serdaru M. Human autonomy and the frontal lobes. Part I: imitation and utilization behavior: a neuropsychological study of 75 patients. *Ann Neurol* 1986;19:326–334.
3. Shimomura T, Mori E. Obstinate imitation behaviour in differentiation of frontotemporal dementia from Alzheimer's disease. *Lancet* 1998;352: 623–624.
4. Ganos C, Ogrzal T, Schnitzler A, Münchau A. The pathophysiology of echopraxia/echolalia: relevance to Gilles de la Tourette syndrome. *Mov Disord* 2012;27:1222–1229.
5. Cho YJ, Han SD, Song SK, Lee BI, Heo K. Palilalia, echolalia, and echopraxia-palipraxia as ictal manifestations in a patient with a left frontal lobe epilepsy. *Epilepsia* 2009;50:1616–1619.
6. Hadano K, Nakamura H, Hamanaka T. Effortful echolalia. *Cortex* 1998;34:67–82.
7. Walusinski O. Georges Gilles de la Tourette. Beyond the eponym. Oxford: Oxford University Press, 2019:175.
8. Pridmore S, Brune M, Ahmadi J, Dale J. Echopraxia in schizophrenia: possible mechanisms. *Aust NZ J Psychiatry* 2008;42:565–571.
9. Seed D (ed.). *American travellers in Liverpool*. Liverpool: Liverpool University Press, 2008:8.
10. Jones G. Echolocation. *Curr Biol* 2005;15:R484–488.
11. Thaler L, Arnott SR, Goodale MA. Neural correlates of natural human echolocation in early and late blind echolocation experts. *PLoS One* 2011;6:e20162.

Echolalia; with a note on some synaesthestic phenomena

Echolalia

Echolalia may be defined as the involuntary automatic repetition of an interlocutor's speech.[1] The involuntary qualification excludes voluntary or wilful repetition, which many of us may have indulged in, perhaps as children, with a view to annoy or ridicule parents or friends.

There may be various clinical causes for echolalia, including autism; transcortical aphasias including dynamic aphasia; Tourette syndrome; neurodegenerative disorders such as some cases of Alzheimer's disease, behavioural variant frontotemporal dementia, and corticobasal degeneration; and focal epilepsy.

Remarkably enough, the word echolalia is used in two classics of the American 20th century literary canon.

In *The Great Gatsby* (1926) by F Scott Fitzgerald (1896–1940), at one of Gatsby's famed and opulent parties:

There was the boom of a bass drum, and the voice of the orchestra leader rang out suddenly above the echolalia of the garden.[2]

The word seems to be used here to describe the babble or chatter of voices, and not a clinical phenomenon.

In *Slaughterhouse-five, or the Children's Crusade* (1969) by Kurt Vonnegut (1922–2007), a more extensive usage of the word echolalia appears. Billy Pilgrim, the book's protagonist, is lying in a hospital bed in 1968 having just survived an aircrash. He shares his hospital room with Professor Bertram Copeland Rumfoord of Harvard, Official Historian of the United States Air Force. Rumfoord is puzzling over how to incorporate in his one-volume history of the Army Air Force in World War Two an account of the bombing of the German city of Dresden on 13th February 1945 in which around 135000 civilians were killed, an event which Billy witnessed as a prisoner of war, locked in Slaughterhouse-five.

"I was there," he said.

It was difficult for Rumfoord to take Billy seriously, since Rumfoord had so long considered Billy a repulsive non-person who would be much better off dead. Now, with Billy speaking clearly and to the point, Rumfoord's ears wanted to treat the words as a foreign language that was not worth learning.

"He's simply echoing the things we say ... He's got echolalia now."

The author then tells the reader that:

Echolalia is a mental disease which makes people immediately repeat things that well people around them say. But Billy didn't really have it.

Rumfoord went on insisting for several hours that Billy had echolalia – told nurses and a doctor that Billy had echolalia now.

Nobody took Rumfoord's diagnosis seriously.[3]

Clearly echolalia is being used in a clinical sense here, although by a non-clinician, to label somebody as mentally deficient.

Another, more recent, literary example of "echolalia" is found in Michel Houellebecq's novel *The possibility of an island* (2005):

For a long time I had been the victim of a sort of mental echolalia, which in my case did not apply to famous songs, but to the phrases used by classic comedians.[4]

This "sort of mental echolalia" sounds perhaps rather more like musical hallucinosis than echolalia.

Jonathan Miller (1934–2019), who had some training in neurology before he became a director in both theatre and opera, identified another example in Anton Chekhov's play *Three Sisters* (1901). Reading from the newspaper, Chebutykin says "Balsac's marriage took place at Berdichev" and repeats this as he jots it down in his notebook. Irena, singing softly to herself whilst playing patience, then repeats the phrase.[5] Miller states that "There is no connection between the two speakers; they are merely talking alongside one another, but people often struggle to find some profound significance in this repetition. It is, in fact, what is called echolalia, and unless it is treated as such, the effect is lost. It is a masterly inclusion of something that gives the genuine rhythm of undirected speech. Irena is preoccupied with turning over a card and the phrase has simply gone in one ear, and she faintly repeats the sound.

Chekhov's plays are simply concerned with showing the chronic coming and going of fairly undirected discourse."[6]

Synaesthestic phenomena

There are some other passages of possible neurological interest in Kurt Vonnegut's novel *Slaughterhouse-five*. Time is an important element in the book, indeed Billy is a traveller in time, as well as space. A passage in which time appears to run backward, such that Billy sees planes taking off backwards (i.e. appearing to land), was apparently a stimulus for Martin Amis's novel *Time's Arrow: or The Nature of the Offence* (1991). Billy is also taken to the planet Tralfamadore (alien abduction phenomenon?) where "the most important thing" he learns is that:

> All moments, past, present, and future, always have existed, always will exist.[7]

This "tenseless" philosophical viewpoint of time is picked up on by Cytowic and Eagleman in their book on synaesthesia. They discuss "number forms" or "spatial sequence synesthesia", a phenomenon reported by some synaesthetes in which number or time sequences are experienced in precise locations in relation to the body.[8]

There are some further passages in Vonnegut's novel which are perhaps suggestive of transmodal sensory experience or cross-modal activation. For example, whilst listening to the singing of a barbershop quartet on his wedding anniversary, an unexpected event occurs:

> as the quartet made slow, agonized experiments with chords ... Billy had powerful psychosomatic responses to the changing chords. His mouth filled with the taste of lemonade, and his face became grotesque, as though he ... were being stretched on ... the rack.[9]

This description includes several of the characteristics ascribed to synaesthetic experience: it was involuntary or automatic; generic or categorical ("taste of lemonade"), and affect-laden, although there is no indication as to whether the experience was consistent (how often do we hear a barbershop quartet?).

In addition, during his wartime experience in Europe, Billy

> had been seeing St Elmo's fire, a sort of electronic radiance around the heads of his companions and captors. It was in the treetops and on the rooftops of Luxembourg, too, it was beautiful.[10]

This might be termed illusory visual spread or visual perseveration, other literary examples of which have been noted.[11] This might also be a synaesthetic phenomenon: Cytowic and Eagleman report a patient who "has emotionally mediated synesthesia causing him to see colored auras around objects".[12]

I do not know whether Vonnegut was synaesthetic, but it is possible he may have suffered from depressive episodes and post-traumatic stress disorder, perhaps related to his war experience in Dresden.[13]

Acknowledgement

Adapted from: Larner AJ. Neurological signs: echolalia; with a note on some synaesthetic phenomena. *Adv Clin Neurosci Rehabil* 2013;13(6):43.

References

1. Larner AJ. *A dictionary of neurological signs* (4th edition). London: Springer, 2016:109–110.
2. Fitzgerald FS. *The Great Gatsby*. London: Penguin [1926] 1990:50.
3. Vonnegut K. *Slaughterhouse-five, or the Children's Crusade*. London: Vintage [1969] 2000:140–141.
4. Houellebecq M. *The possibility of an island*. London: Phoenix [2005] 2006:96.
5. Fen E (trans.). *Chekhov Plays*. Harmondsworth: Penguin, 1954:282.
6. Greaves I (ed.). *Jonathan Miller. One thing and another. Selected writings 1954-2016*. London: Oberon Books, 2017:259.
7. Op. cit., ref. 3:19.
8. Cytowic RE, Eagleman DM. *Wednesday is indigo blue. Discovering the brain of synesthesia*. Cambridge: MIT Press, 2009:124–125.
9. Op. cit., ref. 3:125–126.
10. Op. cit., ref. 3:46.
11. Larner AJ. Illusory visual spread or visuospatial perseveration. *Adv Clin Neurosci Rehabil* 2009;9(5):14.
12. Op. cit., ref. 8:10.
13. Shields CJ. *And so it goes: Kurt Vonnegut, a life*. New York: Henry Holt, 2011.

Gambling

Gambling may be defined as any game of chance involving financial stakes and an element of risk. Such games are common in our society, either using ones own money (e.g. the National Lottery, betting on horse or dog racing, visiting a casino or on-line gambling) or, better, other people's money (e.g. banking, insurance, the Stock Market). Gambling, as a form of risk-taking and decision-making, is of interest to neuropsychologists and may be characterised as an executive function task,[1] amenable to testing with instruments such as the Iowa Gambling Task (IGT)[2] and the Cambridge Gamble Task.[3] The neuroanatomical substrates of such decision making are believed to encompass the prefrontal cortex and the amygdala. Gambling may be defined as pathological when greater risks are taken and potential losses are correspondingly greater.

A famous "sufferer" from this "addiction" was the author Fyodor Dostoevsky (1821–1881), who wrote a novella, *The Gambler* (1866), on the subject in just 26 days (the film *Alex & Emma* is based on the same premise, and is very loosely based on Dostoevsky's novella). Dostoevsky might have been encouraged to write on this topic not only by his own insolvency but also by the example of his countryman Nikolai Gogol (1809–1852) who wrote a play entitled *The Gamblers* (ca. 1840). Dostoevsky's story was the basis for an opera of the same name (1917) by Sergei Prokofiev (1891–1953), and Dmitri Shostakovich (1906–1975) attempted to write an opera based on Gogol's play but never completed it (ca. 1942). Gambling, possibly of an obsessional nature, is a key theme in Alexander Pushkin's (1799–1837) story *The Queen of Spades* (1834), the basis of a later (1890) opera by Pyotr Ilyich Tchaikovsky (1840–1893). Gambling features in many other artistic works. For example, in Maria Edgeworth's (1768–1849) novel *Belinda* (1801), the "heroine ... breaks off her engagement to a kind and virtuous young man on the eve of her wedding and dismisses him from her life for ever because he has been gambling – this with the author's evident approval".[4]

Pathological gambling may also be a reflection of brain disease and its treatment. Reports of pathological gambling in patients with Parkinson's disease initially appeared in the early 2000s, the common factor apparently being treatment with various dopamine agonists.[5,6] It was initially unclear whether the small numbers of patients reported in these case series simply reflected the population prevalence of gambling behaviour, irrespective of treatment, or whether the numbers of PD patients with "problematic gambling" were in fact much higher. Later studies suggested the latter, e.g. 10% of patients prescribed dopamine agonists in the west of Scotland.[7] Certainly such cases were also seen outside dedicated PD treatment centres: I saw two such patients in district general hospital clinics, both with debts exceeding £10000, who were able to conceal their gambling activities from family members for long periods of time.[8] IGT performance may be impaired early in PD, suggesting ventromedial prefrontal cortical dysfunction.[9]

If gambling is an executive function, then one might anticipate that frontal lobe pathology would be associated with impaired performance on tests of gambling.[3] This is the case in patients with behavioural variant frontotemporal dementia (bvFTD) who have been shown to display risky decision-making, even in early disease and without evidence of behavioural disinhibition or impulsiveness.[10] bvFTD presenting with pathological gambling has been reported.[11,12] It has also been reported that risk-taking behaviour in bvFTD may be ameliorated by methylphenidate,[13] and the combination of paroxetine for impulsive behavior and carbamazepine to stabilize mood has also been used.[12] In contrast to bvFTD, successful gambling may be preserved in other focal frontotemporal lobar degeneration syndromes. A patient with semantic dementia continued to bet on the horses with, according to his wife, with whom he shared half his winnings, no tailing off in his success rate despite being essentially mute; the bookies noticed he said little but believed he had had a stroke.[14]

Acknowledgement

Adapted from: Larner AJ. Gambling. *Adv Clin Neurosci Rehabil* 2007;7(1):26.

References

1. Lehto JE, Elorinne E. Gambling as an executive function task. *Appl Neuropsychol* 2003;10:234–238.
2. Bechara A, Damasio AR, Damasio H, Anderson SW. Insensitivity to future consequences following damage to human prefrontal cortex. *Cognition* 1994;50:7–15.
3. Rogers RD, Everitt BJ, Baldacchino A et al. Dissociable deficits in the decision-making cognition of chronic amphetamine abusers, opiate abusers, patients with focal damage to prefrontal cortex, and tryptophan-depleted normal volunteers: evidence for monoaminergic mechanisms. *Neuropsychopharmacology* 1999;20:322–339.
4. Jenkyns R. *A fine brush on ivory: an appreciation of Jane Austen.* Oxford: Oxford University Press, 2004:117.
5. Driver-Dunckley E, Samanata J, Stacy M. Pathological gambling associated

with dopamine agonist therapy in Parkinson's disease. *Neurology* 2003;61:422–423.

6. Dodd ML, Klos KJ, Bower JH, Geda YE, Josephs KA, Ahlskog JE. Pathological gambling caused by drugs used to treat Parkinson disease. *Arch Neurol* 2005;62:1377–1381.

7. Grosset KA, Macphee G, Pal G, Stewart D, Watt A, Davie J, Grosset DG. Problematic gambling on dopamine agonists: not such a rarity. *Mov Disord* 2006;21:2206–2208.

8. Larner AJ. Medical hazards of the internet: gambling in Parkinson's disease. *Mov Disord* 2006;21:1789.

9. Perretta JG, Pari G, Beninger RJ. Effects of Parkinson disease on two putative nondeclarative learning tasks: probabilistic classification and gambling. *Cogn Behav Neurol* 2005;18:185–192.

10. Rahman S, Sahakian BJ, Hodges JR, Rogers RD, Robbins TW. Specific cognitive deficits in mild frontal variant frontotemporal dementia. *Brain* 1999;122:1469–1493.

11. Lo Coco D, Nacci P. Frontotemporal dementia presenting with pathological gambling. *J Neuropsychiatry Clin Neurosci* 2004;16:117–118.

12. Manes FF, Torralva T, Roca M, Gleichgerrcht E, Bekinschtein TA, Hodges JR. Frontotemporal dementia presenting as pathological gambling. *Nat Rev Neurol* 2010;6:347–352.

13. Rahman S, Robbins TW, Hodges JR et al. Methylphenidate ('Ritalin') can ameliorate abnormal risk-taking behavior in the frontal variant of frontotemporal dementia. *Neuropsychopharmacology* 2006;31:651–658.

14. Larner AJ, Brookfield K, Flynn A, Ghadiali EJ, Smith ETS, Doran M. The cerebral metabolic topography of semantic dementia. *J Neurol* 2005;252(suppl2):II106 (abstract P399).

Geophagia (geophagy) and pica (pagophagia)

29th November [1870]. – *Safura* is the name of the disease of clay or earth eating, at Zanzibar; it often affects slaves, and the clay is said to have a pleasant odour to the eaters, but it is not confined to slaves, nor do slaves eat in order to kill themselves; it is a diseased appetite, and rich men who have plenty to eat are often subject to it. The feet swell, flesh is lost, and the face looks haggard; the patient can scarcely walk for shortness of breath and weakness, and he continues eating until he dies.

This extract from the last journals of Dr David Livingstone[1,2] describes geophagia (geophagy), earth or clay eating. This may also fall under the rubric of pica, or pagophagia, a morbid craving for unusual or unsuitable food.

Another example may be found in the novel *One hundred years of solitude* by Gabriel Garcia Marquez (1927–2014), first published in 1967, concerning an eleven year-old girl, Rebeca, who arrives in the town of Macondo carrying a canvas sack which contains her dead parents' bones: "Rebeca only liked to eat the damp earth of the courtyard". The behaviour recurs later in her life when she experiences the passion of unrequited love.[3]

Although one might possibly dismiss the latter account as nothing more than an example of "magic realism", pica is a recognised symptom in childhood, sometimes associated with brain damage, learning disability, and emotional distress. Other inedible items which are sometimes eaten include paper and paint. Sufferers are obviously at risk of infection from contaminated foods, such as soil.[4] An association of pica with iron deficiency is well recognised,[5] as is a link with pregnancy. Livingstone noted that "clay built in walls is preferred, and Manyuema women when pregnant often eat it".[1]

Reports of geophagia have been found dating back to Hippocrates.[6] It was also encountered in the slave states in antebellum America, where "physicians and slaveowners … complained often and bitterly … about its frequency among their patients and wards", where it represented a potential source of roundworm infection.[7]

Geophagia may be associated with neurological complications. Cases have been reported of flaccid quadriparesis[8] and of proximal myopathy[9] associated with profound hypokalaemia in the context of geophagia. Livingstone mentioned weakness associated with clay eating (see above); he also mentioned "A Banyamwezi carrier, who bore an enormous load of copper, is now by safura scarcely able to walk".[1] A previous review of neurological problems described by Livingstone in his many writings failed to note this particular syndrome of geophagia-associated weakness.[10] The loss of flesh associated with geophagia which was noted by Livingstone was re-reported almost a century later as "Cachexia Africana".[11]

Acknowledgement

Adapted from: Larner AJ. Neurological signs: geophagia (geophagy) and pica (pagophagia).. *Adv Clin Neurosci Rehabil* 2009;9(4):20.

References

1. Waller H (ed.). *The last journals of David Livingstone in Central Africa, from 1865 to his death. Continued by a narrative of his last moments and sufferings obtained from his faithful servants Chuma and Susi.* London, 1874 (2 volumes):II83–II84.
2. Gelfand M. *Livingstone the doctor. His life and travels. A study in medical history.* Oxford: Basil Blackwell, 1957:10,256–257.
3. Garcia Marquez G. *One hundred years of solitude.* London: Picador [1967] 1978:42,59,61,79,81–82.
4. Gelder M, Gath D, Mayou R. *Oxford textbook of psychiatry.* Oxford: Oxford University Press, 1983:645.
5. Von Garnier C, Stunitz H, Decker M, Battegay E, Zeller A. Pica and refractory iron deficiency anaemia: a case report. *J Med Case Reports* 2008;2:324.
6. Woywodt A, Kiss A. Geophagia: the history of earth-eating. *J R Soc Med* 2002;95:143–146.
7. Savitt TL. *Medicine and Slavery. The diseases and health care of blacks in antebellum Virginia.* Urbana: University of Illinois Press, 1978:65–66.
8. Trivedi TH, Daga GL, Yeolekar ME. Geophagia leading to hypokalemic quadriparesis in a postpartum patient. *J Assoc Physicians India* 2005;53:205–207.
9. McKenna D. Myopathy, hypokalaemia and pica (geophagia) in pregnancy. *Ulster Med J* 2006;75:159–160.
10. Larner AJ. Dr David Livingstone (1813–1873): some neurological observations. *Scott Med J* 2008;53(2):35–37.
11. Mengel CE, Carter WA, Horton ES. Geophagia with iron deficiency and hypokalemia. Cachexia Africana. *Arch Intern Med* 1964;114:470–474.

Hyperkinetic motor perseverations

Alexander Romanovich Luria (1902–1977) was one of the most celebrated neuropsychologists of the 20th century, noted perhaps particularly for his work on frontal lobe functions. Reading a volume dedicated to his legacy,[1] I was struck by a chapter describing the Executive Control Battery (ECB), developed by Luria's pupil Elkohonon Goldberg and based on Luria's studies.[2] Although not familiar to me as such, clearly the ECB has influenced other tests of executive function, such as the much briefer Frontal Assessment Battery (FAB)[3] (this has been used in some of the clinical work undertaken in Liverpool, either as the main focus of interest[4,5] or as comparator[6]).

ECB consists of four subtests, of which the first is the Graphical Sequences Test. This was designed to elicit perseverations, of which four types are described. The first of these, hyperkinetic perseveration, is described thus:

> Hyperkinetic perseveration ... is defined as an inability to stop a single elementary graphomotor component such as drawing a circle or straight line. ... Here the patient literally continues to draw a circle or straight line over and over.[7]

This account put me in mind of a possible literary example of this phenomenon, a character drawing repeated circles encountered in Joseph Conrad's 1907 novel *The Secret Agent*.[8] (Spoiler alert: if you have read this far and plan to read further, what follows discloses some of the key plot features of Conrad's novel.)

Adolphe Verloc, the titular "secret agent", lives in Soho with his wife, Winnie, her mother, and her brother, Stevie. The latter is "a terrible encumbrance", "delicate and, in a frail way, good-looking too, except for the vacant droop of his lower lip" (ref. 8, p.7). Although he has apparently learned to read and write he is not able to sustain work, for example as an errand boy, although he "helped his sister with blind love and docility in her household duties" (9). Indeed, his most frequent descriptor is docile or docility (47,126,136,182), but "In the face of anything which affected ... his morbid dread of pain, Stevie ended by turning vicious" (134). His future is a source of concern to his mother and sister. Evidently he has a limited verbal output, but feels deeply for the sufferings of poor people and animals. In addition:

His spare time he occupied by drawing circles with compass and pencil on a piece of paper. He applied himself to that pastime with great industry ... (9)

At a meeting of Verloc's small circle of anarchists, they notice:

... the innocent Stevie, seated very good and quiet at a deal table, drawing circles, circles, circles; innumerable circles, concentric, eccentric; a coruscating whirl of circles that by their tangled multitude of repeated curves, uniformity of form, and confusion of intersecting lines suggested a rendering of cosmic chaos, ... (36)

Later, however, Stevie's behaviour changes:

... when discovered in solitude [Stevie] would be scowling at the wall, with the sheet of paper and the pencil given him for drawing circles lying blank and idle on the kitchen table. (148)

This change is a marker of (or metaphor for?) Verloc's increasing influence over Stevie, culminating in his inducing (radicalizing?) his brother-in-law to perpetrate a bombing in Greenwich Park, notionally on behalf of the anarchists. This goes wrong, the bomb explodes before being left, and Stevie is blown to pieces.

The "idiot character as gullible bomber" is picked up on in Patrick McDonagh's cultural history of idiocy (ref. 9, especially at pp.310–8), which examines the "symbolic work of idiocy in this discourse" (23). McDonagh suggests that Stevie's "mystical circles replace language" (317) and that "the novel's conflicting ideological positions lie ... in the eternal chaos of Stevie's circles" (318). The novel itself was based on an 1894 incident, similar in many respects, including the assertion that the bomber was an "idiot".

Is any medical explanation of Stevie forthcoming? From within the text itself, we have this opinion from Comrade Alexander Ossipon, "- nicknamed The Doctor, ex-medical student without a degree", who lectures to working-men's associations on the "socialistic aspects of hygiene" (ref. 8, p.37), i.e. eugenics (ref. 9, p.315). Observing Stevie drawing his circles in the kitchen, Ossipon opines that he is "typical of this form of degeneracy", and that "It's enough to glance at the lobes of the ears. If you read Lombroso – " (ref. 8, p.37). Another anarchist, Karl Yundt, then promptly rubbishes the views of Lombroso.

With the benefit of hindsight, we might perhaps suggest that Stevie has some form of learning disability (without fits; ref. 8, p.8), although if he has acquired the ability to read and write and draw with compasses this may be mild. Another possibility is that repeated head trauma may have contributed to his difficulties, since it is reported that his father called him a "slobbering idjut" and his disciplinary measures included physical blows when he was impatient with his son (8,140,192). Learning disability or mild traumatic brain injury might produce evidence of executive dysfunction, as indicated by hyperkinetic motor perseveration.

Acknowledgement

Adapted from: Larner AJ. Neurological literature: hyperkinetic motor perseverations. *Adv Clin Neurosci Rehabil* 2017;17(2):16.

References

1. Christensen AL, Goldberg E, Bougakov D (eds.). *Luria's legacy in the 21st century*. Oxford: Oxford University Press, 2009.
2. *Ibid.*, pp.122–145.
3. Dubois B, Slachevsky A, Litvan I, Pillon B. The FAB: a Frontal Assessment Battery at bedside. *Neurology* 2000;55:1621–1626.
4. Larner AJ. Frontal Assessment Battery (FAB): a pragmatic study. *Neurodegen Dis* 2011;8(Suppl 1):565.
5. Larner AJ. Can the Frontal Assessment Battery (FAB) help in the diagnosis of behavioural variant frontotemporal dementia? A pragmatic study. *Int J Geriatr Psychiatry* 2013;28:106–107.
6. Larner AJ. FRONTIER Executive Screen (FES). *J Neurol Neurosurg Psychiatry* 2017;88(Suppl1):A21 (PO034).
7. *Op. cit.*, Ref. 1, pp.130–131.
8. Newton M (ed.). *Joseph Conrad. The secret agent. A simple tale.* London: Penguin Classics, [1907] 2007.
9. McDonagh P. *Idiocy. A cultural history.* Liverpool: Liverpool University Press, 2008.

Hypermnesia

Awareness of failure to recall may prompt a complaint of poor memory function without there necessarily being any pathological substrate, and certainly this kind of functional disorder is the bread-and-butter work in the cognitive function clinic. Amnesia in its various forms is less frequently encountered. Some literary accounts of impaired memory have already been presented in the journal.[1] Indeed there are many more, so much so that "the amnesia story" has been claimed as a specific genre of literature.[2]

Conversely, I do not recall ever encountering in clinical practice a complaint of memory being too good, or hypermnesia. This general term, like amnesia, may be further qualified, dependent upon the particular nature of exceptional memory or functional excellence. Hyperthymesia, or the hyperthymestic syndrome, is the ability to remember an abnormally large number of life experiences in vivid detail, and is also known as highly superior autobiographical memory (HSAM).[3] Eidetic, or "photographic", memory is the ability to recall precisely images from memory after a brief or single viewing. Some definitions of eidetic memory exclude use of mnemonic devices, as used by trained mnemonists. However, synaesthesia may be linked to eidetic memory, with synaesthetic experience possibly being used as a mnemonic aid.

The classic account of hypermnesia is that of AR Luria (1902–77), who in *The mind of a mnemonist* described his patient, Solomon Shereshevsky, a journalist with fivefold synaesthesia whose memory was apparently "for all practical purposes ... inexhaustible". Studied over a period of thirty years beginning in the 1920s, Luria noted that Shereshevsky was able to convert information into visual images. In his introduction to the 1968 reprint, Jerome Bruner credited Luria with founding a new literary genre with this book.[4]

Another noted hypermnesic was the Hungarian-US mathematician John von Neumann (1903–57), said by his wife to have an "almost photographic memory",[5] a report corroborated by his colleagues: he could apparently memorise names, addresses, and telephone numbers from a phone book on sight.[6] His work on computers was initially justified by means of biological analogy with the working of neurones (only latterly did the analogy reverse to "brain as computer") although subsequently he came to doubt the parallel, as shown in his posthumously published Silliman lectures of 1957.[7] I do not know whether or not von Neumann's own prodigious memory stimulated his interest in the potential similarities and differences between computers and brains.

The "photographic memory" is also, of course, a trope much resorted to in film and TV. Examples, conjured fairly randomly from my memory, include the film *Carry on Spying* (1964) in which Barbara Windsor (1937–2020), who later developed dementia, plays Agent Daphne Honeybutt; and Sheldon Lee Cooper in the long running TV serial *The Big Bang Theory* (2007–2019). Sheldon may be synaesthetic: in one episode (series 9, episode 12) he reports that prime numbers are red and twin primes are pink, although it is not clear if the presentation of these numbers is visual (non cross-modal) or auditory (cross-modal); the fact that twin primes also "smell like gasoline" obviously is cross-modal.

There are also some literary accounts suggestive of hypermnesia. Perhaps the most notable is that by the Argentine author Jorge Luis Borges (1899–1986) in his short story, *Funes el memorioso*, usually translated as *Funes, the memorious* but also as *Funes, his memory*, which appeared in a collection entitled *Artifices* first published in 1944. In his foreword to this collection, the author calls this story "one long metaphor for insomnia".[8] Set in Uruguay in the 1880s, it describes Ireneo Funes who, having been "hopelessly crippled" after being knocked unconscious when bucked by a half-broken horse, finds that now, in his late teenage years, "his perception and his memory were perfect". However, there is evidence that his perception of time and memory for proper names was "precise" even before the injury. Now "the most trivial of his memories was more detailed, more vivid than our own perception of a physical pleasure or a physical torment".

> He had effortlessly learned English, French, Portuguese, Latin. I suspect nevertheless that he was not very good at thinking. To think is to ignore (or forget) differences, to generalize, to abstract. In the teeming world of Ireneo Funes there was nothing but particulars – and they were virtually immediate particulars.

Oddly enough, given these exceptional memory faculties, Funes also crops up in the aforementioned anthology devoted to amnesia.[2] Oliver Sacks made several references to Funes, finding him to be "uncannily similar" to Luria's patient, and wondering whether he may have been based on a personal encounter between the author and a mnemonist.[9] Unlike the situation of Funes and of Shereshevsky, for von Neumann "the trees did not conceal the forest from him".[6]

The history of prodigious feats of memory is, in fact, ancient. One of the books which Funes reads is the *Naturalis Historia* of Pliny the Elder (AD 23–79) which catalogues (in Book VII, Chapter XXIV) cases of prodigious memory, for example (in the translation of Philemon Holland, 1601):

One Charmidas or Carmadas, a Grecian, was of so singular a memorie, that he was able to deliver by heart the contents word for word of all the bookes that a man would call for out of any librarie, as if he read the same presently within a booke.

A more recent example is to be found in Pascal Mercier's novel *Night train to Lisbon*, set partially in the time of the Portuguese dictatorship in the early 1970s. Estefania Espinhosa "had this unbelievable memory. Forgot nothing, neither what she had seen nor what she had heard. Addresses, phone numbers, faces. We used to joke that she knew the phone directory by heart" (shades of von Neumann?). This "phenomenal memory" is used to retain all the secrets of the *Resistência*: "We didn't have to write anything down, didn't have to leave a paper trail. The whole network was in her head" (in the film version, which differs in many details from the book, Estefania is shown reciting names and telephone numbers of supporters of the resistance). However, the possession of these abilities renders Estefania a liability when the secret police seek to track her down, necessitating her flight from Portugal. As she recalls: "it was about keeping me safe ... but it wasn't only me, it was mainly my memory".[10]

Detrimental effects of these exceptional memory functions are reported. For example, Shereshevsky appeared unable to hold down any job for a prolonged period. There is a quote attributed to Friedrich Nietzsche (1844–1900) to the effect that "Many a man [*sic*] fails as an original thinker simply because his memory is too good". So, perhaps we should not be too harsh on our own memory lapses!

Acknowledgement

Adapted from: Larner AJ. Neurological literature: hypermnesia. *Adv Clin Neurosci Rehabil* 2021;20(2):27–28.

References

1. Larner AJ. *"Neurological literature": cognitive disorders*. Adv Clin Neurosci Rehabil 2008;8(2):20.
2. Letham J (ed.). *The Vintage book of amnesia: an anthology of writing on the subject of memory loss*. New York: Vintage, 2000.
3. Parker ES, Cahill L, McGaugh JL. *A case of unusual autobiographical remembering*. Neurocase 2006;12:35–49.
4. Luria AR. *The mind of a mnemonist. A little book about a vast memory*. New York: Basic Books, 1968.
5. Von Neumann J. *The computer and the brain* (2nd edition). New Haven and London: Yale University Press [1958] 2000:xxiv.

6. Halmos PR. *The legend of John von Neumann.* Am Math Mon 1973;80:382–394.
7. Cobb M. *The idea of the brain. A history.* London: Profile Books, 2020:181–183,187–192.
8. Borges JL. *Fictions.* London: Penguin Classics, 2000:91–99.
9. Sacks O. *The man who mistook his wife for a hat.* London: Picador, 1985:106n,114,191,219–220.
10. Mercier P. *Night train to Lisbon.* London: Atlantic Books [2004] 2009:279,280–281,283,284,415,420.

Lassitude

During my clinical training in the mid-1980s it was possible to subscribe to the *British Medical Journal* (it had not yet metamorphosed into "*BMJ*") at student rates. This was an era when the journal was still largely devoted to clinical matters, unlike now, and hence relevant to clinical training, usually with several editorials. I recently had reason to recall one of these editorials (published 20th April 1985), entitled simply "Lassitude".[1] One of the consultant physicians on the firm I was then attached to, the late (great) clinical pharmacologist David Grahame-Smith, commented that he had seen the title but had not been able to summon the energy to read it.[2]

The cue for this recall came from my experience of COVID-19 in January and February 2021. Initially presenting with monosymptomatic anosmia, my self-isolation period was almost complete when systemic symptoms set in, with swinging pyrexias, non-productive cough, inability to eat, sleep disturbance, and physical and mental prostration, all presumably a consequence of pneumonia (thankfully never bad enough to necessitate hospital admission). Hardly able to do much more than transfer between bed and couch, I wondered how best to describe this sluggishness: Lethargy? Inertia? Lassitude? Even when the call to urinate was apparent, initiating movement off the couch was still difficult: I could not "get moving". "Avolitional" might be the adjective that best captures this, and might also be relevant to the extraordinary inability to countenance eating any food. This was not simply indifference to food as a consequence of anosmia: I had eaten adequately during the monosymptomatic phase. Moreover, I had food cravings (often for childhood treats: Smarties! Lardy cake!). Nor was it a consequence of nausea (only induced by the aloe vera smell of my hand soap, suggesting my anosmia was partial rather than complete), and cognitively I knew I must eat. Nevertheless, foods passed their best before dates and, shamefully, had to be wasted. I lost about 6kg during the course of the illness.

So, what explanation might be advanced for this lassitude? No doubt the interstitial fluids are a veritable soup of cytokines, interferons, and other inflammatory mediators which I have not heard of, as a consequence of the immune response to SARS-Cov-2. But is an explanation along these lines sufficient to satisfy a neurologist's curiosity? It may be the case that the self-styled "coroneurologists" have already solved this particular issue, and I claim no familiarity with the mushrooming literature. In my ignorance (stream of consciousness?), what came to mind was the Bereitschaftspotential. (Justification for this introspective approach, if it be needed, may be derived from Miller Fisher, who opined that "there is a place for the scrutiny of personal experience ... Physicians, particularly neurologists, are in an advantageous position to utilise the analysis of personal events for insights they may provide into the biology of the nervous system".[3])

As an undergraduate I had learned, from the first edition of the textbook by Kandel and Schwartz,[4] of the work of Kornhuber and Deecke in the 1960s which, using back averaging techniques, characterised the Bereitschaftspotential,[5] or "readiness potential", or "premovement potential", occurring in the 1000ms or more prior to voluntary movement (Michael Trimble ascribes its discovery to William Grey Walter in 1964).[6] Different components of the Bereitschaftspotential have subsequently been characterised, an early component thought to originate in the anterior supplementary motor area (SMA) and rostral pre-SMA, and a late phase from the SMA and contralateral primary motor area.[7,8] Both cortical and subcortical (basal ganglia) generators may contribute to the Bereitschaftspotential. Some evidence has subsequently accrued for the absence or diminution of the Bereitschaftspotential in involuntary movement disorders such as Parkinson's disease, but with preservation in (so called) psychogenic movement disorders.

So, I wondered if my COVID-19–related lassitude/inertia/lethargy/avolition might possibly be a consequence of an inability to generate a Bereitschaftspotential, or a component thereof. Interestingly in this connection there was a frontal-subcortical flavour to some of my other symptoms at the time of systemic illness: stooped posture when attempting to walk, slow short-stepped gait, bradykinesia, and bradyphrenia (I couldn't concentrate on daytime TV programmes, let alone read).

If there is any credibility to this suggestion (and it should be noted that cogent conceptual argument may be made that the temporal priority of the Bereitschaftspotential to movement may not be equivalent to causal priority[9]) might it be relevant beyond the specific situation of COVID-19–related symptoms of lassitude? Might such mechanisms contribute to similar age-related symptoms, unmasked in this particular quinquagenerian by superimposed infection? Could difficulties in generating a Bereitschaftspotential, or components thereof, potentially explain clinically defined syndromes such as abulia and akinetic mutism? These syndromes are often associated with frontal lobe damage or pathology. Perhaps some examples of long COVID might also be related to this mechanism.

Acknowledgement

Adapted from: Larner AJ. COVID-19, lassitude, and the *Bereitschaftspotential.* *Adv Clin Neurosci Rehabil* 2021;20(3):33.

References

1. Havard CWH. *Lassitude.* BMJ 1985:290:1161–1162.
2. Aronson JK. *David Grahame Grahame-Smith. Clinical pharmacologist 1933–2011.* Br J Clin Pharmacol 2011;73:830–832.
3. Fisher CM. *Neurologic fragments II: Remarks on anosognosia, confabulation, memory, and other topics; and an appendix on self-observation.* Neurology 1989;39:127–132.
4. Kandel ER, Schwartz JH. *Principles of neural science.* London: Edward Arnold, 1981, p.331.
5. Kornhuber HH, Deecke L. *Hirnpotentialänderungen bei Willkürbewegungen und passiven Bewegungen des Menschen: Bereitschaftspotential und reafferente Potentiale.* Pflügers Archiv 1965;284:1–17.
6. Trimble MR. *The intentional brain. Motion, emotion, and the development of modern neuropsychiatry.* Baltimore: Johns Hopkins University Press, 2016, p.274.
7. Shibasaki H, Hallett M. *What is the Bereitschaftspotential?* Clin Neurophysiol 2006;117:2341–2356.
8. Colebatch JG. *Bereitschaftspotential and movement-related potentials: origin, significance, and application in disorders of human movement.* Mov Disord 2007;22:601–610.
9. Nachev P, Hacker P. *The neural antecedents to voluntary action: a conceptual analysis.* Cog Neurosci 2014;5:193–208 [at 201,202].

Mirror phenomena: clinical catoptrics

"I've had the experience of finding myself unexpectedly before a mirror and not recognising myself ...."

André Malraux *La Condition Humaine* (published in English as *Man's Fate*)[1]

The speaker of these lines is an ageing Chinese academic, Old Gisors, who habitually smokes opium, a habit which might possibly be relevant to his strange sensory experiences. A number of mirror phenomena are described in the neurological literature,[2] of which those with a cognitive flavour are briefly considered here (i.e. neither mirror movements nor the "mirror dystonia" sometimes encountered in writer's cramp are discussed). As catoptrics [sic] is the branch of optics which investigates the formation of images by mirrors, these phenomena might be termed "clinical catoptrics".

Mirror Sign and Mirrored Self-Misidentification

The experience reported by Old Gisors, a failure to recognise ones' own reflection in a mirror, may be described as the "mirror sign". In addition to this failure, patients may sometimes develop a delusional belief that their reflection is in fact that of a stranger, which has been termed "mirrored self-misidentification",[3] a response which might contribute to the "phantom boarder sign" (the belief that there is someone else living in the house).

Rather little seems to have been published on these signs, but the articles which have appeared generally indicate that it is a reflection (no pun intended!) of cognitive decline,[3] for example in Alzheimer's disease (AD)[4,5] or dementia with Lewy bodies.[6] Mirror sign may perhaps be a consequence of visual agnosia, and has been noted in a patient with the posterior cortical atrophy variant of AD who also had visual hallucinations.[7] Unusually mirror sign may occur as a focal deficit at the onset of a progressive dementing illness, indicative of non-dominant hemisphere dysfunction. In addition to perceptual (face processing) impairments, affective and reasoning deficits may also contribute to the pathogenesis of mirror sign.[8] Dementia is not, however, a *sine qua non*: mirrored self-misidentification has also been noted in an elderly patient with a right dorsolateral frontal infarct, bilateral frontal encephalomalacia consistent with previous head trauma, and posterior periventricular ischaemic lesions but without dementia. Based on these observations, the authors suggested that the right dorsolateral prefrontal cortex may be important for self-recognition.[9]

Mirror Agnosia, Mirror Apraxia, Mirror Ataxia

Mirror agnosia and mirror apraxia are related phenomena, as may be mirror ataxia.

Mirror agnosia is a deficit in which patients are unable to use mirror knowledge when interacting with mirrors (a definition which might also encompass mirror sign and mirrored self-misidentification). Also sometimes known as the "looking glass syndrome", or "Ramachandran's sign" after the first description,[10] patients are unable to point to the real object when it is seen in a mirror. They may attempt to reach "into" the mirror even when the actual location of the target has been shown, suggesting an inability to distinguish between the real and virtual images. This reaching for the virtual object has been termed mirror apraxia.[11] Reaching for the real object but with increased errors of direction has been termed mirror ataxia.[12] Parietal lobe lesions with associated hemispatial neglect may underlie these signs, with dissociation of retinotopic (allocentric) space and body schema (egocentric space). A lesion study suggested different areas of parietal lobe might underpin mirror ataxia (postcentral sulcus) and mirror agnosia (posterior angular gyrus and superior temporal gyrus).[12]

Mirror Hallucination

The visual hallucination of seeing ones' own face, autoscopy, has been termed mirror hallucination since there is left-right reversal as in a mirror image. This has been described in association with epilepsy, migraine, and parieto-occipital space-occupying lesions.[13]

Mirror Writing

Mirror writing is a mirror image of normal writing, hence in English it runs from right to left with characters back to front. In double mirror writing (*écriture en double mirroir*) script is also inverted top to bottom (script goes up the page) as well as being mirror reversed. Mirror writing may occur spontaneously, more often in left-handers, as well as in a variety of pathological situations, mostly associated with left hemisphere damage. Leonardo da Vinci is perhaps the most celebrated historical mirror writer.[14]

Mirror writing should perhaps not be included here since it is most probably a motor phenomenon, akin to mirror movements, rather than a cognitive phenomenon, although it is reported to occur on occasion in the context of cognitive impairment or dementia. That said, in my experience of asking people with cognitive complaints to write sentences (e.g. when administering the Mini-Mental State Examination or the Addenbrooke's Cognitive Examination and its subsequent iterations, ACE-R and ACE-III) I do not recall ever having seen a mirror sentence produced.

Mirror synaesthesia

Mirror-touch synaesthesia describes the experience of sensation in the same or opposite body part when another person is touched, hence also known as vision-touch synaesthesia,[15] this latter term emphasizing the cross-modality typical of synaesthetic experience, the most common form of which is the experience of coloured visual sensations in response to an auditory percept. Mirror-pain synaesthesia is also described ("feeling others pain"). Although these phenomena are usually developmental conditions, acquired cases are described in some amputees: touching a normal limb may induce sensation below the stump of the contralateral amputated limb, a phenomenon which, based on my own observations, I ventured to term "phantom alloaesthesia",[16] but which others seem willing to call "mirror synaesthesia".[17] The latter term is questionable since there is no cross-modal component here as both actual and phantom limbs experience touch sensation. However, this phenomenon may be especially pronounced when amputees actually "see" their phantom being touched, courtesy of a vertically placed mirror (or "virtual reality box") which reflects the normal limb in the (approximate) location where the amputated limb should be. In this case the "mirror-touch synaesthesia" terminology is reasonable, although "vision-touch synaesthesia" is preferable as less ambiguous.

Conclusion

In his monumental *The Anatomy of Melancholy*, Robert Burton (1577–1640) observed that "'tis ordinary to see strange uncouth sights by Catoptrics".[18] The same may be said of these clinical catoptrics!

Acknowledgement

Adapted from: Larner AJ. Neurological signs: mirror phenomena. *Adv Clin Neurosci Rehabil* 2015;15(4):14; and Larner AJ. Mirror phenomena: a neurologist's perspective. *The Carrollian (The Lewis Carroll Journal)* 2021;35–36:113–118

References

1. Malraux A. *Man's Fate*. London: Penguin Modern Classics [1933] 2009:42.
2. Larner AJ. *A dictionary of neurological signs* (4th edition). London: Springer, 2016:200–202.
3. Connors MH, Coltheart M. On the behaviour of senile dementia patients vis-à-vis the mirror: Ajuriaguerra, Strejilevitch and Tissot (1963). *Neuropsychologia* 2011;49:1679–1692.
4. Kumakura T. The mirror sign in presenile and senile dementias (especially in Alzheimer-type dementias) [in Japanese]. *Seishin Shinkeigaku Zasshi* 1982;84:307–335.
5. Mulcare JL, Nicolson SE, Bisen VS, Sostre SO. The mirror sign: a reflection of cognitive decline. *Psychosomatics* 2012;53:188–192.
6. Gil-Ruiz N, Osorio RS, Cruz I et al. An effective environmental intervention for management of the "mirror sign" in a case of probable Lewy body dementia. *Neurocase* 2013;19:1–13.
7. Yoshida T, Yuki N, Nakagawa M. Complex visual hallucination and mirror sign in posterior cortical atrophy. *Acta Psychiatr Scand* 2006;114:62–65.
8. Breen N, Caine D, Coltheart M. Mirrored-self misidentification: two cases of focal onset dementia. *Neurocase* 2001;7:239–254.
9. Villarejo A, Martin VP, Moreno-Ramos T et al. Mirrored self-misidentification in a patient without dementia: evidence for right hemispheric and bifrontal damage. *Neurocase* 2011;17:276–284.
10. Ramachandran VS, Altschuler EL, Hillyer S. Mirror agnosia. *Proc Biol Sci* 1997;264:645–647.
11. Binkofski F, Butler A, Buccino G et al. Mirror apraxia affects the peripersonal mirror space. A combined lesion and cerebral activation study. *Exp Brain Res* 2003;153:210–219.
12. Binkofski F, Buccino G, Dohle C, Seitz RJ, Freund HJ. Mirror agnosia and mirror ataxia constitute different parietal lobe disorders. *Ann Neurol* 1999;46:51–61.
13. Brugger P. Reflective mirrors; perspective taking in autoscopic phenomena. *Cogn Neuropsychiatry* 2002;7:179–194.
14. Schott GD. Mirror writing: neurological reflections on an unusual phenomenon. *J Neurol Neurosurg Psychiatry* 2007;78:5–13.
15. Blakemore S-J, Bristow D, Bird G, Frith C, Ward J. Somatosensory activations during the observation of touch and a case of vision-touch synaesthesia. *Brain* 2005;128: 1571–1583.
16. Larner AJ. *A dictionary of neurological signs* (2nd edition). New York: Springer, 2006:19,245.
17. Ramachandran VS, Rogers-Ramachandran D. Synaesthesia in phantom limbs induced with mirrors. *Proceedings. Biological Sciences* 1996;263:377–386.
18. Gowland A (ed.). *Robert Burton. The anatomy of melancholy*. London: Penguin Classics, 2021:413.

Pseudomelia and pseudopolymelia

It is well known that Silas Weir Mitchell (1829–1914), justly regarded as one of the founding fathers of neurology, first published his account of phantom limbs not in a neurological journal but in a popular magazine,[1] apparently fearful that if it appeared in a professional context it might induce ridicule (although earlier accounts of phantom limbs had appeared[2]).

Phantom limbs are most often observed in the context of amputation, but reports of extra limbs occurring without amputation have also appeared. Two brief cases are presented here to illustrate the clinical heterogeneity of the supernumerary limb, the possible pathophysiology of which is briefly considered.

Case 1: A 59 year-old right-handed lady was referred to the neurology clinic with a history of three stereotyped episodes occurring over a 5–month period in which she had the sensation of having two arms and two hands on the left hand side, these symptoms lasting between 30 minutes and 2 hours. She was not aware of any spontaneous movement of this extra limb, which was not visible to her, nor could she move it voluntarily. She had a longstanding history of anxiety and her psychiatrist thought that the symptoms might be a reflection of this. Neurological examination was normal. MR brain imaging showed some high signal white matter changes. As it was not possible to say with certainty whether these changes were ischaemic or inflammatory she underwent lumbar puncture which showed normal CSF contents with no unmatched oligoclonal bands. She was then symptom free for around 18 months, when a further cluster of similar episodes occurred. Repeat MR brain imaging showed no change from previously. In the absence of a structural or inflammatory lesion, the working neurological diagnosis was somaesthetic migraine aura (both her children had migraine). About six months later she started getting multi-coloured flashes in her vision and was seen by an ophthalmologist who found no ocular pathology and thought that the visual symptoms likely to be migrainous.

Case 2: A 55 year-old lady (previously reported in abstract[3]) with acute motor and sensory axonal neuropathy which had required ventilatory support developed the sensation of two extra arms and legs during the prolonged recovery phase. More than 6 months after the acute onset of neuropathy, nerve conduction studies showed uniform absence of sensory responses, and likewise absence of lower limb distal and proximal motor responses. Median and ulnar nerve motor responses were markedly reduced (<1mV) with increased latencies and reduced velocities. Awareness of the phantom limbs could be reduced by visualising her normal limbs.

The phenomenon described in these cases has been known by various names, including supernumerary phantom limb(s) (SPL), reduplication of body parts, and pseudo(poly)melia. As these cases show, the phenomenology of SPL is heterogeneous: symptoms may be transient/episodic or persistent/prolonged, and may involve single or multiple limbs, or even other body parts (such as teeth[4]). In most cases, SPL has only somaesthetic characteristics but in some cases the limb can be seen and voluntarily moved (i.e. multimodal SPL). SPL has been described in association with stroke more often affecting the right than the left hemisphere[5-7] and in episodic form in epilepsy.[8,9] A possible migraine-related case is that of Todd and Dewhurst,[10] although their patient also had a diagnosis of epilepsy. SPL has been described in acute inflammatory demyelinating polyneuropathy.[11] Cancellation of SPL by vision of the real limb is reported.

The pathophysiology of phantom limbs has attracted much attention in recent years. Indeed, Ramachandran informs us that he has "genuinely solved the mystery". Sadly for us, he only mentions supernumerary phantoms in passing, and these in the context of amputation.[12] They have been variously regarded as delusional beliefs or hallucinatory perceptions,[13] or as disorders of the body schema resulting from a failure to integrate neural impulses initiating motor action and from sensory feedback.[14] The profound deafferentation indicated by the neurophysiological findings in Case 2, along with impaired motor conduction, would be in keeping with such an explanation. Spatial distortions of body size occurring in migraine (macro- and microsomatognosia, also known as "Alice in Wonderland" syndrome) have also been attributed to "pathologies of sensory input",[14] so a similar mechanism of failure to integrate motor command and sensory feedback might be occurring in Case 1.

Whilst structural reorganisation, with reinnervation of deafferented sensory cortex from other cortical regions, may occur in persistent cases of SPL associated with brain injury (e.g. after stroke), as has been suggested for phantom limbs in amputees,[15] this may not be a necessary feature for the development of SPL, as suggested by transient forms. Functional neuroimaging (fMRI) in a patient with a poststroke (subcortical capsulolenticular haemorrhage) SPL with somaesthetic, visual and intentional motor components showed modality-specific activations in motor, visual and somaesthetic areas, interpreted as cortical deafferentation from the subcortical lesion.[16] fMRI was also undertaken in Case 2 during a motor paradigm task, which showed activation within the primary motor and supplementary motor areas only,[3] as might be anticipated with an exclusively somaesthetic SPL.

I do not know of any literary examples of pseudomelia or pseudopolymelia.

The American playwright Edward Albee (1928–2016), perhaps best known for *Who's afraid of Virginia Woolf?* (1962), wrote a play entitled *The man who had three arms* (1982), the third arm growing between his shoulder blades.

Acknowledgements

Thanks to Dr Mark Doran and Dr Kumar Das for permission to quote details from their case (reference 3). Adapted from: Larner AJ. Supernumerary phantom limbs. *Adv Clin Neurosci Rehabil* 2020;20(1):27.

References

1. Nathanson M. *Phantom limbs as reported by S. Weir Mitchell.* Neurology 1988;38:504–505.
2. Finger S, Hustwit MP. *Five early accounts of phantom limb in context: Paré, Descartes, Lemos, Bell, and Mitchell.* Neurosurgery 2003;52:675–686.
3. Fulton J, Williamson J, Das K, Doran M. *The phantom menace.* J Neurol Neurosurg Psychiatry 2016;87:e1 (abstract 031).
4 Jacome DE. *Dracula's teeth syndrome.* Headache 2001;41:892–894.
5. Halligan PW, Marshall JC, Wade DT. *Three arms: a case study of supernumerary phantom limb after right hemisphere stroke.* J Neurol Neurosurg Psychiatry 1993;56:159–166.
6. McGonigle DJ, Hänninen R, Salenius S, Hari R, Frackowiak RSJ, Frith CD. *Whose arm is it anyway? An fMRI case study of supernumerary phantom limb.* Brain 2002;125:1265–1274.
7. Miyazawa N, Hayashi M, Komiya K, Akiyama I. *Supernumerary phantom limbs associated with left hemispheric stroke: case report and review of the literature.* Neurosurgery 2004;54:228–231.
8. Weisbord A, Saver JL, Leary MC. *Episodic supernumerary phantom limb due to epileptic disruption of the neural representation of the body image.* J Neuropsychiatry Clin Neurosci 2002;14:109 (abstract P27).
9. Millonig A, Bodner T, Donnemiller E, Wolf E, Unterberger I. *Supernumerary phantom limb as a rare symptom of epileptic seizures – case report and literature review.* Epilepsia 2011;52:e97–e100.
10. Todd J, Dewhurst K. *The double: its psycho-pathology and psycho-physiology.* J Nerv Ment Dis 1955;122:47–55.
11. Melinyshyn AN, Gofton TE, Schulz V. *Supernumerary phantom limbs in ICU patients with acute inflammatory demyelinating polyneuropathy.* Neurology 2016;86:1726–8.
12. Ramachandran VS, Blakeslee S. *Phantoms in the brain. Human nature and the architecture of the mind.* London: Fourth Estate, 1999:3,57
13. Cipriani G, Picchi L, Vedovella M, Nuti A, Di Fiorino M. *The phantom and the supernumerary phantom limb: historical review and new case.* Neurosci Bull 2011;27:359–365.

14. Haggard P, Wolpert DM. *Disorders of body schema.* In: Freund HJ, Jeannerod M, Hallett M, Leiguarda R (eds.). *Higher-order motor disorders. From neuroanatomy and neurobiology to clinical neurology.* Oxford: Oxford University Press, 2005:261–271.
15. Ramachandran VS, Rogers-Ramachandran D. *Phantom limbs and neural plasticity.* Arch Neurol 2000;57:317–320.
16. Khateb A, Simon SR, Dieguez S et al. *Seeing the phantom: a functional magnetic resonance imaging study of a supernumerary phantom limb.* Ann Neurol 2009;65:698–705.

Syllogomania

The novelist Barbara Pym (1913–80) has been called the "Jane Austen of our times" because of her acute and comedic observations of social mores, and her work was admired by Philip Larkin, yet I suspect that today few have heard of her. Her novel *Quartet in Autumn* (1977), set in London in the early 1970s, includes a character whose description seems positively to invite clinical diagnosis.[1] (Spoiler alert: what follows discloses some of the plot features of Pym's novel.)

Miss Marcia Ivory is in her sixties, and thought somewhat peculiar by her fellow office workers, Edwin, Letty, and Norman (they constitute the quartet of the book's title). Marcia lives alone in the house she previously shared with her mother and which nobody else enters; she is "set in [her] isolation" (57). The room where her mother died has been left untouched, used only by the cat, Snowy, until he also died there.

Marcia keeps empty milk bottles in a shed in her garden (2), a "special and rather unusual arrangement" (51), with over 100 of them stacked on shelves (172), and "spotlessly clean" (183). These "needed to be checked from time to time and occasionally she even went as far as dusting them" (55). The bottles are all "United Dairy" bottles, and Marcia is irritated to find one is of an "alien brand", namely "County Dairies", and plans to return it to Letty who gave it to her at the office one day (55). Marcia leaves other types of rubbish, such as "bottles of a certain kind … certain boxes and paper bags and other unclassified articles" on the shelves at the local library, "a good place to dispose of unwanted objects", (2–3) although she is not a reader, indeed Letty wonders whether Marcia "ever read" (152).

In addition, to the milk bottles, Marcia has a collection of tinned foods in a kitchen store cupboard (51): "meat, fish, fruit, vegetables, soup … tomato puree, stuffed vine leaves … tapioca pudding" (54); "spam and stewing steak … prawns and peach halves … sardines, soup, butter beans and … macaroni cheese" (184). The drawer in her office desk also contains several tins (90). Every week she buys more tins which require classifying and sorting: "the tins could be arranged according to size or by types of food … There was work to be done here and Marcia enjoyed doing it." (54). Yet Marcia is repeatedly noted not to be a "big eater", indeed one evening she eats "a small tin of pilchards. It was one left over from Snowy's store, so it was not really breaking into her reserves." (74–5)

Finding a plastic bag in her kitchen, "Marcia took the bag upstairs into …

the spare bedroom where she kept things like cardboard boxes, brown paper and string, and stuffed it into a drawer already bulging with other plastic bags … to be sorted into their different shapes and sizes" (93–4; also 170). Elsewhere she has "a drawer full of new Marks and Spencer nighties … All brand new and never worn" (141).

I suggest that these features merit the designation of syllogomania, a name given to a syndrome of hoarding,[2] sometimes also termed "disposophobia", often of items which may be deemed rubbish. Syllogomania may occur in isolation,[3] or may be part of a broader neurobehavioural syndrome of neglect.

As noted, despite her store of food, Marcia's diet is poor. She is noted to be thin (41), then emaciated (111), clothes hanging on her, and eats little of the salad she orders when the quartet meet at a restaurant for lunch (114). By the end of the novel she weighs "only six stone" (149). Social rules are also transgressed, as when Marcia talks too loudly at the restaurant, attracting the attention of the other diners (115), and when she noisily returns Letty's milk bottle to her in the library (117).

In addition to self-neglect, Marcia's house is also neglected: "The dust on the hall table told its own story" (53) (*cf.* the milk bottles) as well as "other evidences of long neglect" (142). "On the bed cover there was still an old fur ball, brought up by Snowy in his last days, now dried up like some ancient mummified relic of long ago." (26). Marcia declines a neighbour's offer to cut her grass (55) and spurns repeated visits from a social worker.

Whether the character of Marcia was based on the author's own observations, or simply the product of a creative imagination, is not known. Nevertheless, for this clinician, the symptoms described prompt diagnostic speculation, specifically of Diogenes syndrome,[4] sometimes known as "squalor syndrome". Obsessions of saving, with accompanying hoarding, may also occur in the context of obsessive-compulsive disorder.

Although a syndrome characterised by self-neglect, domestic squalor, hoarding behaviour, and social withdrawal with refusal of external help had been previously described, the term Diogenes syndrome was coined in 1975 by Clarke *et al.*, referring to Diogenes of Sinope (*ca.* 412–323 BC), a cofounder of the Cynic school of philosophy in Athens, who was noted for his austere asceticism and self-sufficiency and his disregard for domestic comforts.[5] Notionally he lived in a barrel or tub, and rebuked Alexander the Great for standing in his sunlight. He has proved a frequent subject for allegorical paintings.

Most patients diagnosed with Diogenes syndrome are elderly, single or living alone, of average or above average intelligence, and often with an adequate income (*i.e.* the condition is not the result of poverty).[6] Although cases may be "primary", unrelated to any underlying cognitive or psychiatric illness, the possibility of an underlying dementia,[7] particularly of the frontotemporal type,[8] should always be considered. A variant characterised by the hoarding of animals has been called the "Noah syndrome".[9]

Diogenes of Sinope should not be confused with two other individuals of the same name. Diogenes of Apollonia (*fl.* 5th century BC) was a pre-Socratic philosopher who has been claimed as a pioneer in vascular anatomy and physiology.[10] Diogenes Laertius (*fl.* 3rd century AD) was a biographer of the Greek philosophers who, to my current knowledge, has no connections with medicine, other than to record anecdotes of Diogenes of Sinope.

Acknowledgement

Adapted from: Larner AJ. Syllogomania; with a note on Diogenes of Sinope. *Adv Clin Neurosci Rehabil* 2020;19(4):47.

References

1. Pym B. *Quartet in Autumn.* London: Picador Classic [1977] 2005. All page references cited in the text refer to this edition.
2. Larner AJ. *A dictionary of neurological signs (4th edition).* London: Springer, 2016:309.
3. Zuliani G, Soavi C, Dainese A, Milani P, Gatti M. Diogenes syndrome or isolated syllogomania? Four heterogeneous clinical cases. *Aging Clin Exp Res* 2013;25:473–478.
4. Larner AJ, Coles AJ, Scolding NJ, Barker RA. *A-Z of neurological practice. A guide to clinical neurology (2nd edition).* London: Springer, 2011:191.
5. Clarke ANG, Manikar GO, Gray I. Diogenes syndrome. A clinical study of gross neglect in old age. *Lancet* 1975;i:366–368.
6. Assal F. Diogenes syndrome. *Front Neurol Neurosci* 2018;41:90–97.
7. Cipriani G, Lucetti C, Vedovello M, Nuti A. Diogenes syndrome in patients suffering from dementia. *Dialogues Clin Neurosci* 2012;14:455–460.
8. Finney CM, Mendez MF. Diogenes syndrome in frontotemporal dementia. *Am J Alzheimers Dis Other Demen* 2017;32:438–443.
9. Saldarriaga-Cantillo A, Rivas Nieto JC. Noah syndrome: a variant of Diogenes syndrome accompanied by animal hoarding practices. *J Elder Abuse Negl* 2015;27:270–275.
10. Crivellato E, Mallardi F, Ribatti D. Diogenes of Apollonia: a pioneer in vascular anatomy. *Anat Rec B New Anat* 2006;289:116–120.

What's in a name? A diagnosis by any other name would be as meet?

It is through the agency of Juliet (who, according to the internal evidence of the play, is not yet fourteen years old) that Shakespeare asks:

What's in a name? that which we call a rose
By any other name would smell as sweet.
(*Romeo and Juliet*, Act II, scene II, lines 47–48).

A recent case highlighted the issue of diagnostic naming, prompting my attempted (lame?) revision of Shakespeare's lines.

A 46 year-old lady with longstanding psoriasis was referred to the neurology clinic by her dermatologist for opinion on recurrent episodes of unilateral facial swelling over the previous three years. These occurred around once a month and lasted for about 24 hours. There were no obvious triggers and episodes were self-limiting. There was no history of facial weakness (confirmed by photos of her face when symptomatic), sensory disturbance, or tongue involvement. Previous MR brain imaging was normal. A diagnosis of monosymptomatic Melkersson-Rosenthal syndrome (MRS) was made and the patient reassured that no further neurological investigation was required.

Simultaneously the dermatologist had referred the patient to an allergist. The allergist made a diagnosis of chronic spontaneous angioedema, and checked complement and C1 inhibitor levels which proved normal. The patient was, understandably, confused by the different diagnostic labels.

MRS is defined by the triad of orofacial oedema, recurrent facial palsy and fissured tongue (lingua plicata). Most neurologists will recall MRS amongst the small print causes of recurrent facial nerve palsy but the classical triad is rarely observed, oligosymptomatic and monosymptomatic forms being more common.[1] Facial oedema is the most common initial finding and is an acknowledged mimic of hereditary or acquired angioedema. A possible association of MRS and psoriasis has been described.[2] Allergic diseases (atopic eczema, allergic rhinitis) have been observed concurrently with MRS.[3]

Eponyms may sometimes be memorable, particularly if the name(s) involved seem(s) exotic; MRS may fall into this category, despite its rarity (I believe I have only diagnosed it once before in 20 years as a consultant). Eponyms may prompt those with an interest in history to investigate the originators, if indeed they were the first to describe the disorder. It is possible that neither Ernst Melkersson (1928)[4] nor Curt Rosenthal (1931)[5] were the first to report "their" condition.[6]

Naming may be conceptualised as a form of cross-modal non-contextual paired associate learning, a process which may be challenging for both learning and retention. How often do patients attending the cognitive clinic complain of difficulty remembering people's names? Eponyms may have a certain economy of expression, but risk implying uniformity where there may in fact be heterogeneity, for example at the clinical, investigational, pathological or genetic level ("Pick's disease" might be cited as a good example of this). Moreover, eponyms convey no information on pathogenesis or aetiology, whether defined or suspected, of the disease they denote. The case may therefore be made that this is a situation in which the more descriptive, if prosaic, nomenclature is to be preferred.

Other arguments in favour of abandoning eponyms have been made, for example in cases of misnaming, misattribution, and misuse, and for lacking accuracy.[7] The ethical imperative to expunge from eponymic recognition those involved in Nazi activities is well recognised.[7,8] However, others favour retention,[9] and it seems that *de facto* eponymous labelling will persist, with the potential to confuse patients.

If we agree with Cicero's claim, in his *Tusculan Disputations*, that the "imposition of names on things is the highest part of wisdom,"[10] then care is needed in this exercise since it is more than simply an arid exercise in semantics. Overall, I am sympathetic to the position favoured by Woywodt and Matteson,[7] that medical eponyms should be abandoned in favour of a more descriptive nomenclature. A potential implication of this approach is that nomenclature should be provisional, and hence flexible in the face of new understandings of disease processes.

Acknowledgements

Thanks to Madeleine Fletcher for translating the title of reference 5. Adapted from: Larner AJ. What's in a name? A diagnosis by any other name would be as meet? *Adv Clin Neurosci Rehabil* 2020;19(2):23.

References

1. Larner AJ, Coles AJ, Scolding NJ, Barker RA. *A-Z of neurological practice. A guide to clinical neurology (2nd edition)*. London: Springer, 2011:63,429.
2. Halevy S, Shalom G, Trattner A, Bodner L. Melkersson-Rosenthal syndrome: a possible association with psoriasis. *J Am Acad Dermatol* 2012;67:795–796.
3. Martins JA, Azenha A, Almeida R, Pinheiro JP. Melkersson-Rosenthal syndrome with coeliac and allergic diseases. *BMJ Case Rep* 2019;12(8):e229857.

4. Melkersson E. Ett fall av recidiverande facialspares i samband med ett angioneurotiskt *ødem* [Relapsing facial palsy in conjunction with an angioneurotic oedema]. *Hygiea, Stockholm* 1928;90:737–741.

5. Rosenthal C. Klinisch-erbbiologischer Beitrag zur Konstitutionspathologie. Gemeinsames Auftreten von (rezidivierender familiarer) Facialislähmung, angioneurotischem Gesichtsödem und Lingua plicata in Arthritismus-Familien. *Zeitschrift für die gesamte Neurologie und Psychiatrie* 1931;131:475–501.

6. http://www.whonamedit.com/synd.cfm/9.html (accessed 28/10/19).

7. Woywodt A, Matteson E. Should eponyms be abandoned? Yes. *BMJ* 2007;335:424.

8. Larner AJ. Eponyms revisited. *Prog Neurol Psychiatry* 2018;22(4):22.

9. Whitworth JA. Should eponyms be abandoned? No. *BMJ* 2007;335:425.

10. Roos AM. *Martin Lister and his remarkable daughters. The art of science in the seventeenth century.* Oxford: Bodleian Library, 2019:125.

Miscellany

Neurology and Literature

Abstract

This brief personal view explores some of the interrelationships between the study of neurology and of literature, and the possibilities for cross-fertilization between these disciplines, despite their initially seeming poles apart. Emphasis is given to the narrative structure of both patient/author and neurological accounts. Literary accounts of neurological disease may inform understanding of the patient experience of disease, and the description of neurological disorders may stimulate creative writers. The exchange of ideas in this interdisciplinary subject area may therefore be productive.

Introduction

In the introduction to her edited volume entitled *Neurology and literature, 1860–1920*,[1] Anne Stiles commences by stating that "Neurology and literature are disciplines that initially appear to have little, if anything, to do with one another" (p.1). She points out the dichotomy between neurology-as-science and literature-as-art and contrasts the (ostensibly) objective nature of the former with the subjective nature of the latter, and hence the limited accessibility of neurology to a trained faculty whilst literature is (theoretically) available to any literate individual. Whereas in the time period Stiles considers the rhetorical strategies and cultural assumptions of neurology and literature were largely shared, there has certainly been an increasing divergence since then (the "two cultures" of CP Snow), as reflected in the highly specialised and increasingly technical jargon of neurology which renders such texts difficult to access by lay readers unfamiliar with the language of the discipline.

However, there clearly are points of contact and interchange between neurology and literature. Both are cultural artefacts, whose practitioners may share similar rhetorical strategies. This brief article seeks to explore some of the interrelationships between the two disciplines.

Development

The patient as text

> The sufferers [of epilepsy] therefore I think of not only as sufferers, but as texts; and not only as texts, but as human beings each one with his joys and reliefs as well as pains and pangs.[2]

Clinical practice, as exemplified by the codified processes of taking a history from the patient (anamnesis) and physical examination, is mostly centred around interpretation. Perhaps in no other sphere of medicine is this interpretative process, this focus on pattern recognition, more crucial than in neurology, with its wealth of neurological signs with semiotic value, both in terms of the localization of disease processes within the nervous system and the diagnosis of specific neurological disorders.[3] However, many neurological conditions (e.g. headache disorders, sensory complaints), and all psychiatric disorders, are only discernible through the patient narrative of subjective experience, upon which the clinician is therefore entirely reliant.

Daniel proposed a hermeneutical model of clinical decision making in which the patient may be viewed as a text,[4] and this idea has been taken up by other authors.[5] Although some might see this type of conceptualisation as dangerously reductive, potentially objectifying or ignoring the individuality of the patient and his or her experience of illness (as Sir Henry Harcourt-Reilly suggests, in TS Eliot's play *The Cocktail Party*: "All cases are unique, and very similar to others"[6]), it does nevertheless have some interesting implications. A text ill-attended to is liable to be misread and misunderstood. Misreading and misunderstanding of a patient as text could have unfortunate, or even disastrous, consequences for diagnosis and treatment.

However, the old adage to the effect that all one needs to do in clinical practice is listen and the patient will tell you the diagnosis does not ring true, certainly for this neurologist. Whilst initial, unconditional, attentive listening, a suspension of disbelief, is an appropriate consultation style to ensure that the patient feels he or she is being listened to, the patient narrative thus rendered may be seen as a text which, like all literary texts, needs to be decoded, even deconstructed, since narratives may be elaborated, and narrators may be unreliable (the playwright John Osborne, in his autobiography, suggests that "What we remember is what we become. ... We become resemblances of our past"[7]). The patient with no narrative (because, for example, unconscious, amnesic, or aphasic) presents a particular challenge, requiring the search for collateral or witness history. Hence focused questioning, or interrogation, of the history is required to elucidate those elements key to pattern recognition. Physicians may thus be framed as "clinical historians".[8]

In this respect a distinction must be drawn between literary texts, which are essentially passive, and patients as texts, essentially active and susceptible of disclosing more information. The shortcoming of all literary accounts has been characterised as the "problem of the frame", since they vouchsafe only a limited view over the reality of the past.[9] For example, for want of further, more definitive, information, such as a clinician might be able to obtain through history, examination and investigation, the causes of the inability of children to walk in four fictional cases remain obscure, even to the extent of knowing whether the children described have paraplegia, understood to mean damage to or pathology of the spinal cord.[10] Discussing the same four fictional cases, Lois Keith points out that "drama rather than medical plausibility is the business of the sentimental novelist" who will "ignore medical accuracy in order to allow their characters to walk again".[11] In these books, as elsewhere,[12] illness and recovery may be used as metaphors for transformation and renewal, and inability to walk may be symbolic of psychological distress.

Patient narrative is largely episodic or autobiographical. Although lay explanation of patient symptoms is sometimes attempted, the semantic evaluation of the history is the prerogative of the clinician, based on the assessment and its interpretation,[8] informed by specialised knowledge, training and previous experience. In the words of Kathryn Montgomery Hunter,[13] the clinician's "careful return of the story" (p.xxiii) is an "interpretive retelling that points towards the story's ending" (p.5), be that definitive diagnosis or a plan for future action (observation, investigation, treatment). Literary texts, on the other hand, may contain both episodic and semantic elements, as befits the role of the omniscient narrator.

The doctor as reader
The ineluctable corollary of the formulation of "the patient as text" is "the doctor as reader".[13] This position may encompass not only engagement with the clinical practice of patients as texts but also with literary texts; these two possibilities will be considered in turn.

The clinician's task as a reader of patients as texts is to interpret and shape the autobiographical history: "The patient's story of illness ... is interpreted and shaped into a medically plotted version ... and then compared not only with standardized, textbook plots ... but also with plots of comparable cases in the physician's experience" (p.45).[13] Hence, the gap between individual case and general principle is bridged. Hunter has characterised this as the "meta-story of the illness" (p.13),[13] which facilitates understanding and, hopefully, treatment. Clinical judgement is "the ability to discern a plot" (p.45),[13] the production of a narrative by the clinician based on a reinterpretation of the patient narrative.

Perhaps the key questions when decoding or deconstructing (any) text are: what is the context? And, who is framing the narrative? Informed by a spirit of healthy scepticism, and acknowledging that uncertainty lies at the heart of the medical endeavour, these questions aim to challenge any apparently omniscient narrator (patient or literary text). We are readily familiar with this type of approach when dealing with the statements of self-appointed, self-declared, or self-selected "leaders", generally of the political and managerial (bureaucratic) classes, with their acknowledged tendency to over-valued (non evidence-based) ideas which risk descent into (or may even emanate from) deluding and self-deluding ideology. In other words, in these narratives context is ignored, wilfully or not, so that one particular narrative may be privileged above other narratives which may in fact be more plausible. This is the rhetoric of failure, of epistemological closure, which is anathema to medical scepticism. The management of patients who attend neurology clinics with multiple symptoms for which no neurological explanation is forthcoming despite careful (and sometimes repeated) examination and investigation may be unwilling to accept the clinician's narrative of health anxiety or somatisation, believing against the evidence that there is a serious underlying disorder.

Coming now to literary texts, the reading of such works is, outside of academic circles, a pastime generally undertaken for pleasure, to inform, instruct, and entertain. Nevertheless, as a neurologist, trained in the diagnostic skills of pattern recognition, it is not always possible to switch off and remove ones workaday "neurological spectacles" when reading such texts. (Joost Haan has questioned whether a literary text may be read as a patient, finding that in some respects they belong to the same category.[14]) Hence there is a propensity to find examples of (what seem to be) descriptions of neurological disorders. For example, my initial experience of this type of involuntary (retro-)diagnosis came when reading the description of a character appearing in *The Lazy Tour of Two Idle Apprentices* written by Charles Dickens (and Wilkie Collins), published in 1857, who seemed to have features of parkinsonism with an accompanying eye movement disorder, which seemed highly suggestive of a diagnosis of progressive supranuclear palsy,[15] a condition not formally described in the medical literature until the 1960s.

This approach may be criticised as anachronistic, since it imposes modern concepts of diagnosis or diagnostic criteria on earlier time periods. There is, I think, a tension here between the truism that concepts are historically produced, and that medical discourse should be seen in relation to the ambient culture; and the possibility that diseases of the nervous system are timeless and transcendent categories (the ontological argument). Do we, as neurologists, believe that diseases of the brain and nervous system did not exist before the emergence of neurology as a word (1660s-1670s) or as a clinical discipline (1860s-1870s)? I think most neurologists would answer this question: Clearly not.

Dickens's account also indicates that a lay person possessed of acute powers of observation and adequate descriptive ability may be able to narrate clinical phenomena with sufficient precision to facilitate clinical diagnosis, without the benefit of specific medical training. To a certain extent this is what we rely on in taking a clinical history, in the acknowledgement that some patients are better historians than others.

The more one looks, as a neurologist, the more one sees textual descriptions of (possible) neurological disorders. For example, the occasional "Neurological Literature" series of articles published in the journal *Advances in Clinical Neuroscience & Rehabilitation* (see www.acnr.co.uk) has included contributions on literary accounts of headache, epilepsy, cognitive disorders, and sleep-related disorders. These neurological conditions are common denominators of human experience, likely to be encountered at either first or second hand by many within the population, so it is not surprising that novelists have on occasion used such conditions as source material for elaboration in their narratives. Increasing moves in recent years to include some study of the humanities in medical curricula reflects the way such studies may mutually inform one another.

Neurology as narrative

Patient narratives, as well as being of intrinsic interest, give a patient, as opposed to faculty, perspective on disorders of the nervous system and hence broaden our medical sensibility to, and perception of, the experiential aspects of disease, contributing to what Hunter has termed the narrative structure of medical knowledge.[13] The epistemological importance of narrative in clinical medicine is undisputed, as illustrated by the importance of case reports and case series as pedagogical and heuristic devices.

It is well-recognised that the narrative description of disease in individual patients, the medical case, evolved at about the same time in the nineteenth century as detective fiction, both being examples of case-based inquiry.[13,16] The medical case has been elegantly described as "the retrospective construction of a hypothetical narrative in order to work out the relation of the clues to one another within an acceptable chronology".[13]

These principles continue to inform the production of heuristic texts today. Most case reports by convention follow a fairly standardised linear structure, a fixed regularity which befits this narrative genre, but which may be at odds with lived experience, the sometimes piecemeal haphazard way in which patient diagnosis and management evolves.[17]

The doctor as writer

Since clinical practice is built around the production of narratives by clinicians, it is not surprising that this should sometimes extend to the production of the written word, not only in medical text but also in literary works.

Doctors who were also authors of literary texts are readily familiar,[18] such as Anton Chekhov, Sir Arthur Conan Doyle, Oliver Wendell Holmes, Arthur Schnitzler, AJ Cronin, and W Somerset Maugham, to name but a few. Conan Doyle's approach in the characterisation of the methods of Sherlock Holmes might be seen as particularly "neurological", based as it was on the diagnostic methods of Doyle's teacher at Edinburgh, Joseph Bell.[19] Numerous examples of neurological reference may be found in the Holmes' oeuvre.[20] Holmesian methods of deduction have been cited as analogous to the narrative structure of medical knowledge: "clinical reasoning, like Sherlock Holmes ratiocination, is a ... dialectical process of discovery and understanding ... well suited to narrative representation" (p.68).[13]

In addition to these examples, giants of neurological and neuroanatomical investigation such as Silas Weir Mitchell and Santiago Ramón y Cajal also wrote works of fiction. In this context, Weir Mitchell's work has attracted particular attention.[21,22] His first publication on what he subsequently chose to call "phantom limbs" (the sensations of the presence of an arm or leg following its amputation) appeared in a literary magazine, some five years before his academic publication describing the same.

Literary responses to neurology

Doctors are familiar as characters or subjects within literary texts; many examples may be referenced,[23-26] although few may be specified as neurologists. Medics and medical ideas have long been a stimulus or subject for creative writers, indicating a cultural interplay between medicine and creative literature. HG Wells, Robert Louis Stevenson, and Wilkie Collins have been cited as authors who produced works dramatizing neurological hypotheses (p.2).[1]

An example of this interplay may be afforded by the literary possibilities presented by neurophysiological investigations of the brain. It is perhaps unsurprising that authors within the genre broadly described as "science fiction" have been attracted by the technological implications of electroencephalography (EEG) for recording and/or monitoring the human nervous system. Both Philip K Dick and Ursula K Le Guin, giants in the field of science fiction writing, have explored some of the implications of EEG.[27] The "Penfield mood organ" described in Dick's (1968) novel *Do androids dream of electric sheep?* (on which the 1982 film Blade Runner was based), which permits the user to select their mood state through artificial brain stimulation, is surely a reference to Wilder Penfield (1891–1976), whose work (with Herbert Jasper) stimulating the cortex of awake epilepsy patients undergoing surgery allowed him to map the functions of various regions of the brain.

Conclusions

Both neurology and literature are concerned with narrative, and hence are kindred disciplines which may be subject to the (fruitful) exchange of ideas. This may be seen as an interdisciplinary subject area, transcending the boundaries of professional categories. Neurological practice involves the construction of narratives based upon patient accounts which inform not only patient diagnosis but also the understanding of neurological disease. Literary texts may be seen as "an index of cultural reactions to scientific concepts" (p.165).[28] To return to Anne Stiles,[1] with whom we began, the relationship between neurology and literature is not merely reflective, but may best be described as dialogic or circular (p.2).

Acknowledgements

Thanks to Dr Lauren Fratalia for critical comments on this manuscript. Adapted and extended from: Larner AJ. Neurology and literature. *Neurosciences and History* 2017;5:47–51.

References

1. Stiles A, editor. *Neurology and literature, 1860–1920.* Basingstoke: Palgrave Macmillan; 2007.
2. Pratt J (ed.). *The Nightingale Silenced and other late unpublished writings by Margiad Evans.* Dinas Powys: Honno (Welsh Women's Classics); 2020:133.
3. Larner AJ. *A dictionary of neurological signs* (4th edition). London: Springer; 2016.
4. Daniel SL. The patient as text: A model of clinical hermeneutics. *Theor Med Bioeth.* 1986;7:195–210.
5. Aaslestad P. *The patient as text. The role of the narrator in psychiatric notes, 1890–1990.* Oxford: Radcliffe Publishing; 2009.
6. Eliot TS. *The complete poems and plays of TS Eliot.* London: Faber and Faber; 1969:402.
7. Osborne J. *Looking back. Never explain, never apologise.* London: Faber and Faber; 1999:525.
8. Hughes T. Neurology and the clinical historian. *Medicine.* 2020;48:493–496.

9. Rosetti AO, Bogousslavsky J. Dostoevsky and epilepsy. An attempt to look through the frame. In: Bogousslavsky J, Boller F, editors. *Neurological disorders in famous artists.* Basel: Karger; 2005:65–75.

10. Larner AJ. Some literary accounts of possible childhood paraplegia and neurorehabilitation. *Dev Neurorehabil.* 2009;12:248–252.

11. Keith L. *Take up thy bed and walk: death, disability and cure in classic fiction for girls.* London: Routledge; 2001.

12. Sontag S. *Illness as metaphor.* New York: Farrar, Straus and Giroux; 1978.

13. Hunter KM. *Doctors' stories. The narrative structure of medical knowledge.* Princeton: Princeton University Press; 1991.

14. Haan J. *Migraine, words and fiction.* Newcastle: Cambridge Scholars Publishing, 2022.

15. Larner AJ. Did Charles Dickens describe progressive supranuclear palsy in 1857? *Mov Disord.* 2002;17:832–833.

16. Kempster PA, Lees AJ. Neurology and detective writing. *Pract Neurol.* 2013;13:372–376.

17. Ghadiri-Sani M, Larner AJ. How to write a case report. *Br J Hosp Med.* 2014;75:207–210.

18. Cooper DKC, editor. *Doctors of another calling. Physicians who are known best in fields other than medicine.* Newark: University of Delaware Press; 2014.

19. Godbee DC. Joseph Bell (1837–1911): a clinician's literary legacy. *J Med Biogr.* 1999;7:166–170.

20. Larner AJ. "Neurological literature": Sherlock Holmes and neurology. *Adv Clin Neurosci Rehabil.* 2011;11(1):20,22.

21. Hawgood BJ. Silas Weir Mitchell (1829–1914): toxicologist, neurologist and novelist. *J Med Biogr.* 2000;8:63–70.

22. Satz A. "The conviction of its existence": Silas Weir Mitchell, phantom limbs and phantom bodies in neurology and spiritualism. In: Salisbury L, Shail A, editors. *Neurology and modernity. A cultural history of nervous systems, 1800–1950.* Basingstoke: Palgrave Macmillan; 2010:113–129.

23. Posen S. *The doctor in literature. Volume 1. Satisfaction or resentment.* Oxford: Radcliffe; 2005.

24. Posen S. *The doctor in literature. Volume 2. Private life.* Oxford: Radcliffe; 2006.

25. Surawicz B, Jacobson B. *Doctors in fiction. Lessons from literature.* Oxford: Radcliffe; 2009.

26. Bogousslavsky J, Dieguez S, editors. *Literary medicine: brain disease and doctors in novels, theater, and film.* Basel: Karger; 2013.

27. Larner AJ. "Neurological literature": neurophysiology. *Adv Clin Neurosci Rehabil.* 2017;16(5):14–15.

28. Matus J. Emergent theories of Victorian mind shock: from war and railway accident to nerves, electricity and emotion. In: Stiles A, editor. *Neurology and literature, 1860–1920.* Basingstoke: Palgrave Macmillan; 2007:163–183.

The neuropsychology of board games, puzzles and quizzes

Introduction

A potentially bewildering array of neuropsychological tests exists, examining the various domains of cognitive function, such as intelligence, memory, language, perceptual (especially visuoperceptual) skills, praxis, and executive function. Board games, puzzles, quizzes and other parlour diversions have a number of common features, including being rule bound and subject to the play of chance, and require various degrees of strategy, planning, and flexibility for their execution. Hence, they may be regarded as tapping some of the same functions explored by neuropsychological tests, as examined in the following tentative suggestions. Readers may be able to conjure further examples. Like neuropsychological tests, these diversions are seldom tests of a single function.

Memory

Quizzes are usually tests of semantic (facts) memory. Examples include the board game *Trivial Pursuit*, the long-running radio programme *Brain of Britain*, and TV shows such as *University Challenge*, *Mastermind* and *The Weakest Link*. These are essentially testing recall, although the wording of questions may move questions more toward the recognition paradigm (NB the board game *Mastermind* taps very different cognitive skills). Tests more inclined towards working memory are seldom encountered, although occasional questions in *University Challenge*, of the "Buzz as soon as you know the answer" type, based on mathematical calculations, do occur. A semantic memory test with a forced choice paradigm is presented in *Who wants to be a millionaire*, usually 1 of 4, but occasionally 1 of 2 ("50:50"), and recourse to external memory aids is also possible ("Ask the audience" and "Phone a friend").

Visual memory games often revolve around recalling the locations of matching cards or symbols which are only briefly uncovered, or object shown and then removed (the "tray game"); all may fall under the rubric of Pelmanism. (My personal experience suggests that children are better than this particular adult at these games.)

Language

Many board games are essentially linguistic in the skills they tap, such as *Scrabble* and *Boggle*, where lettered tiles must be used to make words. The latter has a visuospatial element in that letters in the array must be adjacent (vertical, horizontal, or diagonal) to be used to make words, and also there is a fixed time element. The "against the clock" factor for word generation also looms large in the TV show *Countdown*, where word length earns the points rather than number of words generated. Clearly there is an executive function, as well as a linguistic, component to these games, tapping particularly phonemic verbal fluency. Crosswords, depending on their degree of cryptic-ness, probably tax executive function more than simply linguistic skills.

Games involving numerical calculation might be included here, since numbers are a form of language. Certain card games are based on addition (Pontoon, Cribbage). In one form of dominoes, matching of the two end tiles to be multiples of 3 and 5 is the basis of scoring in the game (cf. below). Sudoku obviously tests numerical as well as spatial functions.

Perceptual (especially visuoperceptual) skills

Snap is a classic game of simple visual matching, amenable to even very young children. In one form of dominoes, matching of spots and getting rid of your tiles are the sole objects of the game (cf. above), as in variants such as *Triominoes*. Card games such as Rummy and Patience and even Poker require visual matching, to collect cards with like characterisitics, combined with executive function, with rather more complex rules than snap. Any game involving trumps may also share these cognitive demands.

Visual recognition lies at the heart of Wordsearch puzzles, with visual scanning of an array of letters in search of salience (word recognition). Likewise games such as charades probe visual recognition skills (older readers may recall that this was televised as *Star Turn* on BBC children's TV, before the format was ripped off by ITV as *Give Us A Clue*). *Pictionary* also taxes visual recognition skills. Jigsaw puzzles require matching of visual patterns and colours, but also sometimes shape (e.g. edges, large areas of monochrome sky or grass). Patients with semantic dementia who gradually lose the ability to understand the world around them may nevertheless continue to do jigsaw puzzles successfully, reflecting preserved visuospatial skills and concentration.[1] Playstation and DS are alleged by some to promote visual/manual coordination.

Praxis

Testing of acquired skilled motor movements seems less profitable as a theme for parlour games, as compared to other domains. One might argue that *Jenga* and *Buckaroo* are all about fine motor control, likewise *Operation*.

Executive function

As mentioned, executive function plays a part in many of the games already alluded to. Whereas the throw of the dice determines everything in *Snakes & Ladders* (truly, *alea jacta est!*) and largely so in *Frustration* or *Sorry*, (or its Spanish version, *Parchis*) greater cognitive demands are imposed in dice games such as *Monopoly* and *Careers* (in what proportions do you choose to pursue fame, happiness or fortune?), in which strategy (as well as luck) is important. *Cluedo* requires information to be pursued and inferences to be made. *Risk* is a game of strategy.

Conclusions

In light of these considerations, it may be worth asking patients and carers about facility, or loss thereof, in playing board games and doing puzzles as one element of history taking in the cognitive clinic. However, it must be borne in mind that some games seem largely bereft of all intellectual function: it is hard to see what cognitive functions are tapped in deciding in which order to open a set of boxes (*Deal No Deal*).

Examination of the ability to play games effectively lies at the heart of some existing cognitive tests, such as Wisconsin Card Sorting and tests of gambling such as the Iowa Gambling Task and the Cambridge Gamble Task. Might *Monopoly*, cards, charades, etc., be introduced to the cognitive clinic? Patients might find them less daunting than unfamiliar neuropsychological tests, and it might add some fun to consultations. A loss of enjoyment in such innocent diversions might also be indicative of cognitive disorder with frontal lobe involvement.

Acknowledgement

Thanks to Dr Lauren Fratalia for introducing me to *Parchis*. Adapted from: Larner AJ. The neuropsychology of board games, puzzles and quizzes. *Adv Clin Neurosci Rehabil* 2009;9(5):42.

References

1. Green HA, Patterson K. Jigsaws – a preserved ability in semantic dementia. *Neuropsychologia* 2009;47:569–576.

Scrabble-ing with dementia

Introduction

In a previous article,[1] it was suggested that board games, puzzles, and quizzes might be characterised as neuropsychological tests, probing different domains of cognitive function. One of the board games mentioned, *Scrabble*, was deemed to tap essentially linguistic skills. In recent years I have had the opportunity to witness first-hand the changes in *Scrabble* skills in a previously competent player who developed dementia, namely my mother.

The game

For those unfamiliar with the game, the aim of *Scrabble* (originally marketed as "Criss-Crosswords") is to make words using one hundred letter tiles on a 15x15 board. Individual letters are assigned different values according to the frequency of their use (e.g. in the English version a,e,i,o,u all score 1, whereas q and z score 10). Each player has a hand of seven tiles, picked at random, with which to construct words, which may run either horizontally or vertically on the board, building upon letters already in place on the board. Scores for each turn are the sum of the individual letter scores, and these may be augmented by placing tiles on squares labelled as double or triple letter or double or triple word scores. The player with the highest aggregate score once all the letters are played wins the game. For those unfamiliar and/or curious, the full rules may be consulted.[2]

Although purchased initially for the entertainment of their children, my mother and father continued to play *Scrabble* frequently, often nightly, after we had passed on to other interests, and indeed after we had left home.

The patient

My mother developed cognitive decline in her mid-eighties, having previously been in good health aside from occasional migraine after the onset of menopause[3] and late life hypertension. An elective hip replacement in her eighties was certainly associated with change in cognitive and functional abilities. She was diagnosed with Alzheimer's disease in her early nineties, based on clinical assessment and cognitive testing (ACE-III 49/100) by an old age psychiatrist. She is treated with donepezil. My sister is her named carer and provides resident assistance with all activities of daily living.

Now 94, my mother continues to play *Scrabble* on a daily basis. Although she never initiates the plan to play, she generally expresses willingness if it is suggested, often commenting that it keeps the mind active and provides an opportunity to learn new words. She perseveres at each game, never expressing any wish to stop playing once a game is underway, although on occasion a game has been terminated because she is in pain (particularly from the previous hip replacement).

Observed changes in *Scrabble* skills

My mother is sometimes slow in making words, and certainly her playing vocabulary is impoverished in comparison with her past abilities, now with a predilection for short (usually three- or four letter) words. Nevertheless, she can on occasion "see" words and play immediately (pre-processing?), such that usual turn taking may be overridden in her enthusiasm to play a word, requiring a reminder that "It's not your go yet!".

Difficult letters, such as q, z, j, may be marginalised, literally and physically, and apparently ignored, sometimes for the whole duration of a game. The two blank tiles, which can be used to represent any letter, are often a source of confusion, and may be turned upside down. Nevertheless, she can sometimes surprise us by working out unfamiliar words (e.g. from an opening hand of letters, d,d,e,j,r,s,u, she eventually played all seven as "judders").

On occasion she may play letters in the wrong direction (i.e. backwards), suggesting visuospatial problems, or may attempt to play a word for which she does not have all the letters. She may make a word with the tiles in her hand which cannot be played onto the board for lack of suitable letter/space to which it can be joined.

Playing strategy has also changed in other ways. Whereas in earlier years the opportunity to play on, for example, a triple word score would not be overlooked, this is no longer the case. She does not calculate or keep her own score. Generally her completed game scores are between 100–150, occasionally 200, whereas in her heyday she regularly scored around 300.

The option to replace some or all of a hand of letters in exchange for foregoing a turn of play, which she frequently used in the past if stuck with a handful of vowels, is never now used. The use of a dictionary to check word spelling is eschewed, indeed those availing themselves of this facility, entirely within the rules of the game, may be accused of cheating!

In summary, I suggest that my mother's current standard of *Scrabble* play reflects a general decline in her linguistic skills, perhaps some loss of memory for words, occasional visuospatial errors, and change in executive function as reflected in her less competitive strategy.

Another phenomenon, which seems very curious, occurs on occasion. Despite her experience of playing *Scrabble* over many decades, my mother will sometimes state "I don't think I've played this game before". With encouragement and example she may pick it up again, but on other occasions this is not the case. She may report that she just cannot see how she could play the letters in her hand, sometimes laying them on top of letters already on the board. I wonder if this is a form of "closing in", a term used to describe copying drawings close to or superimposed upon the original, seen in some patients with Alzheimer's disease, and variously interpreted as "constructional apraxia", a visuospatial deficit, or stimulus-boundedness. This fluctuation in the ability to play occurs particularly (but not invariably) in the afternoons, and I think might reflect waning of attentional resources, manifest as an executive deficit of not understanding how the game is played.

Conclusion

My previous judgment that *Scrabble* is essentially a test of linguistic skills[1] has been shown, in part from observation in the change in my mother's play, as far too simplistic. Evidently, *Scrabble* requires the allocation of attentional resources, intact verbal and visual memory, visuospatial skills, and executive function, as well as linguistic abilities, for its successful performance.

Acknowledgements

I thank my mother and sister for permission to report this case. My mother managed a very slow and assisted game on the morning of the day she died (18th January 2020) and she still managed to make a few simple words. Adapted from: Larner AJ. *Scrabble*-ing with dementia. *Adv Clin Neurosci Rehabil* 2019;18(4):25.

References

1.   Larner AJ. The neuropsychology of board games, puzzles and quizzes. *Adv Clin Neurosci & Rehabil* 2009;9(5):42.
2.   https://scrabble.hasbro.com/en-us/rules (accessed 22/04/19).
3.   Larner AJ. Familial migraine without aura with perimenopausal onset. *Int J Clin Pract* 2010;64:128–129.

Dysphonia clericorum: Clergyman's sore throat

REVEREND SAMUEL GARDNER: Good morning, I must apologize for not having met you at breakfast. I have a touch of – of- fell down in the market-place, and foamed at mouth, and was speechless.
FRANK GARDNER: Clergyman's sore throat … fortunately not chronic.

Of the many ailments that may assail the clerical profession, one that is thankfully no longer heard of is clergyman's sore throat, or dysphonia clericorum. However, theatre goers attending the first performance of George Bernard Shaw's (1856–1950) play *Mrs Warren's Professsion* in 1894 would have been familiar with the condition alluded to in this exchange from Act III, here used as a euphemisim by Frank for his father's overindulgence in alcohol when entertaininting his guests the night before: "I never saw a beneficed clergyman less sober" is his comment. But what was clergyman's sore throat? Does it still exist?

Clergyman's sore throat was a slowly developing condition due to constant or increased use of the voice, which caused inflammation of the throat and impairment of speech. The fictitious Reverend Gardner was not the only sufferer. Before he became the famed explorer of Africa, Dr David Livingstone travelled from the arena of his missionary work in southern Africa to Cape Town in 1852 to have his uvula surgically excised. The indication for this operation he subsequently reported in his first "best seller", *Missionary travels and researches in South Africa*, published in 1857:

> Our services having necessarily been all in the open air, where it is most difficult to address large bodies of people, prevented my recovering so entirely from the effects of clergyman's sore throat as I expected, when my uvula was excised at the Cape.

Later he noted:

> I gave many public addresses to the people of Sesheke … They often amounted to between five and six hundred souls, and required an exertion of voice which brought back the complaint for which I had got the uvula excised at the Cape.

And later still:

"Clergyman's sore throat" ... partially disabled me from the work.[1]

The failure of the surgery to cure his problem was no doubt a source of great regret to Livingstone; immediately after the operation he had written in his private journal:

Got my uvula excised, which I hope will enable me more fully to preach unto the gentiles the unsearchable riches of Christ.[2]

(probably a paraphrase of St Paul's Epistle to the Ephesians, 3:8).

Belief in the culpability of the uvula may have been widespread. Describing the symptoms of his tuberculosis around 1884, Robert Louis Stevenson (1850–1894) reported "The cough is from the throat, which is in a state of fine congestion; uvula much elongated".[3]

Livingstone was not only a missionary but also a qualified doctor, and "clergyman's sore throat" was certainly no folk or lay diagnosis. The pioneer American throat specialist Horace Green (1802–1866) published in 1846 a textbook entitled *Treatise on Diseases of the Air Passages, Comprising an Inquiry into the History, Pathology, Causes and Treatment of those Affections of the Throat called Bronchitis, Chronic Laryngitis, Clergyman's Sore Throat, etc.* which ran to a fourth edition by 1858.

It is probable that the term "clerical throat" denoted the same or similar symptoms. The "Ammoniaphone" developed by Dr Carter Moffatt of Glasgow, and used by Lewis Carroll to try to improve his speech impediment (stammering),[4] was advertised as effective for, amongst many other things, "clerical throat".

It was recognised that the disorder was not confined to ordained clergymen, since other public speakers, such as schoolteachers and street hawkers, could also be affected. Being of its time we do not know whether the condition would have affected "women priests", but of possible interest is the comment of George Eliot (1819–1880), in *Impressions of Theophrastus Such* (1879), that:

... the poor curate, equally with the rector, is liable to clergyman's sore throat.

It is of course anachronistic to try to interpret 19th century disease categories in terms of 21st century medical understanding, but such considerations have seldom inhibited amateur medical historians. It might be that many cases of clergyman's sore throat were nothing more than self-limiting episodes of laryngitis; "repetitive strain injury" might be a modern day equivalent label.

Some cases may have resulted from involuntary muscle contraction in the throat, a condition now known as spasmodic dysphonia.

Why has clergyman's sore throat become an archaic, obsolete diagnosis? Again it is speculation, but one might suggest the tendency to briefer sermons, delivered to smaller congregations, with the assistance of electronic amplification, as contributory factors.

Acknowledgement

Adapted from: Larner AJ. "Clergyman's sore throat" Dysphonia clericorum. *Catalyst (Neston Parish Magazine)* 2006;January:16–17.

References

1. Livingstone D. *Missionary travels and researches in South Africa; including a sketch of sixteen years' residence in the interior of Africa, etc.* London: John Murray, 1857:164, 205, 578.
2. Schapera I (ed.). *Livingstone's private journals 1851–1853.* London: Chatto & Windus, 1960:80.
3. Harman C. *Robert Louis Stevenson. A biography.* London: Harper Perennial, 2005:266.
4. Blom JD. *Alice in Wonderland syndrome.* London: Springer, 2020:105n31.

"Holy dementia": religious contributions to understanding brain disease

The clergy are charged, amongst other things, with the cure of the diseased souls of their parishioners. The religious have also made contributions to our understanding of diseased brains, through the findings of studies performed in recent years, particularly in the field of dementia. In the 100th year since Dr Alois Alzheimer originally described the disease which was later to bear his name, it is perhaps worth looking at some of these contributions.

The Nun Study has followed up members of the School Sisters of Notre Dame, a teaching order of nuns in the USA, for many years, testing their cognitive abilities sequentially and then examining their brains after death. These religious are excellent research subjects since they share a relatively uniform environment, stay in the same place and so are not lost to long-term follow-up, and are free from some of the confounding factors (e.g. smoking, drinking alcohol) seen in secular cohorts. This important study has shown, amongst other things, the importance of verbal abilities at an early age, and of mild physical activity, as being protective against later cognitive decline, as well as the role of cerebrovascular disease in enhancing the clinical expression of Alzheimer type change in the brain.[1]

The Rush Religious Orders Study, based at Rush University Medical Center in Chicago, has followed up a large cohort of catholic nuns, priests, and brothers recruited from 40 groups across the USA. Of the many results published from this study, perhaps the most striking is the observation that frequent participation in "cognitively stimulating activities" (it could be something as simple as reading a newspaper) is associated with a reduced risk of developing Alzheimer's disease.[2] So, it may be that attending weekly to a cognitively stimulating sermon (or even, unlikely as it may seem, reading this article) may protect your brain from the consequences of ageing and disease. The age-old dictum of "use it or lose it" may indeed be true of cognitive function.

A recent study from Jerusalem examined religiosity, spirituality, and organizational and private religious practices in a group of patients with probable Alzheimer's disease. The finding, which requires corroboration, was that higher levels of spirituality and private religious practices were associated with slower progression of disease.[3] This is a potentially important finding, since no currently available medications for the treatment of Alzheimer's disease have been shown to slow disease progression.

The need to address the spiritual, as well as physical, emotional, and cognitive, issues in patients with late life cognitive decline is now increasingly recognised. It does not follow that the gradual and inexorable dissolution of personality means that individuals with dementia are non-persons.

Acknowledgement

Adapted from: Larner AJ. "Holy dementia": religious contributions to understanding brain disease. *Catalyst (Neston Parish Magazine)* 2007;August:26–27.

References

1. Snowdon D. *Aging with grace. The Nun Study and the science of old age. How we can all live longer, healthier and more vital lives.* London: Fourth Estate, 2001.
2. Wilson RS, Mendes de Leon CF, Barnes LL et al. Participation in cognitively stimulating activities and risk of incident Alzheimer disease. JAMA 2002;287:742–748.
3. Kaufman Y, Anaki D, Binns M, Freedman M. Cognitive decline in Alzheimer disease: impact of spirituality, religiosity, and QOL. Neurology 2007;68:1509–1514.

Neurological literature: a clinical trial

Clinical trials are an integral part of neurology. Many neurologists will have been involved in their conduct, and all will apply their outcomes to clinical practice. A working knowledge of the methodology of clinical trials is fundamental to their evaluation, and hence a learning objective for neurological trainees.

Sinclair Lewis (1885–1951) was the first American winner of the Nobel Prize for Literature, in 1930, following a series of acclaimed novels published in the 1920s. In one of these, *Arrowsmith* (1925), the protagonist, Martin Arrowsmith, is a doctor (as was Sinclair Lewis's father), whose medical career the novel charts, from medical student, to country doctor, to public health official, to research scientist.[1] In the latter context, a description of a clinical trial is to be found.

Narrative

Aged 34 (p.322), and hence, from internal evidence, in about 1917, Martin discovers "the X Principle" which destroys staphylococcus, but the novelty of his findings is short-lived as his scientist mentor Max Gottlieb finds a report from d'Hérelle of the same phenomena, described as bacteriophage (p.327). Martin's subsequent researches focus on the possibility of curing bubonic plague with phage (p.337). Aged 37 (p.384), and hence around 1920, the opportunity arises to put this laboratory discovery into clinical practice.

The scene is the fictional Caribbean island of St Hubert, a "British possession" (p.355) located in the Lesser Antilles (pp.352,355) between Barbados and Trinidad (p.343) where there is an epidemic outbreak of bubonic plague (p.348). The plan of Max Gottlieb is "to use the phage with only half [of the] patients and keep the others as controls, under normal hygienic conditions but without the phage" (p.348), thus permitting "an absolute determination of its value" (p.348). On departure, he urges Martin: "do not let ... your own good kind heart, spoil your experiment" (p.354).

Martin's co-worker on the trip, Gustaf Sondelius, wants to give phage to everybody (pp.349,381) since "in this crisis mere experimentation was heartless" (p.350) and on principle twice refuses treatment for himself (pp.352,378), but Martin insists on having "real test cases" (p.349), perhaps a reflection of his training from Gottlieb as a medical student in the importance of controls (p.40). Martin's final plan: in "a district which was comparatively untouched by the plague ... one half injected with phage, one half untreated. In the badly afflicted districts, he might give the phage to everyone, and if the disease slackened unusually, that would be a secondary proof" (p.350).

On St Hubert, both the Governor of the island (pp.375–6) and the Board of Health (p.377) object to the plan of "half to get the phage, half to be sternly deprived" (p.375) despite Martin's assertion that the "luckless half would receive as much care as at present" (p.377).

In the village of Carib, where "every third man was down with plague", Martin "gave phage to the entire village" (p.379), following which there is an apparent slackening of the epidemic in the village, observations which Martin hopes will prompt the local bureaucracy to "let me try test conditions" (p.379). Carib village is then burnt in order to kill all the rats, the locals evacuated to a tent village where Martin remains for 2 days giving them phage (p.380).

The opportunity for experiment is provided in St Swithin's Parish, where, unlike Carib, "the plague had only begun to invade" (p.386). Martin "divided the population into two equal parts. One of them ... was injected with plague phage, the other half was left without" (p.386). "The pest attacked the unphaged half of the parish much more heavily than those who had been treated ... These unfortunate cases he treated, giving the phage to alternate cases" (pp.386–7).

However, following a personal bereavement, Martin damns experimenta- tion and "gave the phage to everyone who asked" other than in St Swithin's parish, where "his experiment was so excellently begun ... some remnant of honor [kept] him from distributing the phage universally" (p.392). Unsurpris- ingly people from St Swithin's are seen in the queue for treatment in the main town of St Hubert, Blackwater (p.393). Eventually Martin "went back to the most rigid observation of his experiment in St Swithin's ... blotted as it now was by the unphaged portion of the parish going in to Blackwater to receive the phage" (p.394).

Six months after Martin's arrival, the "plague had almost vanished" (p.395). Martin is lionised by the populace as "the saviour of all our lives" but one local doctor reflects that "plagues have been known to slacken without phage" (p.396). Martin knows that he does "not have complete proof of the value of the phage" (p.397), that "his experiment had so many loopholes" (p.400). He plans to take his data to a "biometrician" who may, he notes, "rip 'em up. Good! What's left, I'll publish" (p.400). Raymond Pearl, the biometrician, "pointed out that his agreeable results in first phaging the whole of Carib village must be questioned, because it was possible that when he began, the curve of the disease had already passed its peak" (p.404). It is evident to Martin's friend, Terry Wickett, that "you bunged it up badly" (p.405).

Comment

Arrowsmith has previously attracted attention for its portrayal of contemporary immunology[2] and public health,[3] and belatedly I discovered a prior commentary related specifically to the details of the clinical trial.[4] Whilst literary accounts of neurological illness are often to be found, I have not previously encountered a fictional account of a clinical trial.

It is not difficult to enumerate the many shortcomings in this clinical trial: no ethics, no planning, no involvement of a statistician from the outset, no patient consent, no blinding of any kind, no randomisation, no matching of cases and controls, no clear definition of outcomes, etc. Indeed this might be better termed a "therapeutic experiment" rather than a clinical trial. Of course, there is no reason why Lewis as author should present the perfect trial, motivated as he was by literary rather than scientific concerns, specifically to illustrate the tension between Martin as clinician-scientist and clinician-humanitarian.[5] Although the randomised clinical trial as we know it was not to evolve for several more decades, clinical trials characterised by "fair allocation" schedules had been undertaken at least from the time of James Lind.[6]

Sinclair Lewis was awarded the Pulitzer Prize for fiction for *Arrowsmith*, but he declined it, his previous novels (*Main Street, Babbitt*) having been passed over. In the same year, 1926, the surgeon Harvey Cushing (1869–1939) also won a Pulitzer Prize for his biography of Sir William Osler (1849–1919). According to another Osler biographer, Michael Bliss (1941–2017), "Cushing wrote friends that he had nothing but contempt for the spirit of Lewis's novel, which had mythologized research and denigrated medical practice. Cushing hoped his Osler biography would be an antidote to *Arrowsmith*".[7] Cushing's objection may have been to the "Literary stereotypes that portrayed surgeons as money-grubbers in novels of the early 20th century":[8] his name appears in the novel (p.85) in a list of surgeons with exceptional surgical technique. He may also perhaps have baulked at a description of one of Martin Arrowsmith's medical student chums "reading a Sherlock Holmes story which rested on the powerful volume of Osler's Medicine which he considered himself to be reading" (p.61; although Holmes' creator was, of course, medically qualified and the Holmes oeuvre features some interesting medical material[9]). Osler is mentioned elsewhere in *Arrowsmith*: as the "god" (p.82) of the professor of internal medicine and Dean of Arrowsmith's medical school who is a "fit disciple of Osler" (p.127), and his treatment of diphtheria is cited (p.158). Lewis had been "fed inside knowledge"[10] for the novel by the microbiologist Paul de Kruif (1890–1971), later to gain fame with his book *The Microbe Hunters* (1926),[11] who is acknowledged at the start of the novel.

This episode in *Arrowsmith* has also been characterised as "the clearest exposition ... in literature" of the dichotomy between "the epistemic value of doing "good science" and the ethical value of administering a potentially useful treatment if the preliminary results look promising."[12]

Acknowledgement

Adapted from: Larner AJ. Neurological literature: a clinical trial. *Adv Clin Neurosci Rehabil* 2019;18(4):18–19.

References

1. Lewis S. *Arrowsmith*. New York: Signet Classics [1925] 2008. All page references cited in the text refer to this edition.
2. Löwy I. Immunology and literature in the early twentieth century: "Arrowsmith" and "The Doctor's Dilemma". *Med Hist* 1988;32:314–332.
3. Markel H. Reflections on Sinclair Lewis's Arrowsmith: the great American novel of public health and medicine. *Public Health Rep* 2001;116:371–375.
4. Löwy I. Martin Arrowsmith's clinical trial: scientific precision and heroic medicine. JLL Bulletin: Commentaries on the history of treatment evaluation 2010 (http://www.jameslindlibrary.org/articles/martin-arrowsmiths-clinical-trial-scientific-precision-and-heroic-medicine/)
5. Fangerau HM. The novel Arrowsmith, Paul de Kruif (1890–1971) and Jacques Loeb (1859–1924): a literary portrait of "medical science". *Med Humanit* 2006;32:82–87.
6. Chalmers I. Comparing like with like: some historical milestones in the evolution of methods to create unbiased comparison groups in therapeutic experiments. *Int J Epidemiol* 2001;30:1156–1164.
7. Bliss M. *William Osler. A life in medicine*. Oxford: Oxford University Press, 1999:483 [index wrongly states 482].
8. Weisz G. *Divide and conquer. A comparative history of medical specialization*. Oxford: Oxford University Press, 2006:198.
9. Larner AJ. "Neurological literature": Sherlock Holmes and neurology. *Adv Clin Neurosci Rehabil* 2011;11(1):20,22.
10. Williams G. *Paralysed with fear. The story of polio*. Basingstoke: Palgrave Macmillan, 2015:129.
11. Summers WC. On the origins of the science in Arrowsmith: Paul de Kruif, Felix d'Herelle, and phage. *J Hist Med Allied Sci* 1991;46:315–332.
12. Matthews JR. *Quantification and the quest for medical certainty*. Princeton: Princeton University Press, 1995:142.

The demise of botany in the medical curriculum

Gardening is one of our most popular pastimes – witness the many newspaper columns, TV programmes, and magazines devoted to it. Even patients with dementia may retain their interests in gardening despite progressive amnesia and agnosia.[1] However, it is many years since the study of botany, let alone horticulture, was required as part of medical student education, a situation which contrasts strongly with the historical tradition.

The *De materia medica* of Dioscorides (ca. 40–90 AD), a herbal dating from the first century AD which described over 600 medicinal plants, based on the author's lifetime study, was available in Latin translation by the 6th century, a translation enlarged and alphabetised in the late 11th century, and became a staple of medical education, alongside Hippocrates and Galen, for centuries. The *Natural History* of Pliny the Elder (ca. 23–90 AD) also offered 900 substances of possible therapeutic use.

The Renaissance brought new developments, perhaps most notably the pharmacopoeia of the German Valerius Cordus (1515–1544) in the 16th century, who described 500 new species. Geographical discoveries also stimulated the founding of botanical gardens whose resources were also used for the teaching of medical students, for example by Jacob Bobart (1599–1680) in his role as Keeper of the Physic Garden in Oxford between 1632–1680. Roger French has grouped medical botany with human dissection as "new departures of the Renaissance" noting that both disciplines were practical rather than theoretical, useful specialisms dependent partly on sensory observation.[2]

The study of plants with medicinal properties was also deemed central to the training of apothecaries, to which end the Society of Apothecaries of London organised, shortly after its establishment (1617), simpling days, later known as herbarizings, to instruct apprentices in botany. Initially these expeditions were on Hampstead Heath or in Greenwich,[3] but later the Society founded a garden of its own, which became the Chelsea Physic Garden.[4] French points out that the "development of botanical gardens is a well-known feature of early modern medicine (botany was one of the several chairs that Boerhaave came to hold) and by the end of the seventeenth century a great deal of thought was being given to how plants should be grouped".[5]

Botany therefore also influenced disease nosology: Thomas Sydenham (1624–1689) famously stated (1676) that "it is necessary that all diseases be reduced to definite and certain species ... with the same care which we see exhibited by botanists and their phytologies". In the eighteenth century,

Linnaeus (1707–1778), whose nomenclature was so successful in classifying plants, also made an attempt on diseases, as did Boissier de Sauvages (1706–1767) in 1731, a physician with strong botanical interests, and William Cullen (1710–1790) in Edinburgh.

Looking to individual medical biography, a number of practitioners have made a mark in both medicine and botany, perhaps most particularly in the eighteenth and nineteenth centuries. The 1785 account of the uses of the foxglove by William Withering (1741–1799) is a medical classic,[6] likewise the celebrated work on *Medical Botany* by William Woodville (1752–1805) published in the 1790s. Contemporaneously Erasmus Darwin (1731–1802) published his didactic scientific poem "Botanic Garden" in 2 parts, "The Economy of Vegetation" and "The Loves of the Plants". Interestingly all of these men had received medical training in Edinburgh where botany was available with materia medica as part of the medical curriculum. However, courses in the knowledge of drugs and of botany were separated in 1768,[7] and although botany was still available, Lisa Rosner's careful analyses suggest that relatively small numbers of students attended these lectures.[8]

Nonetheless, botany remained a useful part of medical education, thought to develop habits of accurate observation, as well as ensuring that prescriptions were properly dispensed. In 1858, John Kirk (1832–1922) was on the point of accepting a chair in botany in Canada before being appointed by David Livingstone as "Economic Botanist and Medical Officer" on the latter's ill-fated Zambesi expedition.[9] In 1860, Bentley published a work outlining the advantages to the student of medicine of a knowledge of botany.[10] Botany remained popular with medical students at Cambridge as part of the Natural Science Tripos into the 1850s, but was perhaps fading by the 1870s.[11] Materia medica was taken out of the prescribed syllabus for medical qualification in 1895.

The demise of botany in the medical curriculum may be regretted by few, but nonetheless the subject may be neglected at our peril, since, as in the past, new and potent therapeutic agents may emerge from the discovery of new species and/or the study of plant biology. For example, in the field of dementia, galantamine, a tertiary alkaloid originally extracted from bulbs of the *Amaryllidaceae* family (e.g. snowdrops, daffodil), is licensed for use in mild-to-moderate Alzheimer's disease; extracts from the maidenhair tree (*Ginkgo biloba*) may have transient benefits and are the non-prescription medication most frequently used by dementia patients; and lemon balm (*Melissa officinalis*) has been suggested as an alternative or complementary therapy.

Acknowledgement

Adapted from: Larner AJ. Demise of botany in the medical curriculum. *J Med Biogr* 2008;16:1–2.

References

1. Larner AJ. Gardening and dementia. *Int J Geriatr Psychiatry* 2005;20:796–797.
2. French R. *Medicine before science. The business of medicine from the Middle Ages to the Enlightenment.* Cambridge: Cambridge University Press, 2003:128,223.
3. Hunting P. *A history of the Society of Apothecaries.* London: Society of Apothecaries, 1998.
4. Minter S. *The Apothecaries' garden. A history of the Chelsea Physic Garden.* Stroud: Sutton, 2003.
5. French (*op.cit.*, ref. 2):229–230.
6. Aronson JK. *An account of the foxglove and its medical uses 1785–1985.* Oxford: Oxford University Press, 1985.
7. Risse GB. *Hospital life in Enlightenment Scotland. Care and teaching at the Royal Infirmary of Edinburgh.* Cambridge: Cambridge University Press, 1986:68.
8. Rosner L. *Medical education in the age of improvement. Edinburgh students and apprentices 1760–1826.* Edinburgh: Edinburgh University Press, 1991.
9. Larner AJ. Charles Meller and John Kirk: medical practitioners and practice on Livingstone's Zambesi expedition, 1858–64. *J Med Biogr* 2002;10:129–134.
10. Bentley R. *On the advantages of a study of botany to the student of medicine.* London, 1860.
11. Weatherall MW. *Gentlemen, scientists and doctors. Medicine at Cambridge 1800–1940.* Cambridge: Boydell Press, 2000:92–93.

Medical memorials in the Linnean binomial taxonomy

Dr Conacher's fascinating account of Dr John Dickinson, and particularly his picture of Dickinson's kestrel (*Falco dickinsoni*),[1] put me in mind of other species of fauna and flora which have been named after medical practitioners in the Linnaen binomial taxonomy.

For example, considering other medically qualified explorers, there were present on David Livingstone's Zambesi expedition of 1858–1864 a number of individuals who would have known John Dickinson, specifically Dr John Kirk (1832–1922), Dr Charles James Meller (1836–1869), and Dr David Livingstone (1813–1873) himself,[2] all of whom have species named for them.

As "economic botanist" as well as medical officer to the expedition, John Kirk identified many plant species and sent a number of communications during his time in Africa to journals such as the *Transactions of the Botanical Society* and the *Journal* and *Transactions of the Linnean Society*. Plant species bearing his name are the *Psychotria kirkii* and *Uapaca kirkiana*. Following the Zambesi expedition, Kirk worked in the Consulate in Zanzibar, during which time he identified the Zanzibar red colobus (*Piliocolobus kirkii*), a small leaf-eating monkey, also known as Kirk's red colobus, found only in Zanzibar and now classified as an endangered species.

Charles James Meller, who succeeded Kirk as medical officer on the Zambesi expedition, afterwards went to Madagascar as Vice-Consul where he identified a species of dabbling duck, now known as Meller's duck (*Anas melleri*). This is now listed as an endangered species.

Livingstone's fruit bat, or flying fox (*Pteropus livingstonii*), is a bat found only on two islands in the Comoros group located off the eastern coast of Africa between northern Madagascar and northeastern Mozambique, whence a number of "Johanna men" accompanied the Zambesi expedition. The rarest and largest of all Comorian bat species, these animals defend themselves by spraying urine at potential predators. Again, this is a threatened species due to destruction of its preferred forest habitat. (Both Meller's duck and Livingstone's fruit bat may be seen at the Durrell Wildlife Conservation Trust in Jersey.) Livingstone's Cichlid (*Nimbochromis livingstonii*) is a freshwater cichlid fish native to Lake Malawi, an area explored by Livingstone and Kirk.

Some other examples of such Linnean medical memorials may be mentioned. The father of medicine, Hippocrates (ca. 460–370 BCE) has a tropical vine (*Hippocratea*) and its family (*Hippocrateaceae*) named after him. Sigmund Freud (1856–1939) is commemorated by two species of scarab beetle (*Cyclocephala freudi, Lepithrix freudi*). Arthur Conan Doyle (1859–1930), remembered for his writing, particularly of Sherlock Holmes, rather than for his medical practice, has a genus of pterosaur from the Early Cretaceous era named after him (*Arthurdactylus conandoylei*), discovered in Brazil in the 1990s in jungle environment similar to that in which Doyle's novel *The Lost World* (1912) is set. Although he did not qualify in medicine, Charles Darwin (1809–1882) was at one time a medical student, and now has more than 120 species and nine genera named after him, many in his honour rather than because they were originally described by him. Likewise John Keats (1795–1821) had some medical training before turning full time to poetry, and has a wasp named for him (*Keatsia*) by Girault, who evidently had literary interests since he named other wasps after Dante Alighieri, Plutarch, Thomas Carlyle, Ralph Waldo Emerson, Johann Wolfgang Goethe, and Henry Wadsworth Longfellow.

Many other species have been named, perhaps fancifully, for celebrities, musicians, philosophers, and writers, many of whom have surely had little or no interest in natural history. Examples include Bill Gates, John Cleese, Frank Zappa, John Lennon, Ringo Starr, Kate Winslet, George Bush, etc., etc., ...[3–5]

Returning to our starting point, one may ask why it is that medical explorers should have achieved eponymous fame in the binomial taxonomy. Megan Vaughan has described the "relentless empiricism of the early tropical doctor",[6] which encompassed not only medical issues but also ethnography, anthropology and geography, as well as botany and zoology, in which latter two domains many of these individuals would have received some instruction as part of their medical training, unlike the situation today.[7] One may also see the desire to describe and classify, the scientific objectification of the otherness of foreign landscapes and their natural inhabitants, as not only advancing scientific knowledge but also as one element in the exertion of colonial power.

Acknowledgement

Adapted from: Larner AJ. Medical memorial in the Linnean binomial taxonomy. *J Med Biogr* 2010;18:123.

References

1.   Conacher ID. John Dickinson MB (1832–1863), Chikwawa, Malawi. *J Med Biogr* 2010;18:174. See also Conacher ID. John Dickinson MB (1832–1863): the man behind the bird. *J Med Biogr* 2016;24:339–350.

2. Larner AJ. Charles Meller and John Kirk: medical practitioners and practice on Livingstone's Zambesi expedition, 1858–64. *J Med Biogr* 2002;10:129–134.

3. www.CuriousTaxonomy.net/etym/people.html (accessed 30/01/2010).

4. http://en.wikipedia.org/.../List_of_animals_named_after_celebrities (accessed 30/01/2010).

5. www.freebase.com/view/user/arielb/.../views/animals_named_after_people (accessed 30/01/2010).

6. Vaughan M. *Curing their ills. Colonial power and African illness.* Cambridge: Polity Press, 1991:32.

7. Larner AJ. Demise of botany in the medical curriculum. *J Med Biogr* 2008;16:1–2.

Osler centenary

29th December 2019 marked the 100th anniversary of the death of Sir William Osler (1849–1919), an anniversary already celebrated, very prematurely, elsewhere.[1]

Few clinicians of the modern era can have had greater lasting impact on the profession of medicine than Osler. His most evident contributions relate to his emphasis on bedside clinical teaching, his acute descriptions of many clinical disorders, and the influence of his textbook, the *Principles and Practice of Medicine* which was pre-eminent in its day.[2] However, there is also a "charge sheet" against Osler.

He was a persistent and determined "practical joker".[3] My understanding of this terminology suggests its meaning to be along the lines of having fun for personal gratification at the expense of unwitting others. Whilst this might work with your close friends, it may cause embarrassment and distress to others, and, like most such jokers, Osler was less enthusiastic when the joke was at his expense (e.g. when given incorrect information on ergotism which was nearly included in *PPM*; see ref 2, p.185). This "practical joking" also extended for Osler to a wilful and persistent perversion of the medical literature with publications under his alias of Egerton Yorrick Davis (EYD).

Whilst it is not appropriate to judge a historical figure by the mores of later times, since we are all of us more or less prisoners of the cultural assumptions of our times, it is likely that such behaviours today would be viewed with opprobrium and might prompt sanctions, possibly even expulsion, for transgressing codes of professional and ethical behaviour.

Osler's views on women in medicine were not entirely progressive. He advised Dorothy Reed to go home before commencing her medical studies at Johns Hopkins,[4] although later was a supporter, as for other female students. Again this behaviour may be viewed as typical of his age.

I do not doubt that such comments may provoke howls of protest from those who regard Osler as little less than a (secular) saint. But since no one now has direct experience of Osler, the man or the clinician, some, perhaps particularly those now entering the profession, may ask the question as to why he is so sanctified when the circumstances of clinical practice have changed so significantly. It remains to be seen if his ability to inspire medical practitioners persists into a second century after his death.

Acknowledgement

Adapted from: Larner AJ. Editorial. *J Med Biogr* 2019;27:185.

References

1. Becker RE. Remembering Sir William Osler 100 years after his death: what can we learn from his legacy? *Lancet* 2014;384:2260–2263.
2. Bliss M. *William Osler. A life in medicine.* Oxford: Oxford University Press, 1999.
3. Wright JR, Jr. "Osler warned": was William Osler a grave robber while at McGill or was he a victim (or perpetrator) of one final practical joke? *Clin Anat* 2018;31:632–640.
4. Dawson P. *Dorothy in a man's world. A Victorian woman physician's trials and triumphs.* North Charleston, South Carolina: CreateSpace Independent Publishing Platform, 2017, pp.1–3.

Sherlock Holmes as "an exact embodiment of somebody or other"

It is probable that every reader of the Holmes canon develops their own personal mental image of Sherlock Holmes, a visualisation or imagining which is perhaps now more likely to be coloured by the many film and television portrayals of the great consulting detective. For example, it is well known that the deerstalker and Inverness cape are entirely absent from the canon. One sees this influence, for instance, in Jon Dressel's poem *Note to a Character*:

> ... I saw this gaunt black dog half
> wolfhound half god knows what coming on it was
> strange and fierce and flashing tongue
> and fang for a moment i thought i was in
> an old sherlock holmes movie ...[1]

But how might early readers, naive to film and television portrayals, have envisaged Sherlock Holmes? One possible insight may be found in a work by the Anglo-Welsh author Margiad Evans (1909–1958).

Evans, the pseudonym of Peggy Whistler, published a number of highly acclaimed novels in the 1930s and 1940s which have recently been the subject of renewed critical attention.[2] Her collection of short stories entitled *The Old And The Young* was published in 1948,[3] one story in which, *Miss Potts and Music*, dating from 1944–5, features a character:

> [Miss Potts'] aunt who looks an exact embodiment of somebody or other
> – or rather two somebodies as it has taken me years to realize. Combining
> [Dante Gabriel] Rosetti's Beata Beatrix and my own idea of Sherlock
> Holmes, I have the most perfect projection of her. A long, long throat, a big
> clever nose, a thin ethereal face with ascetic and romantic eyes, that was
> B.B.S.H. when I was ten. She looked a saint of music and her niece was her
> novice. But with her nostrils down on her fiddle she became pure Sherlock
> Holmes.

Elsewhere BBSH is said to have a "peculiar ecstatic smile" and a "frail profile".[4]

Margiad Evans is recognised to have "had a strongly visual imagination, through which she saw distinctly the people ... she described".[5] She had some training at art college and drew illustrations for some of her works, under her real name of Peggy Whistler, including *The Old And The Young*, but regretably no image of BBSH. The quoted passage has been described as indicative of the "imaginative and associative nature of the narrator's mind".[6] Whilst it cannot be said with certainty which attributes of BBSH pertain to Rosetti's Beata Beatrix and which to Sherlock Holmes, some speculations might be permitted.

The link with playing the violin is obvious enough. Watson assessed Holmes as playing the violin well in the list of "his limits" in *A Study in Scarlet*, and also that his powers were "very remarkable". BBSH is described as "pure Sherlock Holmes" when she has her "nostrils down on her fiddle". Margiad Evans also aspired to play the violin well, owned a violin in the years that she was writing the stories in *The Old And The Young*, had lessons at various times in her life, and wrote an article on violin makers and violinists.[7]

Physiognomy may also have contributed to Evans's mental linkage between Miss Potts' aunt and Sherlock Holmes. Also in *A Study in Scarlet*, Watson describes Holmes as, *inter alia*, "excessively lean", with eyes that were "sharp and piercing", and with a "thin, hawk-like nose". Moreover, another medical man, Dr James Mortimer, notes, in *The Hound of the Baskervilles*, Holmes's dolichocephalic skull. Hence, "A long, long throat, big clever nose, a thin ethereal face" may all conceivably be a reflection of long-headedness, and this might be accompanied by leanness and a hawk-like nose, but whether "ascetic and romantic eyes" can be equated with "sharp and piercing" eyes is perhaps in the eye of the beholder.

GK Chesterton, an author who might be acknowledged to know something about fictional detectives, opined in his study of Charles Dickens, published in 1906, that:

> there is one figure in our popular literature which would really be recognised by the populace. Ordinary men would understand you if you referred currently to Sherlock Holmes. Sir Arthur Conan Doyle would no doubt be justified in rearing his head to the stars, remembering that Sherlock Holmes is the only really familiar figure in modern fiction. But let him droop that head again with a gentle sadness, remembering that if Sherlock Holmes is the only familiar figure in modern fiction Sherlock Holmes is also the only familiar figure in the Sherlock Holmes tales.

This familiarity is also taken up by Michel Houellebecq:

> In every Sherlock Holmes story you immediately recognise the characteristics of the character; but, as well as that, the author never fails to introduce some new peculiarity ... Conan Doyle succeeded in creating a perfect mixture of the pleasure of discovery and the pleasure of recognition.[8]

Use of Sherlock Holmes as a comparator, a touchstone, a reference point, for the description of others – as "an exact embodiment of somebody or other" – is thus perhaps not surprising. That said, each age and discipline may adopt Holmes for their own purposes. For example in my own field of clinical medicine, he is cited as an exemplar of the narrative structure of medical knowledge[9] and of the discipline of evidence-based medicine.[10]

Acknowledgement

Adapted from: Larner AJ. Sherlock Holmes as "an exact embodiment of somebody or other". *The Sherlock Holmes Journal* 2017;33:60–61.

References

1. Lloyd D (ed.). *Imagined Greetings. Poetic Engagements with RS Thomas.* Llanrwst: Carreg Gwalch, 2013:38.
2. Bohata K, Gramich K (eds.). *Rediscovering Margiad Evans. Marginality, gender and illness.* Cardiff: University of Wales Press, 2013.
3. Lloyd-Morgan C (ed.). *Margiad Evans. The Old and the Young.* Bridgend: Seren [1948] 1998.
4. Ibid., pp.108,110,114.
5. Ibid., p.13.
6. Brown T. Time, memory and identity in the short stories of Margiad Evans. In: Bohata K, Gramich K (eds.). *Rediscovering Margiad Evans. Marginality, gender and illness.* Cardiff: University of Wales Press, 2013:69–85 [at 84n3].
7. Evans M. The man with the hammer. *Life and Letters including the London Mercury* 1948:59(134):11–27.
8. Houellebecq M. *Platform.* London: Vintage Books, 2003:96.
9. Hunter KM. *Doctors' stories. The narrative structure of medical knowledge.* Princeton: Princeton University Press, 1991.
10. Nordenstrom J. *Evidence-based medicine in Sherlock Holmes' footsteps.* Oxford: Blackwell, 2007.

Anthony Trollope (1815–1882) and headache

Introduction

Few lives remain undisturbed by even the occasional headache: it has been estimated that three billion individuals worldwide were affected by headache in 2016. In many cases headaches are recurrent or even chronic, contributing to a substantial global health burden and a significant cause of time lost from work and recreational activities,[1] not least because of the systemic upset often accompanying headaches. For example, migraine is often attended with nausea, vomiting (hence "sick headache" or "bilious headache"), vertigo or dizziness, visual disturbance such as light sensitivity (photophobia), impaired concentration, and even prostration.

It therefore comes as little surprise to find such a mundane experience as headache mentioned in works of literature. Examples have been noted in the works of several 19th century authors of fiction who undoubtedly (Charlotte Brontë,[2] Elizabeth Gaskell[3]) or possibly (Jane Austen,[4] Anne Brontë[2]) suffered from headaches themselves.

If we accept Henry James's view that Trollope had a "complete appreciation of the usual"[5] then it might be anticipated that instances of such a prevalent experience as headache would be found in his fiction. Moreover, it is known that Trollope had close knowledge of the effects of headache, based on his father's experience. In *An Autobiography*, he reports of Thomas Anthony Trollope:

> My father's health was very bad. During the last ten years of his life, he spent nearly half of his time in bed, suffering agony from sick headaches. But he was never idle unless when suffering.[6]

Even this brief passage indicates the potential severity of headache and its consequent effects on social and occupational function. More detail is afforded in Victoria Glendinning's biography, indicating that Trollope's father had a long-standing headache disorder. During their courtship, Thomas Anthony wrote to Fanny about his "dreadful headaches which sometimes lasted for days". After marriage, "family life did nothing for his bilious headaches". "Calomel [mercurous chloride] was what Mr Trollope ... habitually took, in large quantities, in an attempt to relieve his chronic headaches." Referring to the passage in *An Autobiography*, Glendinning specifies "bilious headaches" as keeping Trollope's father half the time in bed.[7]

Whilst Trollope's fictional doctors have received attention,[8,9] the ailments they might have been called upon to attend have been less noticed.[10] The purpose of this article is to collate and examine instances of headache mentioned in the six Barsetshire novels (all page citations are to Penguin Classics editions).

The evidence base: descriptions of headache in the Barsetshire novels

I find no references to headache in *The Warden*. In *Barchester Towers*, Bishop Proudie, arguing with his wife about Mr Slope, "felt himself not very well just at present; and began to consider that he might, not improbably, be detained in his room the next morning by an attack of bile. He was, unfortunately, very subject to bilious annoyances." (143). Sure enough, when Mr Slope calls the next morning "His lordship complained of being rather unwell, had a slight headache, and was not quite the thing in his stomach" (146), meaning that he avoids a potentially difficult meeting with Archdeacon Grantly.

At Miss Thorne's entertainment, the Ullathorne Sports, Mr Thorne's tenant farmer, Mr T. Lookaloft, does not attend with his family, because, as Mrs Lookaloft informs him, "Such a headache, Mr Thorne! ... in fact, he couldn't stir, or you may be certain on such a day he would not have absented hisself [*sic*]. ... It is only bilious you know, and when he's that way he can bear nobody nigh him." Trollope as narrator informs us that "The fact, however, was that Mr Lookaloft ... had not chosen to intrude on Miss Thorne's drawing room" (342).

In *Doctor Thorne*, Frank's intention to marry Mary Thorne prompts argument between his father and Lady Arabella, but eventually she "was driven to retreat in a state of headache, which she declared to be chronic; and which, so she assured her daughter Augusta, must prevent her from having any more lengthened conversations with her Lord – at any rate for the next three months" (246).

In *Framley Parsonage*, Lucy Robarts, inattentive to the ongoing conversation, confesses to her sister-in-law, "Oh dear, Fanny, my head does ache so, pray don't be angry with me" and then throws herself on the sofa. Mrs Robarts asks, "Dearest Lucy, what is it makes your head ache so often now? You used not to have those headaches", but Lucy must keep secret her love for Lord Lufton (315).

In *The Small House at Allington*, Lily Dale tells her mother she has a headache after Adolphus Crosbie has told her that although he plans to stand by their engagement it will ruin his prospects (156). (This is the event upon which Pamela Blake chose to focus when exploring what Trollope can tell us about headaches.[10])

A few weeks after her wedding, Lady Alexandrina De Courcy has a headache following Adolphus's shouted refusal of her suggestion to invite her brother George and his wife as house guests (529). The headache is still present the next morning ("My head is splitting"), so that Adolphus breakfasts alone (530), and it persists into the evening: "He went home, and his wife, though she was up, complained still of her headache" which has prevented her from going out of the house (533). I find, *contra* Blake,[10] no report that Alexandrina's wedding day draws to a close with headache, although it is said that "she is very tired, and will lie down till dinner-time" (499).

In conversation with Hopkins as the time to leave Allington approaches, Lily Dale reports that her mother has a headache, to which Hopkins replies "Got a headache, has she? I won't make her headache no worse. It's my opinion that there's nothing for a headache so good as fresh air" (631). He later asserts that "I don't believe she got no headache at all" and muses on the differences between gentlefolks and a poor man telling lies (632).

In *The Last Chronicle of Barset*, the elder of the Miss Prettymans, Annabella, who keep a girls' school at Silverbridge and with whom Grace Crawley is living, is described as "subject to racking headaches, so that it was considered generally that she was unable to take much active part in the education of the pupils. ... She could not even go to church, because the open air brought on neuralgia." (49).

Dining with Archdeacon Grantly and Mr Harding shortly after the former has subtly pressured him to give up his desire to marry Grace Crawley, Major Henry Grantly has little to say and confesses to his father "I've got rather a headache this evening, sir." (218).

Miss Madalina Demolines reports to John Eames that her mother, Lady Demolines is unable to appear for a variety of passing maladies, including "a nervous headache" (457) but latterly discontinues these references (775).

Bishop Proudie, after his wife has effectively ejected Dr Tempest, says to her "Perhaps you will go away now and leave me to myself. I have got a bad headache, and I can't talk anymore." (480).

Discussion

This does not claim to be an exhaustive account of headaches in the Trollope canon: certainly there are other examples, such as Lady Laura Kennedy in *Phineas Finn*. Victoria Glendinning mentions Jemima Stanbury's relief, in *He Knew He Was Right*, that her niece Dorothy wears no chignon, since "How is a woman not to have a headache, when she carries a thing on the back of her poll as big as a gardener's wheelbarrow?".[11] Trollope also recognised the possible effect of alcohol in the genesis of headaches, speaking in his essay on *The genius of Nathaniel Hawthorne* of "yesterday's tipsy man with this morning's sick-headache".[12]

Nevertheless, these examples from Barsetshire give some insight into Trollopes uses of headaches as a literary device, of which two seem prominent to me.

Firstly, individuals, both women and men, with amatory difficulties may succumb to headaches: examples include Lucy Robarts, Lily Dale, and Major Henry Grantly. Emotionally charged encounters may also be a trigger for headache, in which category one might include Lady Arabella, Lady Alexandrina, and Bishop Proudie following the contretemps between his wife and Dr Tempest (*The Last Chronicle of Barset*), all leading to avoidance of the person involved in the argument. These might all be deemed "stress triggers" or "life events with emotional impact,"[10] and such literary usage of headache is familiar from the works of many other 19th century novelists.[2-4]

Secondly, there are usages where the presence of headache is in fact uncertain or unlikely, although implied, but results in behavioural change which is potentially to the advantage of the reported sufferer: Bishop Proudie (*Barchester Towers*), Lady Arabella, and Lady Alexandrina use headache as an excuse to avoid unpleasant encounters and conversations. In the cases of Mr Lookaloft, Mrs Dale, and Lady Demolines, their headaches are reported by others (Mrs Lookaloft, Lily Dale and Madalina Demolines respectively). It might be surmised that these are examples of feigned illness. Trollope's playful account of Mr Lookaloft suggests this possibility, and in his Introduction to the Penguin Classics edition of *The Small House at Allington* Julian Thompson labels Mrs Dale's headache as "specious" (xxviii), hence agreeing with the view of Hopkins the gardener. Such illness behaviour may result in what medical sociologists term "secondary gain", here avoidance of awkward situations or discussions on the plea of illness. If this analysis is credible, it may be a further example of how Trollope's "dialogue ... shows a penetration into human psychology"[13] and of his "comic pleasure".[14]

Acknowledgement

Adapted from: Larner AJ. Headaches in Trollope. *Trollopiana. The Journal of the Trollope Society* 2020;116:13–18.

References

1. GBD 2016 Headache Collaborators. Global, regional, and national burden of migraine and tension-type headache, 1990–2016: a systematic analysis for the Global Burden of Disease Study 2016. *Lancet Neurol.* 2018;17:954–976.
2. Larner AJ. Charlotte Bronte's headaches: fact and fiction. *Bronte Studies* 2012;37:208–215.
3. Larner AJ. "A habit of headaches": the neurological case of Elizabeth Gaskell. *Gaskell Journal* 2011;25:97–103.
4. Larner AJ. "A transcript of actual life": headache in the novels of Jane Austen. *Headache* 2010;50:692–695.
5. Smalley D (ed.). *Anthony Trollope. The critical heritage.* Abingdon: Routledge, [1969] 2013:527.
6. Trollope A. *An Autobiography.* Oxford: Oxford World's Classics, [1883] 2008:13.
7. Glendinning V. *Trollope.* London: Pimlico, 2002:6,11,14,34.
8. Smithers DW. The Barsetshire doctors. *BMJ.* 1982;285:1806–1808. Reprinted in *Trollopiana* 1997;39:17–22.
9. Taylor R. Trollope and his doctors. *Trollopiana* 2007;77:pagination not known.
10. Blake P. What Anthony Trollope can teach us about headaches. *Headache* 2017;57:637–640. Reprinted in *Trollopiana* 2019;114:5–11.
11. Glendinning V. *Trollope.* London: Pimlico, 2002:267.
12. Trollope A. The genius of Nathaniel Hawthorne. *North American Review* 1879;274:203–222 [at 213].
13. Curtis Brown B. *Anthony Trollope* (2nd edition). London: Arthur Barker, 1969:63.
14. Herbert C. *Trollope and comic pleasure.* Chicago and London: University of Chicago Press, 1987.

Kraepelin's analogy: the brain as a pipe organ

To describe the brain as an "organ" is entirely unobjectionable in a physiological sense, indeed it is a commonplace, in keeping with the description of the heart, lungs, kidneys and liver as organs of the body. However, to compare the workings of the brain to the workings of an organ, specifically a pipe organ, may occasion some surprise and hence require further explanation. The history of this analogy affords links with a previous report suggesting that evidence from organists may prompt questions about brain function and organisation.[1]

Emil Kraepelin (1856–1926) was a German neuropsychiatrist who is best remembered for his attempts to develop a classification, or nosology, of psychiatric disorders. This is principally manifested in his *Textbook of Psychiatry* which went through several editions in the late 19th and early 20th centuries; the 8th edition, of 1910, for example, first introduced the term "Alzheimer's disease" to denote the dementia syndrome described by Alois Alzheimer in 1906–7.

In one of Kraepelin's later articles, dating from 1920,[2] he "compared the brain to an organ".[3] There are three specific references, all to organ stops. Firstly, Kraepelin states: "We may compare the clinical signs [of psychiatric disorders] with the different stops on an organ. They can be set in motion according to the severity and extent of the pathological changes." This was Kraepelin's attempt to reconcile the empirical clinical observation that similar features sometimes occur in different psychiatric disorders, such as manic depression and schizophrenia. This leads to his second reference to organ stops: "At best one could say … that one pathological process has a preference for this or that organ stop, or even confines itself to one stop." Finally, Kraepelin summarizes by saying that "we can distinguish three main groups of manifestations of insanity, or organ stop, so to speak."

Kraepelin's pipe organ analogy may have been informed by some personal knowledge of music. His father worked as both an opera singer and a music teacher. Whether Emil had direct links or friendship with an organist who could demonstrate the workings of a pipe organ is not known. In his own "self-assessment", written after the end of the First World War,[4] Kraepelin states that:

As for music: I was really only interested in it during my childhood and student days; I sang for many years in the church choir and was also later

involved in sacred music concerts. Playing the piano afforded me no pleasure and I was allowed to give it up in response to my urgent pleas. Things
might well have proved different with the violin, but when I first became
acquainted with it my time totally precluded me from taking any more
thorough instruction. My understanding of more intricate compositions
was slight; I soon grew weary of listening to them and could not follow
them for long. Consequently, I mainly preferred music I already knew well.
Most pleasing to my ear were the simple, melodious compositions of
Haydn and Mozart, but also those of Beethoven and Brahms, and moreover the songs of Schubert, Schumann and Brahms. As a rule Wagner left
me cold, and Liszt I found downright boring. My musical horizons were
fairly restricted and I lacked the desire to broaden them, because
completely new compositions rarely gave me any pleasure at first. In my
later years I considered that the most perfect combination of music and
drama was to be found in Beethoven, whose music I could listen to only
with the deepest emotion. Wagner's late operas struck me, as far as my
acquaintance with them permits me to say, as an artistic aberration.

Many analogies have been called upon, over millennia, to serve as possible
explanations for brain function and dysfunction: hydraulic, mechanical, electrical, and, most recently, computational.[5] Little subsequent attention seems to
have been given to Kraepelin's pipe organ analogy, until quite recently.

Lobo & Agius noted that "chords constructed from a multitude of 'pipes'
that can be blended together to create different mixtures of sound illustrates
well the concept of disorders with multifactorial origins". Psychiatric disorders
may thus be characterised by a "multitude of symptoms … that may be present
in different combinations, much like Kraepelin's organ pipes",[6] hence their
classification as heterogeneous syndromes (analogous to multiple stops)
rather than categorical disorders (single stops).

Kraepelin's pipe organ analogy may therefore inform modern, dimensional,
as opposed to categorical, classifications of psychiatric disorders.[7] We suggest
this is another example of the versatility, literal as well as figurative, of the
organ!

Acknowledgement

Thanks to Ms Amalie Fisher (former Organ Scholar, Fitzwilliam College,
Cambridge) and Dr Crispin Fisher for advice on the pipe organ.

References

1.   Larner AJ, Fisher CAH. Amazing brains: Questions arising from the neurological histories of two blind organists. *Organists' Review* 2009; November: 38–39.
2.   Kraepelin E. Die Erscheinungsformen des Irreseins. *Zeitschrift für die gesammte Neurologie und Psychiatrie* 1920; 62: 1–29. I have used the English translation by Beer D. The manifestations of insanity. *History of Psychiatry* 1992; **3**: 509–529.
3.   Blom JD. *Alice in Wonderland syndrome*. London: Springer, 2020: 164.
4.   Engstrom EJ, Burgmair W, Weber MM. Emil Kraepelin's "Self-Assessment": clinical autography in historical context. *History of Psychiatry* 2002; 13: 89–119.
5.   Cobb M. *The idea of the brain. A history*. London: Profile Books, 2020.
6.   Lobo DM, Agius M. The mental illness spectrum. *Psychiatria Danubina* 2012; 24Suppl1: 157–160.
7.   Regier DA. The Kraepelinian pipe organ model (for a more dimensional) DSM-5 classification. In: Kendler KS, Parnas J (eds.). *Philosophical issues in psychiatry. II Nosology*. Oxford: Oxford University Press, 2012: 95–98.

"Neurological literature": Headache 10

Those familiar with neurological consultations will know from experience that patients referred with headache may sometimes (but not always!) struggle to describe their symptoms, requiring some semi-structured promptings from the clinician to draw out the salient features (it makes no sense, conceptually, to speak, as some do, of "featureless" headaches).

Many years ago, the neurologist JN ("Nat") Blau (1928–2010) reported that in his clinics most patients (70%) spoke for two minutes or less when invited to describe their symptoms, indeed 42% spoke for less than 1 minute.[1] Although not all were headache patients (although that was Blau's area of specialist interest, and some of the patients were seen in a dedicated migraine clinic), the findings may nevertheless support the idea that, without interruptions or promptings, patient accounts are generally brief. It would be interesting to know, more than 30 years after Blau's report, if this is still the case.

Blau noted that those with experience of speaking in public spoke the longest. How might professional writers, whose metier is dependent on words, describe headache?

Previous instalments in this series of occasional pieces published in *ACNR* (and now conveniently collected elsewhere[2]) documenting accounts of headache encountered in literary or biographical material have provided some examples, but whether or not these are based on personal experience, or simply products of the writerly imagination, is seldom disclosed.

AS Byatt (b. 1936) won the 1990 Booker Prize for her novel *Possession*.[3] In a correspondence purportedly dating to the mid-nineteenth century, one of the characters, Christabel LaMotte, reports to the poet, Randolph Henry Ash,

> I write to you from an unhappy House ... for I have an invalid dependent upon me – my poor Blanche – quite *racked* with hideous headaches – and nausea – quite prostrated – and unable to pursue the work which is her life. ... she is too ill and cannot go on. I am not in much better case myself – but I make *tisanes*, which I find efficacious. (172–3)

Christabel's correspondent responds:

> I do have the clearest olfactory ghost of yr [sic] tisanes – though they hesitate between verveine and lime and raspberry-leaves, which my own dear mother found most efficacious in case of headache and lassitude. (177)

Tisanes are herbal teas, made from the infusion or decoction of herbs, spices, or other plant material. Verveine, or vervain, also known as lemon verbena, is a type of herbal tea. In the circumstances of the developing relationship between Christabel and Ash, it may be a signifier: according to Nicholas Culpeper's (1616–1654) *The English Physitian* (1652), vervain is "an herb of Venus" as well as a treatment for headache: "applied with some oil of roses and vinegar unto the forehead and temples, it eases the inveterate pains and ache of the head."[4] Other literary examples of tea used as a headache treatment may also be noted, for example in Jane Austen's *Mansfield Park* (1814), and in Thomas Mann's *Doctor Faustus* (1947) where "real strong tea made real sour with lots of lemon" is suggested. Caffeine, of course, may be the active ingredient in these remedies.

Christabel later reports to Ash that:

> I see whole bevies of shooting stars – like gold arrows before my darkening eyes – they presage Headache … The headache proceeds apace. Half my head – is merely a gourd full of pain – . (194–5)

In the novel, these old letters only come to light in the late twentieth century when two academics, respectively researching LaMotte and Ash, collaborate. They also view the journal of Ash's wife, Ellen, who, it turns out, also had headaches:

> June [1859]

> I felt a headache coming on … I retired to my room and slept for two hours, waking somewhat refreshed, though with a vestigial headache. (227)

> A worse day. The headache seized me and I lay all day in a darkened bedroom, betwixt asleep and wake. There are many bodily sensations that are indescribable yet immediately recognisable … which could never be conveyed to one who had no previous experience of them. Such is the way in which the preliminary dizziness or vanishing incapacitates the body and intimates the headache to come. It is curiously impossible – once entered into this state – to imagine ever issuing out of it – so that the Patience [sic] required to endure it seems to be a total eternal patience. Towards evening it lifted a little.

> Worse still. Dr Pimlott came and prescribed laudanum, which I found some relief in. (230)

Much of the typical migraine symptomatology is to be found in these letters and journal entries: their severity, accompanying nausea and visual symptoms, hemicranial involvement, interruption of occupational function, recourse to treatment. All contribute to the authenticity of the account. The report that these "sensations … could never be conveyed to one who had no previous experience of them" might be pertinent to the brevity of patients' accounts of their headache symptoms (and also of other neurological symptoms).

Interestingly, Ellen Ash's sister, Patience, also complains of "incessant … headaches" (225). A family history of migraine is, of course, not uncommon, and may be associated with a lower age of onset.[5] As is well-known, AS Byatt's younger sister, Margaret Drabble (b. 1939), is also a writer. If we accept the premise that AS Byatt is writing from personal experience of migraine with aura in *Possession*, it might be interesting to know if her sister may be similarly afflicted, perhaps assessed by any reference to headaches in her literary works.

Although I claim no familiarity with Drabble's extensive oeuvre, I think there is some subtle evidence to answer this question. For example, in what may be her first written short story, *A Pyrrhic victory* (although not the first published, appearing in 1968),[6] the central character, Anne, is described at the outset as "exhausted: her head ached with the sun, she felt both sick and hungry" (49). In *A day in the life of a smiling woman* (1973), the title character, Jenny Jamieson, has a headache when tired on returning late from her work one evening (111). In *The merry widow* (1989), an offstage character, Harriet, is described as "always ill … what stories of migraines" (151). No detailed account of symptoms is provided in any of these passing references.

Despite featuring scenes set in both primary and secondary medical care settings, no headaches occur in Drabble's novel *The millstone* (1965). However, in *Jerusalem the golden* (1967), the central character, Clara Maugham, a student in London, encounters the Denham family, whose attitudes and behaviour differ greatly from her own restricted upbringing in "Northam".[7] At the end of a visit to the Denham household in Highgate, Clara "began to feel a sense of overwhelming fatigue. Her head ached … her mind would no longer pay attention. Whole concepts, whole reorganizations of thought swam drunkenly through her head … when she got home she was suddenly and violently sick" (106). Subsequently Clara finds that "she grew accustomed to leaving their house with a headache" (107) and later discloses that this was because the experience was "so marvellous I couldn't take it" (167).

These brief descriptions of headache in some of Drabble's works may lack the richness of the material in Byatt's novel, but nonetheless suggest a familiarity with headache symptomatology. The brevity of Drabble's portrayals may be typical of patient accounts before the clinician draws out additional details. To paraphrase, it may indeed be the case that even with the word skills of a professional writer "many bodily sensations … are indescribable" and cannot therefore "be conveyed to one who had no previous experience of them".

Acknowledgement

Adapted from: Larner AJ. Neurological literature: Headache 10. *Adv Clin Neurosci Rehabil* 2022;21(1):28–29.

References

1. Blau JN. *Time to let the patient speak.* BMJ 1989;298:39.
2. Larner AJ. *Neuroliterature: Patients, doctors, diseases. Literary perspectives on disorders of the nervous system.* Gloucester: Choir Press, 2019:241–271.
3. Byatt AS. *Possession. A romance.* London: Vintage [1990] 1991.
4. Arikha N. *Passions and tempers. A history of the humours.* New York: Harper Perennial, 2008, p.204.
5. Hsu YW, Liang CS, Lee JT et al. *Associations between migraine occurrence and the effect of aura, age at onset, family history, and sex: a cross-sectional study.* PLoS One 2020;15(2):e0228284.
6. Drabble M. *A day in the life of a smiling woman. The collected stories.* London: Penguin, 2011.
7. Drabble M. *Jerusalem the golden.* Harmondsworth: Penguin [1967] 1969.

A short history of neurology in a short neurological history

Older neurologists will know, and younger neurologists will learn, that clinical practice in the early years of ones career may differ markedly from clinical practice in the later years. A nice illustration of this occurred in the context of taking a neurological case history.

In the mid-1970s, when the patient was in his early twenties, he suffered a severe headache requiring admission to his local general hospital (no longer extant, its site now the location of an Asda superstore). This was before the widespread availability of CT brain scanning so he underwent lumbar puncture which confirmed a subarachnoid haemorrhage. As a consequence, he was briefly transferred to the regional neurosurgical centre for bilateral carotid and right vertebral catheter angiography which was reported to show no aneurysm or arteriovenous malformation. Conservative and expectant management was therefore pursued. At discharge, the patient was left with the uncertainty as to whether or not there would ever be a recurrence.

Just over twenty years later, in the mid-1990s, when the patient was in his mid-40s, a similar severe headache occurred, waking him from sleep. On this occasion, four vessel catheter angiography revealed a bilobular aneurysm at the division of the right middle cerebral artery. At craniotomy this aneurysm was clipped and he made an excellent recovery from the surgery.

A further ten years later, in the mid-2000s, and now in his late 50s, the patient had a further sudden onset severe headache. At the local general hospital CT brain scan and lumbar puncture were reportedly normal but, following referral to the regional neurosciences centre, CT angiography showed a pericallosal aneurysm, 2–3 mm in diameter. This was subsequently coiled.

This brief neurological case history gives a brief history of the evolving management of subarachnoid haemorrhage over a period of little more than 30 years. Before the widespread availability of CT brain scanning diagnosis depended on CSF analysis for xanthochromia and catheter angiography to detect any underlying aneurysm. If found, surgery might be undertaken, the procedure having been pioneered by Norman Dott (1897–1973) in the 1930s.[1] However, by the early 2000s surgical aneurysm clipping procedures were being rendered obsolete by the better outcomes of interventional radiological coiling techniques.[2]

Some historians have become sceptical of ideas of "progress". Nevertheless, one such sceptic admits that "In science progress is a fact. ... The accelerating advance of scientific knowledge fuels technical innovation, ... Post-modern thinkers may question scientific progress, but it is undoubtedly real".[3] As shown in this short neurological history, the same may be said of the history of neurology (sometimes, at least!).

References

1. Dott NM. Intracranial aneurysms: cerebral arteriography: surgical treatment. Edinb Med J 1933;40:219–240.
2. Maurice-Williams RS, Lafuente J. Intracranial aneurysm surgery and its future. J R Soc Med 2003;96:540–543.
3. Gray J. *Heresies. Against progress and other illusions.* London: Granta Books, 2004, p.3.

"Idiots" and "naturals": contextualising Elizabeth Gaskell's portrayals of intellectual disability

Abstract

Recent publications on the history of intellectual disabilities have noted the account of Willie Dixon in Elizabeth Gaskell's 1855 short story *Half a life-time ago* as a cultural exemplar of this clinical phenomenon. However, this is far from the only occurrence of characters described as "idiots" and "naturals", as they were then called, in Gaskell's oeuvre. This article attempts to collate these various instances of intellectual disability, and then to consider the contexts in which these portrayals were composed. These are suggested to include: Elizabeth Gaskell's personal encounters with individuals with intellectual disability; the medical context of new ideas about the care and training of idiots as conveyed through the activities of her brother-in-law, Dr Samuel Gaskell; and the literary context as reflected most particularly in accounts of intellectual disability in the works of Charles Dickens and Charlotte Brontë. These fictional examples and factual contexts prompt the view that Gaskell's approach to the care of idiots focused on the importance of female caregivers outside the institutional framework of the asylum or workhouse, at a time when professional discourses were more oriented to the need for male authority to manage these individuals in institutional settings.

1. Introduction

In his publications on the cultural history of idiocy, Patrick McDonagh cites Elizabeth Gaskell's short story *Half a life-time ago* amongst various literary sources which portray individuals with intellectual disability.[1] More recently, Simon Jarrett's study of the idea of the disabled mind references the same Gaskell story.[2] These critical works reflect an increasing interest in the study of the history of intellectual disability which has occurred in recent times.[3] Analysis of contemporary works of literature has informed these studies through their portrayals of afflicted individuals and the reactions and responses of society to them, and hence both the narrative and symbolic uses to which intellectual disability has been put. A deeper study of those works by Elizabeth Gaskell which feature characters with intellectual disability, extending beyond *Half a life-time ago*, may further contribute to this field.

By the mid-nineteenth century the distinction was being drawn by contemporary commentators between idiocy and lunacy, the latter corresponding to what might now be termed mental or psychiatric illness, characterised by psychosis (hallucinations and delusions sufficient to compromise social and occupational functions) and mood disorders. The definition of idiocy was somewhat flexible but generally incorporated the notion of defective mental understanding from the time of birth (i.e. a congenital disorder). However, individuals with either lunacy or idiocy, falling into the undifferentiated category of "insanity", might be found amongst the heterogeneous populations of inmates found in Poor Law workhouses or county asylums, along with people with epileptic seizures and with cognitive decline resulting from dementing disorders of later life.

Just as many names have been used to describe "madness",[4] so various terms have been used over the years to describe the clinical phenomena under consideration here, by both professional and lay observers. This rich vocabulary, much of it jargon and slang, includes idiocy, imbecility, dull-wittedness, feeble-mindedness, mental deficiency, mental retardation, and intellectual deficiency. Other nouns include: fool, natural, simpleton, innocent, half-wit, imbecile, moron. Other adjectives include: silly, simple, foolish, dull-witted. The almost invariably pejorative connotations of these terms preclude their usage now, with "learning disability" or "intellectual disability" the currently most favoured appellations. However, the older terms are used here in the appropriate contexts (e.g. direct quotations) and to avoid ahistoricism.[5]

The purpose of this article is to examine in more detail Elizabeth Gaskell's portrayals of "idiots" and "naturals" and to consider the contexts, personal, medical, and literary, in which these portrayals were written.

2. Elizabeth Gaskell's portrayals of "idiots" and "naturals"

Before considering *Half a life-time ago* and its cultural historical readings advanced by McDonagh and Jarrett, further accounts of, or references to, "idiots" or "naturals" in Elizabeth Gaskell's oeuvre are briefly reviewed here, presented in chronological order of publication. This collation does not claim to be exhaustive. Possible accounts suggestive of lunacy or insanity in Gaskell's works (e.g. Alice Carr in *Morton Hall* (1853)) are eschewed, but, as for accounts of idiocy, some have been previously noted.[6]

Mary Barton, A Tale of Manchester Life (1848)
Jem Wilson's younger brothers, Joe and Will, are described as "helpless, gentle, silly children, but not the less dear to their parents and to their strong, active, manly, elder brother. They were late on their feet, in talking, late every way;

had to be nursed and cared for when other lads of their age were tumbling about in the street, and losing themselves, and being taken to the police-office miles away from home".[7] As previously mentioned, "silly" was a recognised descriptor of learning disability, as is evidenced by the account of Joe and Will's delayed motor and linguistic milestones and their inability to keep up with their peers. The contrast with Jem ("strong, active, manly") is typical of 19th century definitions of idiocy according to its otherness, and hence the early demise of these children is to some degree anticipated.

Martha Preston (1850)

The eponymous heroine of this story, from a Lakeland Statesmen family, has a younger brother, Johnnie, who at about the age of 16 suffers a raging fever, possibly typhoid, for a period of 20 days, but "as he recovered, his wandering lost senses were not restored" and "stupor remained still upon his poor brain". "Martha knew the truth in her heart, that her brother was an idiot." Martha's intended husband, Will Hawkshaw, suggests that Johnnie be "shut up in an asylum", the phraseology suggesting the institution has a custodial rather than a therapeutic function, but Martha refuses, knowing the asylum to be a "madhouse", a decision which causes the loss of her marriage prospects.[8] This story was later revised by Gaskell as *Half a life-time ago* (vide infra).

The Well of Pen-Morfa (1850)

Set in a village in north Wales, this is the story of Nest Gwynn, who takes in Mary Williams, variously described as "the half-witted woman – the poor crazy creature", and a "poor idiot".[9] Mary has been beaten and underfed by John Griffiths with whom she had previously been boarded by the parish. Nest receives the same money from the parish but pursues a more caring approach. Local attitudes to Mary are of note. Mrs Thomas tells David Hughes that "half-wits ... take more to feed them than others", and Nest tells him that when Mary's paroxysms of wild mood are coming on "she would kneel and repeat a homily rapidly over, as if it were a charm to scare away the Demon in possession".[10] Following Nest's death, Mary goes to the workhouse.

The precise chronology of this story (which is also cited by McDonagh in his cultural history, as "The Well at Pen-Morfa" [sic]),[11] is uncertain. The character of David Hughes, aged 81 at the time of the story, is said to have first encountered John Wesley (died 1791) as a "white-haired patriarch",[12] facts which could conceivably locate the story in the present (1850), were it not for the author prefacing the story as occurring "Many, many years back – a life-time ago"[13] (so perhaps twice as distant as *Half a life-time ago* which can be accurately dated from internal evidence – (vide infra)?). Evidently the account given is one of outdoor relief, the idiot maintained in the community at the

expense of the parish, with indoor relief (incarceration in the workhouse) as
the last resort. These are provisions of the Poor Law, dating from Elizabethan
times (1601) which underwent various amendments prior to the Poor Law Act
of 1834.[14]

A number of stereotypical features of the idiot are encountered in the
portrayal of Mary Williams: the neighbour's report of excessive appetite; her
characterisation as "a dumb animal",[15] although evidently from the text she has
some verbal abilities; and the allusion to demonic possession as a cause of her
behavioural disturbance, although the text suggests the possibility that Mary,
in her recourse to prayer, has some religious sensibility.

North and South (1855)
Mr Bell, Fellow of an Oxford college, makes two allusions to issues of mental
insufficiency. Speaking to Mr Hale on the night before the latter's untimely
death whilst visiting his old friend in Oxford, he opines "… men set me down
in their fool's books as a wise man. … The veriest idiot who obeys his own
simple law of right … is wiser and stronger than I."[16] Speaking to Mr Thornton
in Milton, he compares the way different men die, opining that "the poor idiot
[dies] blindly, as the sparrow falls to the ground, the philosopher and idiot …
all eat after the same fashion".[17] This indirect knowledge of idiots may be
contrasted with that of Nicholas Higgins, a Milton mill worker, who, speaking
of the Union, tells Margaret Hale that "Government takes care o' fools and
madmen",[18] implying an institutional locus of care.

The Half-Brothers (1859)[19]
Gregory is described as "lumpish and loutish, awkward and ungainly", and is
labelled "stupid" by his aunt and stepfather; furthermore "every one [sic] said
he was stupid and dull, and this stupidity and dullness grew upon him". At
school he can "never be made to remember his lessons" and the schoolmaster
advises he be taken out of school. He proves more successful as a shepherd,
and performs a self-sacrificing act to save his half-brother.[20]

Sylvia's Lovers (1863)
Sylvia's father complains of being "shut up wi' women these four days and a'm
a'most a nateral [natural] by this time".[21] Presumably he is likening women's
talk to that of naturals, meaning deficient in content or sense.

Cousin Phillis (1863–4)
Timothy Cooper is described as a "half-wit"[22] and makes errors in his labours
causing Ebenezer Holman to dismiss him, yet Timothy has the insight to
divert carts on Hornby market day so that the sick Phillis is not disturbed by

their noise.[23] This ability may perhaps render the label of "idiot"[24] inappropriate.

The idiot revised: *Half a life-time ago (1855)*

Whilst the idiot character(s) and mention of idiots appear to be incidental and largely peripheral to the narrative demands of several of Gaskell's aforementioned portrayals (e.g. *Mary Barton, Cousin Phillis*), they are necessary and indeed central in others (e.g. *The Well of Pen-Morfa, Martha Preston*). Perhaps Gaskell's fullest account of intellectual disability is to be found in *Half a life-time ago*, the revision of *Martha Preston* which appeared in Dickens's *Household Words* in October 1855.[25] The subject of intellectual disability is central to the iterations of this story.

The heroine in *Half a life-time ago* is Susan Dixon, some ten years older than her brother, "a boy named after his father", William Dixon.[26] The family reside at Yew Nook, a farm in the Westmoreland dales. When Susan's mother, Margaret, is dying, she says of "lile Will" that "Father's often vexed with him because he's not a quick, strong lad" and extracts a promise from Susan to be a mother to the boy.[27] Later, a feverish illness, possibly typhus fever according to the doctor from Coniston, kills William Dixon senior and nearly Susan too. On her recovery she is told that the illness has also affected Willie: "People began to say, that the fever had taken away the little wit Willie Dixon had ever possessed, and that they feared that he would end in being a 'natural', as they call an idiot in the Dales".[28] He is described as having "restless eyes and ever-open mouth, and every now and then setting up a strange kind of howling cry, and then smiling vacantly to himself at the sound he had made", and attempts at verbalisation are described as "idiotic sound".[29] It becomes apparent that Willie "had to have the same care taken of him that a little child of four years old requires".[30]

Michael Hurst, Susan's intended husband, opines of Willie that "the fever has left him silly".[31] Unbeknownst to Susan, he takes Willie to see a Dr Preston, "the first doctor in the county", in Kendal, who is reported by Michael to think that Willie "will get badder from year to year" and advises "he would send him off in time to Lancaster Asylum. They've ways there both of keeping such people in order and making them happy".[32] Michael attempts to console Susan but she says "It's no use trying to make me forget poor Willie is a natural", meaning that "she could not forget what the doctor had said about the hopelessness of her brother's case; Michael had referred to the plan of sending Willie to an asylum, or madhouse, as they were called in that day and place".[33] Susan is aware of "stories of the brutal treatment offered to the insane; stories that were, in fact, but too well founded", and of "horrible stories... about madhouses",[34] and so rejects Dr Preston's advice, to Michael's irritation. He "will not be with a natural who may turn into a madman some day",[35] but Susan has pledged herself to look after her brother, and so her chance of marriage to Michael Hurst is lost. She continues to look after Willie alone for the rest of his life.

The chronology of *Half a life-time ago* is made explicit by internal evidence: the story begins "fifty or fifty-one years ago".[36] Thus, considering the publication date of 1855, this places the story in the first decade of the nineteenth century, in 1804 or 1805, a dating which incidentally renders anachronistic the reference to Lancaster Asylum, which was only opened in 1816.[37]

Neither McDonagh nor Jarrett mentions *Martha Preston*, the adaptation of which resulted in *Half a life-time ago*. McDonagh reads *Half a life-time ago* as a critique of patriarchal authority and an account of masculine folly, and notes that in agreeing to care for her brother Susan Dixon defers to matriarchal authority. In doing so, she is "masculinized" just as Willie is "feminized", a reversal of then typical gender roles,[38] as evidenced by the comment of Susan's father that there is "more of a man in her ... than her delicate little brother ever would have".[39]

Jarrett describes Willie as "another idiot laden with deeply symbolic meanings". Susan's sacrifice of marriage and children and her refusal to commit Willie to Lancaster Asylum is characterized as the loss of "all else from her life. The emasculated idiot is again presented as an obstacle to progress. His presence ... brings to an end a bloodline, prevents new birth and blocks the agricultural progress Susan's fiancé would have brought".[40] Once again the issue of patrimony is raised, a characteristic of the idiot being his [sic] inability to handle money and assume responsibility for his inheritance. The naming of both fictional father and son as William would have been redolent with personal significance for Elizabeth Gaskell.

One might contest Jarrett's particular reading: Michael Hurst's subsequent career, dogged by alcohol misuse, does not necessarily suggest that he would have brought agricultural progress to Yew Nook (one commentator explicitly states that "Michael is a failure"[41]), and moreover Susan proves a canny enough farmer without his assistance. Furthermore, it does not adequately explain why Susan resists sending Willie to Lancaster Asylum: her promise to her mother, and her knowledge of the workings of asylums and madhouses. Fictionally this knowledge is said to come from stories circulating in the "countryside",[42] but whence might this factual knowledge have come to inform the author? Here we must consider possible contexts for Elizabeth Gaskell's fictional creations.

3. Contextualising Gaskell's portrayals of "idiots" and "naturals"

The collated examples indicate that the portrayal of idiots and naturals was a recurrent feature in Elizabeth Gaskell's writings, appearing throughout most of her publishing career (from *Mary Barton* in 1848 to *Cousin Phillis* in 1863–4). Hence it is reasonable to ask what prompted and informed these portrayals. Three possible sources, influences, or stimuli are suggested and explored here: Mrs Gaskell's own personal encounters; the medical context; and the literary context. Although presented separately, these are likely to be interrelated.

Personal encounters
On the basis of her extant correspondence, the evidence for Elizabeth Gaskell's personal encounters with individuals with intellectual disability is slight. Indeed, only a single letter explicitly refers to this. Written to Agnes Sandars from Plymouth Grove and dated Wednesday 11th February 1852, Gaskell describes the present-giving at Capesthorne. Amongst the servants was "a poor idiot to whom Mrs D[avenport] had been very kind. "Silly Billy" dancing along the park dressed in a gay horse-cloth, …".[43]

One further letter might also be pertinent. Writing to Marianne Gaskell on 17th April 1851 (Letter 94) Gaskell tells of a visit to "Deaf & Dumb Asylum" at Swinton.[44] It is possible that some of the children resident in this institution might have had learning disability (recall the description in *The Well of Pen-Morfa* of Mary Williams as a "dumb animal"), but no specific mention of idiocy is made. Moreover, the boy of 16 who was taken off from the Asylum by Gaskell's party to see Schwabe's print works, in view of his being brought up to be a calico printer, was due to write an account of his visit, a skill beyond that which would be accorded to those labelled as idiots.[45]

It is of course possible, if not indeed probable, that in her role as clergyman's wife visiting her husband's parishioners in Manchester Gaskell may have encountered children with intellectual disability, perhaps like Joe and Will Wilson. Hence her recurrent accounts of idiots and naturals might stem from personal encounters, in a manner perhaps similar to her recurrent accounts of headache which, it has been argued, may be based on both her own personal experience and that of other family members.[46] However, other contexts, perhaps more compelling, are to hand.

The medical context
Idiocy had increasingly come under the gaze of the medical profession in the mid-nineteenth century, in contrast to the situation in the 18th century. These developments impinged directly on the Gaskell family, specifically upon Elizabeth's brother-in-law, Samuel Gaskell (1807–1886), a medical doctor who was a

significant figure in the asylum movement from 1840 onwards.[47] In February of that year he was appointed medical superintendent of the Lancaster County Asylum, following election by the county magistrates. This appointment potentially provides a direct link with Elizabeth Gaskell's *Half a life-time ago*.[48]

Samuel Gaskell is credited with ending the system of physical restraint of patients in Lancaster Asylum, one element of the system of "moral treatment" which he promoted, along with Dr Edward de Vitre (1806–1878), also appointed to the Lancaster Asylum (as Visiting Physician) in 1840.[49] This was part of a revolution in the care of lunatics during this period, instigated in England by the work of the Tuke family at the York Retreat,[50] and in France by Philippe Pinel (1745–1826) working at the Bicêtre hospital in Paris.[51] This approach, which sought not only to abolish physical restraint but also to encourage recovery from mental illness through the provision of adequate care, diet, and employment, in a therapeutic (i.e. clean) environment with access to exercise and recreation, was subsequently promoted within the British medical profession by Dr John Conolly (1794–1866), the doyen of English asylumdom, at the Middlesex County Asylum at Hanwell.[52]

A detailed study of the Lancaster Asylum records by John Walton reached the conclusion that "[t]he overall impression is of a genuine attempt by the medical officers [Gaskell and de Vitre] to introduce a system of "moral treatment" in the fullest sense, and to change the whole spirit in which the asylum was conducted. There is sufficient evidence to suggest that, up to a point, they succeeded".[53] A further innovation at Lancaster Asylum, credited to Gaskell, was the allocation of young orphan children to the care of female patients. Gaskell's rationale, as recalled years later by Lord Shaftesbury (1801–1885), who visited Lancaster Asylum in his role as the head of the Lunacy Commission, was "Here are several women wanting occupation, and there are several children wanting care. So these women have the exclusive care of the children day and night". Shaftesbury further recalled that it was Gaskell's aim "to develop in the women the great principle of maternal love".[54]

From the vantage point of his superintendency at Lancaster Asylum, Gaskell was aware of the "large fraction of the inmate population who were idiotic".[55] In his annual report in 1846 he stated that "a very large majority of the patients now admitted into this asylum are imbeciles".[56] These observations are seemingly contradicted by the view developed by historians of the asylum movement that few idiots were sent to county asylums in this period,[57] but the timing of Gaskell's comments may be significant. The 1845 Lunacy Act had obliged Poor Law Guardians to send all patients deemed "insane", a terminology encompassing both those classed as lunatics and idiots, to county asylums. Although many idiots remained in workhouses or in the community, it is possible that there was a genuine increase in the number of idiot patients in Lancaster Asylum at this time. Walton corroborates the increase in congenital patients, albeit temporary,[58] but it was sufficient to prompt Gaskell to undertake a survey of the likely numbers of individuals with idiocy in Lancashire.[59]

Gaskell's observations occurred at a time when ideas were changing about the appropriate care of idiots. Once again, these developments largely originated from the Bicêtre hospital in Paris. Although Pinel had been equivocal about the potential for treating idiots,[60] one of his successors at the Bicêtre, Édouard Séguin (1812–1880), had revolutionised their care and training, experience documented in his various publications.[61] John Conolly was a visitor to the Bicêtre,[62] and Gaskell followed suit in October 1846. He recorded his impressions in three (unsigned) articles which appeared in *Chambers's Edinburgh Journal* in early 1847.[63] Therein he did not mention Séguin by name, and as his visit was "unannounced" there may be no reason to believe that he intended to "learn from the famous physician of the Bicêtre",[64] but rather to observe the various exercises, physical and mental, which the young patients demonstrated.

According to David Wright, it was the reading of Gaskell's articles in *Chambers's Edinburgh Journal* that prompted Mrs Anne Serena Plumbe to contact her minister, the Reverend Andrew Reed, to enquire about the possibility of starting a home for the education of idiots in England.[65] With the assistance of Conolly, this appeal eventually culminated in Reed opening Park House in Highgate in April 1848, later called the National Asylum for Idiots.[66] Further accommodation was opened at Essex Hall, Colchester, and subsequently a purpose-built asylum was constructed at Earlswood near Redhill in Surrey, opening in 1855. John Langdon Down (1828–1896), known to posterity for his description of "mongoloid idiots", now known as Down syndrome, was superintendent at Earlswood from 1858 to 1868.[67]

If Samuel Gaskell harboured hopes for a dedicated institution for the care of idiots in Lancaster, he was to be disappointed, since this did not come to fruition until long after his departure from Lancaster in 1849 to become one of the Commissioners in Lunacy based in London.[68] The Royal Albert Asylum, also known as the Royal Albert Asylum for Idiots and Imbeciles for the Seven Northern Counties, had its origins in 1864 when De Vitre was offered £2000 by James Brunton towards its foundation. The building was completed in 1868, admitted its first patient in 1870, and received a visit from Séguin in 1873. The first superintendent of the Royal Albert Asylum was Dr George Edward Shuttleworth (1842–1928), a protégé of Langdon Down at Earlswood.[69] All these events postdated Gaskell's cessation of medical work following a road accident in 1865 which forced his early retirement the following year due to "mental infirmity".

It has previously been suggested that Samuel Gaskell's work at Lancaster Asylum and as a Lunacy Commissioner may have exerted an influence on his sister-in-law's portrayals of mental illness.[70] A case may also be made that the same holds true with respect to Elizabeth Gaskell's portrayals of idiocy. Although Samuel is only ever briefly mentioned in her correspondence, it is evident that he was involved in advising on care of the Gaskell children, and it is apparent that she found it easy to converse with him: "I believe I am more open with Sam than I dare to be with William, and I love Sam as a dear brother" (Letter 13).[71] It is thus possible that he may have shared with her, within the bounds of medical confidentiality, some aspects of his medical work, including the care of idiots. In addition, European travel was not so common in this era that his visit to Paris was likely to go unremarked in the family, particularly in light of Elizabeth's interest in France.[72]

The literary context

In addition to these developments in medical concepts and management, the subject of idiocy had also come increasingly under the literary gaze in the nineteenth century. Existing literary accounts of intellectual disability would in all likelihood have been familiar to Elizabeth Gaskell, such as William Wordsworth's *The Idiot Boy* (1798), and Dickens's portrayals of Smike in *Nicholas Nickleby* (1839) and of the title character of *Barnaby Rudge* (1841).[73]

Her friendship with Charlotte Brontë may also have influenced Elizabeth Gaskell in this context. In her biography, she transcribes a letter sent from Haworth dated 6th August 1851 in which Charlotte comments on Charles Kingsley's *Saint's Tragedy* (1848) concerning St Elizabeth of Hungary:

> We see throughout (I *think*) that Elizabeth has not, and never had, a mind perfectly sane. From the time that she was what she herself, in the exaggeration of her humility, calls "an idiot girl," to the hour when she lay moaning in visions on her dying bed, a slight craze runs through her whole existence. ... Only a mind weak with some fatal flaw *could* have been influenced as was this poor saint's. (italics in original).[74]

A further example appears in Brontë's novel *Villette* (1853), the "imbecile" pupil, Marie Broc.[75] Whether Gaskell was aware of Charlotte's rueful name of "Idiot Child" for her first novel, *The Professor*,[76] which failed to find a publisher in her lifetime, is not recorded, but considering the intimacy of their conversations and correspondence it is a possibility.

The specific developments in the medical care and training of idiots also impacted on the literary sensibility. In the 4th June 1853 issue of *Household Words*, Dickens (with WH Wills) wrote a piece entitled "Idiots", documenting his visit to Park House in Highgate.[77] The following year Harriet Martineau revisited the subject in the pages of Dickens's journal although there was no specific mention of Park House or Essex Hall.[78]

4. Discussion

Idiocy was evidently a subject of ongoing discourse in both medical and literary circles, particularly during the late 1840s and early 1850s when there was optimism that the alleviation of such deficits was possible within dedicated institutions, which might in turn permit afflicted individuals to return to society with enhanced skills. Elizabeth Gaskell was ideally placed to appreciate these intersecting contexts, both through her literary contacts (Dickens, Brontë) and her medical (family) contact with Samuel Gaskell. Inclusion of idiot characters in her stories is thus unsurprising. She was able to contribute to contemporaneous debates through her narrative and symbolic use of the idiot character. Because of his occupational involvement with the care of the insane, including idiots, throughout the 1840s and 1850s, I suggest that Samuel Gaskell was probably pivotal in raising his sister-in-law's awareness of these issues.

In this context, Erica Larsen has recently suggested that *Half a life-time ago* is a refutation by Elizabeth Gaskell of the moral treatment of the insane championed by, amongst others, Samuel Gaskell, and specifically at Lancaster Asylum. She states that Susan Dixon "models her homecare [of Willie] around the principles of moral management that Dr Gaskell used to reform Lancaster Asylum".[79] But this is to ignore the chronology of the story, based on its internal evidence and writ large in its title. As has been shown, moral treatment had not been introduced to Lancaster Asylum at the time the story is set, the first decade of the nineteenth century, because this institution did not then exist, far less in a state reformed by Samuel Gaskell (and Edward de Vitre). Moreover, Larsen couches her argument in terms of "insanity", and does not differentiate between lunacy and idiocy, following the conflation enshrined in the 1845 Lunacy Act.[80] Whilst, to be sure, it subsequently proved true that "no amount of moral management can successfully treat Willie's insanity",[81] or anyone else's for that matter, this realisation postdated both Elizabeth Gaskell's story (fictionally and factually) and Samuel Gaskell's superintendency of Lancaster Asylum.

I suggest, contra Larsen, that there is no specific criticism of Samuel Gaskell or of his approach to moral management in *Half a life-time ago*, indeed the opposite may be true. At the time of its publication, much of the discourse about the appropriate management of idiots emphasized the need for paternal guidance, particularly for incapable (feminized) idiot males. Elizabeth

Gaskell's most detailed portrayals, on the contrary, emphasize rather the importance of female caregivers (Susan Dixon, aka Martha Preston; Nest Gwynn), be the idiot male (Willie Dixon, aka Johnnie Preston) or female (Mary Williams). Women taking on the care of orphaned children (*Half a lifetime ago*) or those otherwise abandoned (possibly orphaned? – *The Well of Pen-Morfa*) is a feature in these stories. This might perhaps be seen as a call to the instinct of maternal love, and as stressing "the values of a gynecratic system",[82] and hence reminiscent of Samuel Gaskell's innovation in the care of young orphans by female patients at the Lancaster Asylum.[83]

References

1. Patrick McDonagh, Diminished men and dangerous women: representations of gender and learning disability in early- and mid-nineteenth-century Britain, *British Journal of Learning Disabilities*, Vol. 28 (2000), pp.49–53; Patrick McDonagh, *Idiocy. A cultural history* (Liverpool: Liverpool University Press, 2008).

2. Simon Jarrett, *Those they called idiots. The idea of the disabled mind from 1700 to the present day* (London: Reaktion Books, 2020).

3. For example: David Wright, Anne Digby (eds.), *From idiocy to mental deficiency. Historical perspectives on people with learning disabilities* (Abingdon: Routledge, 1996); Patrick McDonagh, CF Goodey, Tim Stainton (eds.), *Intellectual disability. A conceptual history, 1200–1900* (Manchester: Manchester University Press, 2018).

4. Alex Leff, Clean round the bend – the etymology of jargon and slang terms for madness, *History of Psychiatry*, Vol. 11 (2000) pp.155–162.

5. Jarrett, *Those they called idiots. The idea of the disabled mind from 1700 to the present day*, pp.18, 59–62.

6. AJ Larner, Dr Samuel Gaskell (1808–1886): a brief biography, and thoughts on his possible influence on Elizabeth Gaskell's writings, *Gaskell Society Newsletter*, Vol. 62 (2016), pp.11–18.

7. MacDonald Daly (ed.), *Elizabeth Gaskell. Mary Barton: A tale of Manchester life* (London: Penguin Classics, 2003 [1848]), pp.74–78.

8. The story was originally published in *Sartain's Union Magazine of Literature and Art*, Vol. 6 (1850), pp.133–138. It may also be found at http://victorian-studies.net/EG-Martha.html (accessed 10/03/22).

9. Elizabeth Gaskell, *The Well of Pen-Morfa* (Kessinger Legacy Reprints, undated [1850]), pp.17, 18.

10. Gaskell, *The Well of Pen-Morfa*, p.18.

11. McDonagh, *Idiocy. A cultural history*, p.229n12.

12. Gaskell, *The Well of Pen-Morfa*, p.14.

13. Gaskell, *The Well of Pen-Morfa*, p.4.

14. For details on the provisions of the Poor Law, see Peter Rushton, Lunatics and

idiots: mental disability, the community, and the Poor Law in Early Modern England, 1600–1800, *Medical History*, Vol. 32 (1988), pp.34–50.

15. Gaskell, *The Well of Pen-Morfa*, p.19.

16. Patricia Ingham (ed.), *Elizabeth Gaskell. North and South* (London: Penguin Classics, 2003 [1855]), p.341.

17. Ingham, *Elizabeth Gaskell. North and South*, p.354.

18. Ingham, *Elizabeth Gaskell. North and South*, p.286.

19. I have followed the dating on The Gaskell Society website listing of Works compiled by Mitsuhara Matsuoka (https://www.gaskellsociety.co.uk/elizabeth-gaskells-works/, accessed 10/03/22) which states that *The Half-Brothers* was published in the *Dublin University Magazine* in November 1859. However, my search of this journal (https://catalog.hathitrust.org/Record/008696315, accessed 10/03/22) finds no Gaskell contribution in that issue (323), nor in any other issue for 1859. In Mitsuhara Matsuoka, Gaskell's strategies of silence in "The Half-Brothers", *Gaskell Society Journal*, Vol. 17 (2003), pp 50–58, a publication date of 1858 is given (p.53). To be sure, there is "a tale" entitled "The Half-Brothers" in the November 1858 issue of the *Dublin University Magazine*, Vol. 52 (1859), pp.586–598, but this is not Gaskell's story. In Shirley Foster, Elizabeth Gaskell's shorter pieces, in Jill L. Matus (ed.), *The Cambridge Companion to Elizabeth Gaskell* (Cambridge: Cambridge University Press: 2007), pp.108–130, it is stated that "The Half-Brothers" was "written in 1859 specifically for *Round the Sofa*" (p.116). The available evidence thus suggests that the Gaskell Society website attribution is incorrect.

20. The story may be found at https://www.gutenberg.org/files/2532/2532-h/2532-h.htm (accessed 10/03/22).

21. Shirley Foster (ed.), *Elizabeth Gaskell. Sylvia's Lovers* (London: Penguin Classics, 2004 [1863]), p.50.

22. Heather Glen (ed.), *Elizabeth Gaskell. Cousin Phillis and other stories.* (Oxford: Oxford World's Classics, 2010), p.233.

23. Glen, *Elizabeth Gaskell. Cousin Phillis and other stories*, pp.242–243.

24. Jenny Uglow, *Elizabeth Gaskell. A habit of stories* (London: Faber and Faber, 1999 [1993]), p.543.

25. Details of this revision may be found in Larry K Uffleman, From "Martha Preston" to "Half a Life-time ago": Elizabeth Gaskell rewrites a story, *Gaskell Society Journal*, Vol. 17 (2003), pp.92–103.

26. Glen, *Elizabeth Gaskell. Cousin Phillis and other stories*, p.90.

27. Glen, *Elizabeth Gaskell. Cousin Phillis and other stories*, p.93.

28. Glen, *Elizabeth Gaskell. Cousin Phillis and other stories*, p.105.

29. Glen, *Elizabeth Gaskell. Cousin Phillis and other stories*, pp.105, 106.

30. Glen, *Elizabeth Gaskell. Cousin Phillis and other stories*, p.107.

31. Glen, *Elizabeth Gaskell. Cousin Phillis and other stories*, p.106.

32. Glen, *Elizabeth Gaskell. Cousin Phillis and other stories*, pp.107, 108.

33. Glen, *Elizabeth Gaskell. Cousin Phillis and other stories*, pp.108–109.

34. Glen, *Elizabeth Gaskell. Cousin Phillis and other stories*, pp.109, 111.
35. Glen, *Elizabeth Gaskell. Cousin Phillis and other stories*, p.110.
36. Glen, *Elizabeth Gaskell. Cousin Phillis and other stories*, p.90.
37. For details on Lancaster Asylum, see John Walton, The treatment of pauper lunatics in Victorian England: the case of Lancaster Asylum, 1816–1870. In: Andrew Scull (ed.), *Madhouses, mad-doctors, and madmen. The social history of psychiatry in the Victorian era* (Philadelphia: University of Pennsylvania Press, 1981), pp.166–197; Peter Williamson, From confinement to community: the story of "The Moor", Lancaster's County Lunatic Asylum. In: S Wilson (ed.), *Aspects of Lancaster. Discovering local history* (Barnsley: Wharncliffe Books, 2002), pp.123–138; H Shaw, Q Wessels, AM Taylor, E Chin-Quee, The asylums and pioneers of psychiatric care. In: Quenton Wessels (ed.), *The medical pioneers of nineteenth century Lancaster* (Berlin: epubli GmbH, 2016), pp.99–121.
38. McDonagh, *Idiocy. A cultural history*, pp.97–99.
39. Glen, *Elizabeth Gaskell. Cousin Phillis and other stories*, p.92.
40. Jarrett, *Those they called idiots. The idea of the disabled mind from 1700 to the present day*, pp.172–173.
41. Uffleman, *Gaskell Society Journal*, p.100.
42. Glen, *Elizabeth Gaskell. Cousin Phillis and other stories*, p.109.
43. *Further letters of Mrs Gaskell* ed. by John Chapple and Alan Shelston (Manchester: Manchester University Press, 2003 [2000]), p.63.
44. *The letters of Mrs Gaskell* ed. by J.A.V. Chapple and Arthur Pollard (Manchester: Mandolin, 1997 [1966]), p.150.
45. The labelling of idiot children as "dumb" is reported to be relatively uncommon in this period by David Wright, *Mental disability in Victorian England. The Earlswood Asylum 1847–1901* (Oxford: Clarendon Press, 2001), pp.54n38, 64n86, although the conflation of the two is possible.
46. AJ Larner, "A habit of headaches": the neurological case of Elizabeth Gaskell, *Gaskell Journal*, Vol. 25 (2011), pp.97–103; AJ Larner, Headache in the works of Elizabeth Gaskell (1810–1865), *Journal of Medical Biography*, Vol. 23 (2015), pp.191–196.
47. For biographical details of Samuel Gaskell, see Anonymous, Samuel Gaskell F.R.C.S. Eng., *British Medical Journal*, 1 (1886), p.720; Anonymous, The late Samuel Gaskell, Esq., *Journal of Mental Science*, 32 (1886), pp.235–236; HL Freeman, Samuel Gaskell. In: Willis J Elwood, A Félicité Tuxford (eds.), *Some Manchester doctors. A biographical collection to mark the 150th anniversary of the Manchester Medical Society 1834–1984* (Manchester: Manchester University Press, 1984), pp.89–92; Digby Tantam, So you've heard of the Gaskell medal: but who was Gaskell? *Psychiatric Bulletin*, 13 (1989), pp.186–188; Hugh Freeman and Digby Tantam, Samuel Gaskell. In: German E Berrios and Hugh Freeman (eds.), *150 years of British Psychiatry 1841–1991* (London: Royal College of Psychiatrists, 1991), pp.445–451; Andrew Scull, Charlotte Mackenzie, Nicholas Hervey, *Masters of Bedlam. The transformation of the*

mad-doctoring trade (Princeton: Princeton University Press, 1996), pp.161–186; Larner, *Gaskell Society Newsletter*, Vol. 62 (2016), pp.11–18; Shaw et al., The asylums and pioneers of psychiatric care, pp.105–115. Whilst Scull et al. correctly state that Samuel, like his brother William, was born in Warrington, they locate this town on "the coast of Lancashire" (p.161); certainly it is located on the river Mersey, but around 20 miles from the estuary at Liverpool.

48. I am not aware of any evidence to suggest that Elizabeth ever visited Lancaster County Asylum, nor expectation that she would have done so. Dickens, on the other hand, did visit, along with Wilkie Collins, during their tour of the North, in September 1857; see Peter Williamson, From confinement to community: the story of "The Moor", Lancaster's County Lunatic Asylum, p.128. In Dickens and Collins's fictionalised account of this trip, *The lazy tour of two idle apprentices*, "Francis Goodchild" (Dickens's alias) reports to "Thomas Idle" (Collins) on his visit to Lancaster Asylum; see Charles Dickens and Wilkie Collins, *No Thoroughfare & other stories* (Stroud: Alan Sutton, 1990), pp.190–192.

49. Anonymous, Edward Denis de Vitre, *British Medical Journal*, 2 (1878), pp.711–712; Shaw et al., The asylums and pioneers of psychiatric care, pp.117–119.

50. The definitive history of the York Retreat is Anne Digby, *Madness, morality and medicine. A study of the York Retreat, 1796–1914* (Cambridge: Cambridge University Press, 1985).

51. An interesting recent account of Pinel and his work may be found in Kenneth S Kendler, Philippe Pinel and the foundations of modern psychiatric nosology, *Psychological Medicine*, Vol. 50 (2020), pp.2667–2672.

52. For Conolly, see Scull et al., *Masters of Bedlam. The transformation of the mad-doctoring trade*, pp.48–83.

53. Walton, The treatment of pauper lunatics in Victorian England: the case of Lancaster Asylum, 1816–1870, p.177.

54. Scull et al., *Masters of Bedlam. The transformation of the mad-doctoring trade*, pp.169, 322n61 (citing *Journal of Mental Science*, Vol. 27 (1881), pp.444–445).

55. Scull et al., *Masters of Bedlam. The transformation of the mad-doctoring trade*, p.169.

56. Scull et al., *Masters of Bedlam. The transformation of the mad-doctoring trade*, p.171 (citing Lancashire Record Office, QAM 5/1846/7).

57. Wright, *Mental disability in Victorian England. The Earlswood Asylum 1847–1901*, pp.13, 19–20. Writing from the West Riding Pauper Lunatic Asylum in Wakefield in 1872, the superintendent James Crichton-Browne noted that "Idiots are detained at their homes or workhouses, or are boarded out in much larger proportion than the insane". Crichton Browne J. Cranial injuries and mental diseases. *West Riding Lunatic Asylum Medical Reports*, Vol. 2 (1872), pp.97–136 [at 132].

58. Walton, The treatment of pauper lunatics in Victorian England: the case of Lancaster Asylum, 1816–1870, pp.176, 189.

59. Anonymous, The Report of the Medical Officers of the Lunatic Asylum for the County of Lancaster. 1848. *Journal of Psychological Medicine and Mental Pathology*, Vol. 1 (1848), pp.580–582. Note incorrect pagination given for this reference in Wright, *Mental disability in Victorian England. The Earlswood Asylum 1847–1901*, p.28n26.

60. McDonagh, *Idiocy. A cultural history*, pp.58–59.

61. Perhaps most notable of these publications was Édouard Séguin, *Traitment moral, hygiène et éducation des idiots et des autres enfants arrières* (Paris, 1846). See also Murray K Simpson, The moral government of idiots: moral treatment in the work of Séguin, *History of Psychiatry*, Vol. 10 (1999), pp.227–243.

62. John Conolly, Notices of the lunatic asylums of Paris, *British and Foreign Medical Review*, Vol. 19 (1845), pp.281–298. Wright, *Mental disability in Victorian England. The Earlswood Asylum 1847–1901*, p.169.

63. Samuel Gaskell's three articles, all published without attribution, are: Visit to the Bicêtre. *Chambers's Edinburgh Journal*, Vol. 7, No. 158 (9th January 1847), pp.20–22; Education of Idiots at the Bicêtre. Second article. *Chambers's Edinburgh Journal*, Vol. 7, No. 161 (30th January 1847), pp.71–75; Education of Idiots at the Bicêtre. Third article. *Chambers's Edinburgh Journal*, Vol. 7, No. 163 (13th February 1847), pp.105–107. All are available online at https://archive.org/details/chambersedinburg7818cham/page/n33/mode/2u p. (accessed 10/03/22). Peculiarly Scull et al., *Masters of Bedlam. The transformation of the mad-doctoring trade*, p.317n2 and p.323n86, refer to only two of Gaskell's articles, omitting the third. Of note, Gaskell's account of his Bicêtre visit follows many of the patterns of the Earlswood travelogues identified by Patrick McDonagh, Visiting Earlswood: the asylum travelogue and the shaping of "idiocy", in: P McDonagh, CF Goodey, T Stainton (eds.), *Intellectual disability. A conceptual history, 1200–1900* (Manchester: Manchester University Press, 2018), pp.211–237.

64. Wright, *Mental disability in Victorian England. The Earlswood Asylum 1847–1901*, p.27.

65. Wright, *Mental disability in Victorian England. The Earlswood Asylum 1847–1901*, p.28.

66. Freeman and Tantam, Samuel Gaskell, p.448 state that "in collaboration with … Conolly and … (Read) [sic], Gaskell founded … Park House, Highgate", but Wright's account has no mention of Gaskell playing a role in this foundation other than the effect of his articles on Mrs Plumbe.

67. Wright, *Mental disability in Victorian England. The Earlswood Asylum 1847–1901*, pp.155–176.

68. For Samuel Gaskell's work as a Commissioner in Lunacy, see Anonymous, Biographies of Medical Lunacy Commissioners 1828–1912, http://studymore.org.uk/6biom.htm#M11 (accessed 10/03/22).

69. See Shuttleworth's obituary, *British Medical Journal*, Vol. 1 (1928),

pp.1004–1005. He also contributed to the medical literature on idiocy during his long tenure (until 1893) at Lancaster e.g. GE Shuttleworth, Intemperance as a cause of idiocy, *British Medical Journal*, Vol. 2 (1877), pp.308–309.

70. Larner, *Gaskell Society Newsletter*, Vol. 62 (2016), pp.11–18; AJ Larner, Dr Samuel Gaskell at Lancaster Asylum: a medical and literary legacy? *Morecambe Bay Medical Journal*, Vol. 7/7 (2016), pp.177–178.

71. *The letters of Mrs Gaskell*, p.34.

72. Philip Yarrow, Mrs Gaskell and France, *Gaskell Society Journal*, Vol. 7 (1993), pp.16–36.

73. For Dickens's portrayals of intellectual disability see P Marchbanks, From caricature to character: the intellectually disabled in Dickens's novels, *Dickens Quarterly*, Vol. 23 (2006), pp.3–24, 67–85, 169–181. A further, later, example is Maggy in *Little Dorrit* (1857); and perhaps also Sloppy in *Our Mutual Friend* (1865).

74. Elizabeth Gaskell, *The life of Charlotte Brontë* (Oxford: World's Classics, [1857] 2009), pp.388–389.

75. McDonagh, *Idiocy. A cultural history*, pp.121–122.

76. Juliet Barker, *The Brontës* (London: Abacus, [1994] 2010), p.787; John Sutherland, *The Brontësaurus. An A-Z of Charlotte, Emily & Anne Brontë (& Branwell)* (London: Icon Books, 2016), pp.67–69.

77. Charles Dickens and WH Wills, Idiots, *Household Words*, Vol. 8, No. 167 (4th June 1853), pp.313–317. See https://djo.org.uk/household-words/volume-vii/page-313 (accessed 10/03/22).

78. Harriet Martineau, Idiots again, *Household Words*, Vol. 9, No. 212 (15th April 1854), pp.197–200. See https://djo.org.uk/household-words/volume-ix/page-197 (accessed 10/03/22).

79. Erica Larsen, "Strength both of mind and body": asylum reform and the failure of moral management in Elizabeth Gaskell's "*Half a life-time ago*", unpublished MA thesis, Brigham Young University (2020), p.6. See https://scholarsarchive.byu.edu/etd/8667 (accessed 10/03/22).

80. Larsen, "Strength both of mind and body": asylum reform and the failure of moral management in Elizabeth Gaskell's "*Half a life-time ago*", p.7, states "Nor have any critics examining *Half a life-time ago* considered how the story intersects with Dr Gaskell's work at the asylum featured in the story." Again, this is anachronistic, and moreover the author is evidently unaware of previous publications on this potential linkage, viz. Larner, *Gaskell Society Newsletter*, Vol. 62 (2016), pp.11–18; Larner, *Morecambe Bay Medical Journal*, Vol. 7/7 (2016), pp.177–178.

81. Larsen, "Strength both of mind and body": asylum reform and the failure of moral management in Elizabeth Gaskell's "*Half a life-time ago*", p.6.

82. Matsuoka, Gaskell's strategies of silence in "The Half-Brothers", p.51.

83. Peter Carpenter, The role of Victorian women in the care of "idiots" and the "feebleminded", *Journal on Developmental Disabilities*, 8(2) (2001), pp.31–43, has documented examples of the care in small scale institutions initiated and managed by women during this era.

Book reviews

1. Neuroarthistory

The relationship between art and neurology may be described as bidirectional: the art of neurology, and the neurology of art; and also as multifaceted.[1]

The practice of clinical neurology has sometimes been described as, or likened to, an art, although in our current era of guidelines, "guidance" (for which read coercion), and practice parameters, some clinical neurologists may feel themselves to be little more than technicians, and consequently to a greater or lesser extent demoralised in the practice of their art. "Art" may be deemed to carry with it notions of freedom, autonomy, vision.

The "Neurology of Art" is a subject of increasing interest, for example commanding a regular and well-attended session at the annual meeting of the European Federation of Neurological Societies (EFNS). A number of analyses of the influence of neurological disorders, such as neglect, aphasia, and dementia, on the output of creative artists, including those working in the visual arts, haas been published.[2] Vincent van Gogh has been a particularly favoured subject in this regard, with suggested diagnoses including epilepsy and bipolar disorder. The neuroscientist Semir Zeki has stated that "most painters are neurologists" (191); it would be interesting to learn if any saw themselves as such. While the converse of Zeki's statement is obviously not true, there certainly have been neurologists who were able draughtsmen, not least Jean-Martin Charcot, as shown at a special session during the EFNS meeting in Paris in 2004.

Of perhaps even greater current interest than the effect of brain disease on the output of established artists are rare reports of autistic savants who display outstanding artistic skills inconsistent with their general level of intellectual functioning, and of the emergence of artistic talent ("sudden artistic output" syndrome) in individuals without any or only limited prior evidence of such abilities, most particularly in the context of frontotemporal lobar degeneration (FTLD) syndromes, in which there may be concurrent dissolution of language function and increasing behavioural symptomatology.[3,4] One possible explanation for the rare emergence of these abilities in FTLD is the facilitation or disinhibition of non-dominant right parieto-temporal neocortical networks, "liberated" following left anterior temporal lobe dysfunction. The contrast between the accuracy of reproduction and the lack of symbolic elements observed in the visual art of such FTLD patients may be congruent with this observation. Such cases may elucidate some of the brain substrates of artistic ability, but not necessarily the source of creative ideas or drive. Metrics for creativity remain, at best, rudimentary.[5]

Since visual art is a universal human activity, with a history dating back at least 30000 years, it may be ascribed to universal attributes of human biology. Art "processes necessarily depend to some extent on the properties of our biological make-up" (28), with particular preferences (e.g. symmetry, closed forms) and reactions being inborn (82). It may therefore be argued that if brain function is regulated by rules, so may be its artistic products, such that it is our biological nature which shapes our culture. Kant's argument for inherent mental properties was philosophical, but it is implicitly biological (79), as recognised by Peter Medawar, who spoke of "the most breathtaking conceptual exploit in the history of philosophy: Kant's suggestion that instead of acquiescing in the ordinary opinion that our sensory intuitions are patterned by "objects" – by that which is perceived – we should take the view that the world of experience is patterned by the character of our faculties of sensory intuition".[6]

Although some may view science as the very antithesis of art, objecting to any such attempt at mechanical reductionism, nonetheless a discourse of "art as biology", and specifically neurobiology, ignoring as it does any utilitarian considerations of the function of art, may be informative. The neuroscientific approach to art has perhaps been most successsful in the field of aesthetics,[7,8] indeed spawning the term "neuroaesthetics" (5, 191). Hence, an attempted neural approach to art history seems not unreasonable, since cross fertilization between disciplines is often productive of new insights.

The book is thus made up by "sketching the intellectual biographies" (xiii) of 25 individuals who have written something about the possible biological underpinnings of artistic endeavour. These individuals form a heterogeneous group. They cover the 25 centuries from Ancient Greece (Aristotle) to the late 20th century (Zeki). Most are from the European literary tradition, the only exception being the 11th century Arabic scholar al-Haytham. Some names will be familiar to most readers (e.g. Leonardo, William Hogarth, Kant, Marx, Ruskin), others were certainly unfamiliar to me, and may possibly be so to others (e.g. Vischer, Göller, Wölfflin, Riegl). Not all have necessarily written about visual art (e.g. Montesquieu); few have any specific training in the fields of medicine and/or science (Winckelmann, Freud, Zeki). The focus is on original written sources, with an explicit avoidance of secondary literature, in order, it is argued, to be closer to learning from experience rather than interpretation: seeing is deemed more important than reading and, the author's broad erudition notwithstanding, book learning is largely disdained. The substrate of this book may therefore be seen as the "great writings of great men" (since all are men), an approach to the subject which might be deemed "whiggish" by medical historians. The book's broad sweep encompasses not only art history, aesthetics, and neuroscience, but there are also occasional nods to ethology, evolutionary theory, and psychology. This breadth may explain the long gestation of the work, apparently first pondered by the author some 15 years ago.

What kind of discipline is neuroarthistory, as envisaged by Onians? I find no entry for "neuroarthistory" in the OED (accessed online 05/03/08) so presume that this term must be a neologism of the author's own creation. Endeavours to link art and biology seem prone to this new minting of blend words: in addition to neuroaesthetics, one may also encounter "Sciart" (166) and "ArtScience" (*sic*).[9] I find no specific definition of neuroarthistory in this book but, in adducing Freud as a "true neuroarthistorian", it would seem to reflect attempts to "apply the theories ... based on ... neuroscientific knowledge to the study of the works of ... artists" (138). This may be a legitimate premise: neuroscience contributions to understanding the history of art might include insights into the neural substrates of colour vision, imitation and empathy (mirror neurones are frequently mentioned), habituation (to account for changes in artistic styles and fashions between different eras and cultures), and maybe even visual pleasure. However, as the author wisely notes, the "path from hard science to the interpretation of art is extremely risky and the closer the art is to the science the better" (143–4).

For this particular workaday non-academic NHS neurologist, this book proved a challenging but enjoyable read. I am entirely unqualified to say how the book will be received by the art history community, and can only comment from the perspective of a student of the clinical neurosciences. As far as I can tell, this aspect is handled appropriately, I detected only one lapse ("rods, which are the colour sensors in the retina", 23). Peculiarly, Kant's year of birth is wrongly given as 1728 rather than 1724 (79). However, at risk of being branded one of the "pitiless ... practitioners" of scientific method (160), I think a number of objections might be raised to the author's methodology.

Lord Brain once described the 18th century Scottish judge and classicist Lord Monboddo (1713–1799) as an "evolutionist".[10] This was based on Monboddo's interest in the detailed account of a dissection of a chimpanzee published by Edward Tyson (1699), showing that the creature's vocal organs did not differ from those of a man. Monboddo's reasoning, later accorded the status of a "doctrine", was that since the animal possessed all the organs necessary for speech, their use was simply a matter of appropriate training, a view later ridiculed by Samuel Johnson and alluded to in the novel *Martin Chuzzlewit* by Charles Dickens.[11] Neither Monboddo nor Tyson foreshadowed evolution, since both believed in a divinely-ordained chain of being rather than a transformation of species under evolutionary pressures, but even had they held such a belief it may be deemed anachronistic to label them as "evolutionist" before Darwin published and elaborated upon his theory of evolution from 1859 onwards. By the same token, I would question whether there can there be "neuroarthistorians before neuroarthistory" (10), since before any theory of neuroarthistory is advanced this would surely be anachronistic. The author himself may recognise this since, although he sees himself as the latest in a long line of neuroarthistorians (xiii), he describes his wife as a neuroarthistorian *avant la lettre* (xiv).

This objection may be deemed mere sophistry, a semantic nicety, but perhaps a more pressing question relates to the issue of anticipation (could one call it "protoneuroarthistory", the prehistory of neuroarthistory?) which recurs again and again in Onians' book. The bold claim is made, directly following Zeki, that writers on art are often neuroscientists without knowing it (13). The suggestion that certain individuals sound (Burke, 65), or even think (Hogarth, 57), like scientists surely cannot be accepted, since the term "scientist" was not coined until the 19th century by Whewell (the moreso in the case of Burke who of course took great pains to goad public opinion into destroying the house and laboratory of Joseph Priestley, the outstanding British chemist of his day, prompting his emigration to America, an early example of brain drain as a consequence of interference by politicians). Use of the word "theory" in the context of these individuals' ideas is also probably overstating the case (63,65). More examples of this propensity to see the future in the past may be cited: Pater is "startlingly close to modern understanding of the brain's plasticity" (97); Taine's writing "corresponds with the science of today" (100); some of Freud's early, pre-psychoanalysis, work shows a "remarkable correspondence with modern neuroscience" (135). The distinguished art historian Ernst Gombrich, Onians' mentor, and whose presence looms throughout the book, is described as "informally an experimental scientist" (176). Such retrospective judgments of significance may allow the author to succumb to the privileges of hindsight and, possibly, the temptations of bias. For many of the cited authors, their writing had no empirical basis: one interesting exception is the work of Herskovits who tested whether seeing is culturally influenced by examining the cross-cultural susceptibility to visual illusions such as the Müller-Lyer diagram. Though some authors' insights were "purely theoretical" (113), this contrasts with the largely or entirely speculative nature of most contributions, their "findings" having no other basis than assertion. Surely for every such "anticipation" retrospectively identified to be correct, one could locate one or more speculations which have proven incorrect (indeed the author cites a few)? But if our understanding of the visual brain changes, as Onians himself acknowledges that it will (17), might not these apparently prescient statements seem to be less so, or even be rejected altogether?

A third, and related, objection arises in Onians' dealings with his "neural subjects". He claims for neuroarthistory the "ability to reconstruct the unconscious intellectual formation of the makers, users and viewers of art" (13). The "neural history" of his selected protoneuroarthistorians pays "particular attention to the more unconscious formation of their minds, focusing on the uniqueness of their experiences, especially those of a visual kind" (14), such that "the subjectivity they produce can be reconstructed hundreds or even thousands of years after the person in question has died" (15). Whilst it is undeniable that "our mental apparatus is shaped by our experience" (29), and that we each have a "unique neural history" (52) it is surely another, and unwarrantable, step to infer that specific and identifiable experiences can account for the ways in which the selected individuals wrote about seeing, or about art, as allowing them "access to privileged perceptions" (52) or "privileged insights" (100).

A contrast is drawn, for example, between Aristotle's upbringing in a medical family and his peripatetic lifestyle, and Plato's aristocratic origins and fixed metropolitan career. Can this difference really be adduced to explain their different perspectives on art? Widespread travels to differing environments are repeatedly cited (e.g. Aristotle, al-Haytham, Alberti, Leonardo, Ruskin and, thanks to rail travel, Göller and Wölfflin) as influencing subjects' analytical skills and reconfiguring their neural networks, perhaps through enhanced connectivity, on the premise that this allowed these individuals to see more images than any of their predecessors. If true, one might argue that the future for neuroarthistory will be extremely productive since a child of today sees more images in one day on television and the internet than earlier generations saw in a lifetime. However, it should be remembered that Kant, of course, achieved what he did without ever leaving provincial Königsberg (79).

Likewise, one has doubts about the relevance of other possible influences. Illegitimacy is twice cited as favouring intensive reflection on the nature of art (by Alberti, 43,46; and by Leonardo, 47). Since these individuals were children "by nature not by law", they are deemed to have been resistant to authority and hence apt to pay less attention to bookish learning and more to what could be learned from the inner being, in contrast to those with an assured inheritance who were/are apparently less competitive and less reliant on personal mental resources. Their illigetimacy is thus credited as a possible source of profound creative effects or a stimulus to new questioning. Understanding of the variances in wine is also adduced as a stimulus to original ideas on cultural difference (Montesquieu, Ruskin). Since the known history of any historical subject is partial (and if autobiographical partially fictive), this sounds like special pleading; witness the use of qualifiers such as "must have", "may well have", and "likely to". It seems to me that these are views are speculative, being unverifiable but, more importantly, falsifiable, a distinction of which the author is surely aware since he is, through his teacher Gombrich, familiar with Popper and his work (160). Perhaps it may be no more than a reflection of my own impoverished mental powers, but I am uncomfortable with this willingness to think oneself able to reconstruct or read other peoples' minds. If neologisms are to be permitted, I call this "hypermentalising",[12] as the converse of the defect in mentalising reported in autism.

It is furthermore suggested that such neural formation may have helped these individuals "to surprisingly anticipate [sic] modern science" (15). The danger of teleology (function as final cause) seems all too evident in this formulation, as acknowledged, and apparently welcomed, by Gombrich (168). Gombrich seems to have been much given to introspection or self-reflection, and according to Onians was particularly alert to his own experiences. That knowledge of another's experiences might permit reconstruction of their neural networks and their operation and hence explain their behaviour remains, it would seem to me, a belief rather than an empirical fact. Moreover, the assertion, a propos the selected individuals, that "their sensitivities were so heightened that they could identify neurally based phenomena that are only now surrendering their secrets to the latest technology" (15) seems to imply an ability to intuit mental structure, an approach which has been largely eschewed if not entirely discredited by empirical modern neuropsychology. It is moot to what extent understanding of human neural resources can be acquired by experiencing our own body and behaviours.

The blurb claims neuroarthistory as "one of the newest ... human sciences". One should be rightly sceptical of blurb, since it may well have been written by the publisher rather than the author. The discipline of a science suggests an empirical body of knowledge, a methodology, hypotheses, theories, testable predictions. Neuroarthistory, as far as I read this book, has none of these elements at present, although this work may well be seen as a source book for would-be neuroarthistorians. The dedication to "the art historians of the future who have the courage also to be neuroarthistorians" may suggest a manifesto, rather than a monograph. Onians himself suggests that neuroarthistory is "not a theory" but an "approach. ... a readiness to use neuroscientific knowledge to answer any of the questions that an art historian may wish to ask" (17), and hence this will be ever evolving as neuroscience itself develops. So, ultimately, the validity of this endeavour may depend upon whether the human brain can ever understand itself.

The book is the first of a projected trilogy: subsequent volumes will apply a neuroarthistorical approach to the art of Europe and then of the whole world (xiii). Maybe, then, one should suspend judgment at present, and look forward to seeing how things develop.

Note

This book review was written in 2008 at the invitation of the then editor of *Brain*, but never published.

References

1. Onians J. *Neuroarthistory. From Aristotle and Pliny to Baxandall and Zeki.* New Haven and London: Yale University Press, 2007. All page references cited in the text refer to this edition.
2. Bogousslavsky J, Hennerici MG (eds). *Neurological disorders in famous artists Part 2.* Basel: Karger; 2007.
3. Miller BL, Cummings J, Mishkin F, Boone K, Prince F, Ponton M, et al. Emergence of artistic talent in frontotemporal dementia. Neurology 1998; 51: 978–82
4. Seeley WW, Matthews BR, Crawford RK, Gorno-Tempini ML, Foti D, Mackenzie IR, et al. Unravelling Boléro: progressive aphasia, transmodal creativity and the right posterior neocortex. Brain 2008; 131: 39–49.
5. Griffiths TD. Capturing creativity. Brain 2008; 131: 6–7.
6. Medawar PB. *Advice to a young scientist.* New York: Harper Row; 1979: 73.
7. Zeki S. *Inner vision: an exploration of art and the brain.* Oxford: OUP, 1999.
8. Ramachandran VS. *The emerging mind. The Reith Lectures 2003.* London: Profile Books, 2003: 46–69.
9. Espinel CH. Memory and the creation of art: the syndrome, as in de Kooning, of "creating in the midst of dementia". An "ArtScience" study of creation, its "brain methods" and results. In: Bogousslavsky J, Hennerici MG (eds). *Neurological disorders in famous artists Part 2.* Basel: Karger; 2007: 150–68.
10. Brain R. Lord Monboddo: evolutionist and anti-Johnsonian. In: *Some reflections on genius and other essays.* London: Pitman Medical; 1960: 101–12.
11. Larner AJ. Dickens and Monboddo. The Dickensian 2004; 100 (462): 36–41
12. Larner AJ. "Asperger's syndrome and high acheivement: some very remarkable people" by Ioan James; "Different like me. My book of autism heroes" by Jennifer Elder. Advances in Clinical Neuroscience & Rehabilitation 2006;6(5):36.

2. Confabulation

Two books on confabulation published within a year by OUP: one thinks, perhaps, of London buses, but, by contrast, these books are an experience well worth waiting for.[1,2] For example, did you know that in German, WIGAN is a non-word (Schnider, p.149)?

Schnider's monograph is suffused with his clinical experience of trying to rehabilitate confabulating patients: even in the midst of the science he acknowledges that this is a "gruelling experience" (p.243). A review of the history of confabulation, including translations from the early works of Korsakoff, Kraepelin, Pick and others, is followed by the thorny issue of classification, with Schnider developing a 4-fold schema of intrusions, momentary confabulations, fantastic confabulations, and behaviourally spontaneous confabulations (pp.63–4), of which the latter form his main area of study. The aetiology is examined, with anterior limbic structures thought culpable, and the pathogenesis, including a wide variety of diseases, along with associated disorders (amnesia, disorientation, false recognition syndromes including the Capgras delusion, and anosognosia). Mechanisms are elucidated by means of psychophysical and neuroimaging studies, leading to the proposition that confabulators have reality confusion and a failure to integrate contradictory information due to the failure of a filtering process, 200–300 ms after stimulus presentation and before recognition and re-encoding, which normally permits suppression of currently irrelevant memories. This is a fascinating book, systematic in its approach. For those disinclined to battle through the detail, the conclusions to each chapter are excellent.

Hirstein's multi-author volume is, as expected, more diffuse than Schnider's but none the less stimulating. False memories, only briefly touched on by Schnider, are described at greater length here, in two chapters (from Loftus and Zaragoza) the import of which I found rather chilling: our brains have a surprising cognitive vulnerability to forced fabrication (I would be interested to know if this also applies to eidetics). Coltheart & Turner present evidence that the normal response to questions we don't know the answer to is not, as might be imagined, to admit ignorance with an "I don't know" response, but to indulge in confabulation, a tendency exacerbated in certain brain disease states. Wheatley, in what is the best chapter (or worst, depending on your degree of concreteness) I have read in many moons, demolishes the notion of the brain as veridical. The book is more philosophically oriented than Schnider's, and perhaps more peripheral to clinical interests, though still grounded in clinical neuroscience.

In summary: in the human brain, memory is a construction, confabulation is normative, perception is illusion, and "meaning" is privileged over accuracy.

A nihilist might conclude that life mediated through such a prism is an essay in futility, and aporia the only tenable neurophilosophy.

Acknowledgement

Adapted from: Larner AJ. *Adv Clin Neurosci Rehabil* 2010;10(2):31.

References

1. Schnider A. *The confabulating mind. How the brain creates reality.* Oxford: Oxford University Press, 2008.
2. Hirstein W (ed.). *Confabulation. Views from neuroscience, psychiatry, psychology, and philosophy.* Oxford: Oxford University Press, 2009.

3. History of British Neurology

The approach to neurological history adopted in this handsome volume[1] is to present a number of brief biographies, usually no more than a page in length, of neurologists and practitioners in allied neuroscientific disciplines who have made "significant neurological contributions" (p.2). Particularly renowned individuals merit longer entries, such as Thomas Willis, John Hughlings Jackson, William Gowers, Henry Head, and Charles Sherrington. In addition to a summary of their contributions, a brief flavour of personality is also sometimes added to the portrait. Since "history" may also encompass institutions as well as individuals, it comes as little surprise that the development of the National Hospital at Queen Square is discussed. The chapters are largely arranged chronologically, but there are also chapters devoted to neuropathology, neurophysiology, and other neurosciences. Citations are largely to the secondary literature, but there are a few primary references.

The approach is unrelentingly "whiggish", according to the usage coined by the historian Herbert Butterfield (1900–1979). This is apt in some ways, since British neurology has unequivocally made major advances since Willis, but inevitably results in a deeply gendered account: only one woman, Dorothy Russell (pp.269–70), makes the cut, all other females who appear are either patients (Anne Green, pp.22–3; Anne Conway, p.44) or a discredited assistant to a male protagonist (Kathleen Chevassut, pp.168, 201). The specified parameter "British" sometimes breaks down: although one can accept Brown-Séquard (pp.152–5) as born in a British colony (Mauritius), and I suppose historically Ireland did not have home rule at the time of Graves (p.101) and Bentley Todd (p.102), no amount of special pleading can explain Hans Berger (p.295) however great his contribution (EEG). If "contribution" is a prerequisite, the place of Edinburgh's Alexander Monro *tertius* (p.61–2) must also be dubious.

Many neurologists take an interest in the history of their specialty, perhaps most particularly in the lives and discoveries of their predecessors in the discipline, and hence will take a delight in this book. Since numbers of neurologists in the UK have traditionally been few, most practitioners can trace back a "neurological family tree", as it were, to distinguished figures through a fairly circumscribed number of degrees of separation. Clifford Rose himself does this, with his first-hand accounts of Charles Symonds (pp.199–200) and Henry Miller (p.209), amongst others. It is not difficult to think of particular individuals who might also have been included in such a volume as this, and to my way of thinking neuropsychology seems a particular omission.

Reviewing this book shortly after the author's death (1 November 2012), it is appropriate to say that it will stand as a monument to one of Clifford Rose's longstanding interests and endeavours, and will be enjoyed by many readers. However, though not wishing to seem unduly critical, it would be remiss of any reviewer not to mention the lapses in chronology which are by no means infrequent and do detract from the overall enjoyment of reading, likewise the inadequacy of the index.

Acknowledgement

Adapted from: Larner AJ. *Adv Clin Neurosci Rehabil* 2013;13(5):25.

Reference

1.   Rose FC. *History of British neurology*. London: Imperial College Press, 2012.

4. The neurological patient

The history of neurology has typically been told by neurologists about neurologists (their biographies, research, institutions, treatments) – what may be termed a "top down" approach. In contrast, the voice of neurological patients has been largely neglected in the written histories of neurology, paradoxically so in one sense since the neurological encounter is (ideally) dominated by hearing the patient's account, but understandably so in another sense since written patient narratives do not typically enter the historical record. This "bottom up" approach to medical history was advocated most cogently by Roy Porter (1946–2002) some 30 years ago now, and his plea may ultimately have been the stimulus for the current volume examining the neurological patient in history.[1] The editors are well-known historians: Stephen Jacyna co-authored with Edwin Clark the seminal *Nineteenth-century origins of neuro-scientific concepts* (Berkeley: University of California Press, 1987) and has written a biography of Henry Head, whilst Stephen Casper wrote his PhD on British Neurology and has spoken on historical topics at meetings of the Association of British Neurologists.

The book is divided into several sections which examine various ways in which the neurological patient is constructed, for example by medical practice, by patient groups, by historians, and by patients themselves. The latter section is the only one in which the authentic patient voice is truly heard (for example the "psychasthenia" of the poet Robert Nichols, sometime patient of Henry Head, and based on his letters to the neurologist after his retirement), although even here that voice is sometimes mediated by others, for example Gwen Raverat's letters about her husband Jacques' experience of multiple sclerosis. Ballenger documents the evolution of ideas about dementia, from its representation as the entire loss of selfhood through to the assertion of selfhood by "famous" AD patients such as Ronald Reagan. Howard Kushner gives a fascinating account of views on Tourette's syndrome, in particular its psychoanalytic representations, which sometimes directly contradicted patient reports. Casper's chapter on the evolution of the neurological examination is probably the most pertinent for practitioners of the clinical art of neurology.

This is a book for medical historians by medical historians (to my knowledge Kushner is the only medically qualified contributor), and this leads to some pretty semantically dense material which may not be quite the most suitable reading matter for the interstices of the outpatient clinic (my favourite: "Each of these chapters is a register of the historically constituted episteme of its author", p.215; I have absolutely no idea what that means!). Moreover, there are some astonishing errors for which authors and editors must take responsibility: two of the giants of neurology are credited with wrong middle initials (William Gowers given as A instead of R, p.41; William Lennox given as J instead of G, pp.52,55), and one of the most famous neurological patients, the amnesic HM, is given the wrong year of death (2009 rather than 2008, p.223). Nevertheless, some parts of this book will be of interest to clinical neurologists, demonstrating as it does that the neurological patient is a cultural construct which is context (time, location) dependent.

Acknowledgement

Adapted from: Larner AJ. *Adv Clin Neurosci Rehabil* 2014;14(3):23.

Reference

1.   Jacyna LS, Casper ST (eds.). *The neurological patient in history.* Rochester: University of Rochester Press, 2012.

5. Neuroethics of biomarkers

Biomarkers have become an integral part of clinical practice in some spheres of neurology, such as dementia where they are enshrined in diagnostic criteria for Alzheimer's disease as part of a clinico-biological, as opposed to an older clinico-pathological, definition of disease. The hope is that identification of disease in preclinical phases using predictive biomarkers may facilitate preventative treatment. But objections may be raised, for example to medical-ising those who are currently well. The ethics of biomarker use in neurological and psychiatric disorders is explored in this volume,[1] written by Matthew Baum, a Harvard MD-PhD trainee.

Addressing the bioprediction of brain disorder, the author argues for a reorientation of the medical concept of "disorder", rejecting the old binary or categorical formulation (disorder/normalcy) in favour of a probabilistic model based on present and future risks of harm. This is justified in part by the belief, undoubtedly true, that "There is no a priori justification for believing that biomarkers will map cleanly onto diagnostic categories arrived at by historical accident" (p.46). The result is a proposal for a "probability dysfunction" model in which disorders are conceptualised as graphs of probability over time, the area under which would help to separate out self-limiting disorders from those with low probabilities of harm over longer time periods.

"Risk banding", based on the shape of the probability function, is the strat-egy advocated to determine the necessity or otherwise for response. This is illustrated with respect to bioprediction of future psychotic episodes and dementia (Chapter 5). This "risk of harm" approach is not seen as a fracture with past practice, since "Diagnosis is application of heuristic categories that capture a risk of harm associated with biological variation" (p.125). The prob-abilistic claims of biomarkers may be used as a form of Bayesian updating. But will patients accept this reformulation?

This thought-provoking book will particularly appeal to those of a philo-sophical bent, rather than those who just want to know about biomarkers. It is not a book for dipping into during the interstices of the outpatient clinic, although the author must be commended for making the material accessible, his text is highly readable (and sometimes funny). Some clinicians will perhaps have little interest in the ramifications of predictive biomarkers for legal practice and societal distributive justice (when is biopredicted risk morally significant?), although even here there are interesting learning points: the discussion of prediction of seizures and driving is particularly pertinent. Furthermore, I was amazed to learn that in law the appeal to the "reasonable man" is regarded as an "objective" test, although the author rightly points out that this is almost always subjective in that it relies "almost exclusively on common sense and the persuasion of skilled law professionals to do this Bayesian updating" (p.138). Whatever deficiencies there may be in medical (neurological) practice, at least we are attempting to put it on a research-based evidential footing.

Acknowledgement

Adapted from: Larner AJ. *Adv Clin Neurosci Rehabil* 2017;16(4):20.

Reference

1.   Baum ML. *The neuroethics of biomarkers. What the development of biopredic-tion means for moral responsibility, justice, and the nature of mental disorder.* Oxford: Oxford University Press, 2016.

6. Representing epilepsy

A few moments of cogitation and everyone can recall examples of epilepsy as portrayed in works of literature[1] or film.[2] But what relationship do these cultural representations bear to medical representations, and vice versa? This is the issue explored in Jeanette Stirling's book *Representing Epilepsy.*[3] She shows that notions of hereditary taint, degeneration, criminality, and of the epileptic as "disordered other", existing beyond acceptable social boundaries, have accreted to the category of epilepsy not only in literary works but also in medical texts, notably that of Gowers, although Hughlings Jackson seems largely exempted of this kind of statement. The "technically mediated and disembodied modes" (p.18) of medical discourses on epilepsy are not free of cultural bias, however much medics might wish to believe that they are.

Analysis of material falling within this "circuit of culture" includes the familiar, such as "epileptic" characters in works of Dickens and Dostoevsky,[4] George Eliot's *Silas Marner*, and Thomas Hardy's *The Mayor of Casterbridge* (Lucette Le Sueur), as well as publications in the *Lancet* and *British Medical Journal* from the late 19th and early 20th centuries. Much of the latter makes sobering reading for a clinician, with the advocacy of isolation and even steril-isation for epileptics. Do we now advocate policies on medical grounds which will cause posterity to blanch? There is a Liverpool connection here: Francis

Imlach (perhaps familiar from Alan Sykes's recent articles on Birkbeck Nevins[5] and William Carter[6]) undertook hystero-oophorectomy as a treatment for epilepsy (p.60), predicated on 19th century beliefs of a link between disordered sexuality (e.g. Hardy's Lucette Le Sueur) and epileptic seizures.

Nineteenth century social responses to the "problem" of epilepsy included the development of dedicated epileptic "colonies", an international phenomenon which saw epileptics physically removed beyond the boundaries of normal social interaction, to endure a seemingly enlightened (but gender segregated) regime of ergotherapy (pp.131–177). Editorials in the medical journals debated the alleged benefits of these colonies. Stirling rightly regrets the absence of patient narratives from these institutions specifically (p.173), and of epilepsy more generally (p.189), there being perhaps no such accounts until the mid-20th century (e.g. by the author Margiad Evans[7]).

One stimulus for Stirling's book derives from the fact that she experienced a medically provoked seizure in 1972 and was on anti-epileptic drugs until 1990 when she stopped medication, suffering no further seizures thereafter (pp.186–187). Whether or not this change in medication occurred under medical supervision is not stated, but a rider would have been advisable, since not all individuals with epilepsy will benefit from medication withdrawal. Perhaps based on this experience, and on the historical record of the adverse effects of bromides, the first widely used treatment for epilepsy dating from the 19th century, Stirling seems to portray anti-epileptic medications as frankly dangerous, and as a cause of epilepsy, figuring them as partly causal in the suicide of Ian Curtis of the band Joy Division in 1980 (pp.192–193).

The dyad of epileptic as creative genius/mental defective is also explored, with possible examples of the former including van Gogh (p.xix), St Paul, Mahomet, Julius Caesar, Napoleon (p.168), and Dostoevsky (p.98). Voskuil's observation that Dostoevsky did not take medication is cited as an indicator of his awareness (unsubstantiated) of the cost to creativity of contemporary drugs.

From my own medical cultural perspective, I have some disagreements with Stirling's assertions and conclusions. For example, it is stated that Othello's "epilepsy is implicated in the murder of Desdemona" (p.4). From my reading of the play, it is far from certain that Othello has epilepsy, other than Iago's assertion to that effect (and how much weight can be placed on that?).[8] Stirling seems to accept without question Freud's 1927–8 analysis of Dostoevsky's "hystero-epilepsy" (p.44), although this formulation was questioned, if not entirely demolished, as early as 1931 by the historian EH Carr (1892–1982). Some of the Dickensian examples of epilepsy also fail to convince, perhaps through an overreliance on the paper on this subject by Cosnett.[9] For example, Bradley Headstone's attack on Eugene Wrayburn in *Our Mutual*

Friend seems to be ascribed to his epileptic nature (pp.106–107), with Stirling apparently willing to accept a category of "epileptic furore" (pp.118, 214) as well as grand mal seizures and automatisms. The epileptic patient as no more than symptomatology (p.184), the pressure for doctors to medicate epileptics regardless of drug side effects (p.188), and an uncompromising model of epilepsy that demands nothing less than aggressive medical response (p.196), are paradigms which I do not recognise from my clinical experience.

Lyndall Gordon's fascinating account of the life of Emily Dickinson (1830–1886), *Lives like loaded guns*, details what is known of the life of one of America's greatest poets, and the subsequent machinations amongst family members in bringing her to public attention (only 10 of her poems were published during her life time).[10] It contains the suggestion that the poet may have suffered from epilepsy (p.116), a claim not made hitherto to my knowledge, but with a careful and appropriate rider about the dangers of attempting retrospective diagnosis (p.115). The formulation is based on a close reading of some of the poems, and on evidence of the prescription of glycerine, then used, among other indications, for epilepsy. This illness may be one explanation for Dickinson's withdrawal from public life, and even from normal social intercourse. Her earliest editor, Isabel Loomis Todd, lover of Emily's brother Austin, never saw her in the 5 years she was in Amherst, and in close contact with the Dickinson family, prior to the poet's death.

If one accepts Gordon's suggestion (since it is not amenable to refutation, it cannot be called an hypothesis), it begs the question as to what impact epilepsy had on Emily Dickinson's creative output. Gordon notes, alluding to Dostoevsky, that epilepsy may open a "range of experience ... to the gifted" (p.123), and that the freedom the diagnosis gave Dickinson from domestic chores and attendance at social gatherings (pp.121,124–125) may have facilitated her work. The author guesses that Dickinson's four most productive years, 1861–1864, coincided with the sickness being at its height (p.123).

Like Jeanette Stirling's book, the centenary history of the International League Against Epilepsy (ILAE) shows that the outlook for epileptics at the time of Emily Dickinson was bleak, with the expectation of inevitable intellectual decline, and the association of epilepsy with ideas of degeneration and criminality.[11] Indeed, the ILAE took shape from a precursor organisation, never realised, for the Study of the Causes and Prevention of Insanity.

The book documents the successive vicissitudes of the ILAE, its progress fractured soon after birth by the First World War, and its rebirth in 1935 shortly preceding the Second. During the latter, it was largely sustained by the American chapter and in particular through the efforts of Dr William Lennox. The evolution of bureaucratic structures and increasing professionalism in the organisation of ILAE conferences and in the running of its journal, *Epilepsia*, are apparent. The history of this journal in its various incarnations, four in all, is also covered at some length.

Commissions appointed to address specific issues of relevance to epilepsy are also discussed, perhaps most importantly those which have helped to establish classifications of the epileptic seizures and epilepsy syndromes, an endeavour in which Henri Gastaut played a significant role (he also wrote extensively, but with varying conclusions, on Dostoevsky's epilepsy). More recently, the Global Campaign Against Epilepsy, a joint endeavour with the World Health Organisation and the International Bureau for Epilepsy (IBE), an organisation for lay individuals which has shared many of the goals of ILAE, has been of major significance. The ILAE history is closely bound up with that of IBE. Amalgamation of the two bodies was planned for many years, the joint organisation to be called Epilepsy International, but when it came to a vote of the membership in Kyoto in 1981, the proposal was rejected.

Perhaps it is inevitable that all institutional histories run some risk of self-indulgence, perhaps because of limited general interest (only 1000 copies of this book were printed). Nonetheless, one admires the level of scholarship devoted to this book, in terms of searching through the existing archives, in which endeavour one intuits that Simon Shorvon, a prolific author on the subject of epilepsy, has taken the leading role. He and his colleagues are to be congratulated on a beautifully produced volume, undoubtedly a labour of love rather than a potential bestseller.

Acknowledgement

Adapted from: Larner AJ. *Medical Historian* 2009–2010;21:93–97.

References

1. Larner AJ. "Neurological literature": epilepsy. *Adv Clin Neurosci Rehabil* 2007;7(3):16.
2. Ford SF, Larner AJ. Neurology at the movies. *Adv Clin Neurosci Rehabil* 2009;9(4):48–49.
3. Stirling J. *Representing epilepsy. Myth and matter.* Liverpool: Liverpool University Press, 2010.
4. Larner AJ. Dostoevsky and epilepsy. *Adv Clin Neurosci Rehabil* 2006;6(1):26.
5. Sykes AH. Dr J Birkbeck Nevins – sage of Liverpool. *Medical Historian* 2008–2009;20:85–101.
6. Sykes AH. Dr William Carter – a medical life in Victorian Liverpool. *Medical Historian* 2009–2010;21:49–61.
7. Larner AJ. Margiad Evans (1909–1958): a history of epilepsy in a creative writer. *Epilepsy Behav* 2009;16:596–598.

8.   Larner AJ. Has Shakespeare's Iago deceived again? http://bmj.com/cgi/elet-
     ters/333/7582/1335, 2 January 2007.
9.   Cosnett JE. Charles Dickens and epilepsy. *Epilepsia* 1994;35:903–905.
10. Gordon L. *Lives like loaded guns: Emily Dickinson and her family's feuds.*
     London: Virago Press, 2010.
11. Shorvon S, Weiss G, Avanzini G et al. *International League Against Epilepsy
     1909–2009. A centenary history.* Chichester: Wiley-Blackwell, 2009.

7. Histories of Scottish medicine

During a visit to Aberdeen to lecture at the Royal Infirmary, I chanced upon *A
surgical revolution. Surgery in Scotland 1837–1901* by Peter Jones,[1] a retired
Aberdeen surgeon and medical historian. His book covers the period of Queen
Victoria's reign, 64 years which saw a transformation in the practice of surgery,
principally through the advent of anaesthesia and of antisepsis. The infre-
quency of surgical operations before this time (e.g. two per week on average at
Aberdeen Royal Infirmary in the early 1840s; p.14) is testament to the hazards
involved and the unwillingness of both surgeons and patients to risk the knife
in all but the most desperate of circumstances.

The development of anaesthesia in the late 1840s and early 1850s, and the
role of James Young Simpson of Edinburgh in the development of chloroform
anaesthesia, is carefully contextualised, including the role of David Waldie, by
then practising in Liverpool.[2] In this discourse I was intrigued to learn of the
use of ether by a Dr Scott in Dumfries, even before Liston's more celebrated
public demonstration in London (p.34). Scott apparently learned of the
Boston trials of ether from a Dr William Fraser who had witnessed its use, and
who travelled on the *Acadia* which first brought the news of anaesthesia to the
United Kingdom, docking in Liverpool on 16 December 1846. It is of course
well known that the first announcement of Morton's demonstration of ether in
Boston is to be found in the weekly supplement to the *Liverpool Mercury* of
Friday 18 December 1846 ("A method of mitigating pain in surgical operations
by inhalation of certain ethers has been discovered in America, and it is said
that successful experiments have been made") and that use of ether had been
demonstrated in Liverpool by December 1846–January 1847.[3,4]

Antisepsis attracts more extensive coverage than anaesthesia, principally
because this revolution began north of the border through the work of Joseph
Lister, initially in Glasgow and later in Edinburgh. Even before this, however,
there were surgical "advocates of cleanliness" including Thomas Keith (1827–
1895) in Edinburgh who became a skilled ovariotomist in the early 1860s.
Through his careful recording of all his patients, he is also accorded
the distinction of being a forerunner of surgical audit (pp.62–65), as is the

unrelated William Keith of Aberdeen who developed the operation of lithotomy for bladder stone (pp.16–23).

Lister's work is carefully documented, not only antisepsis but also the experimental researches conducted with his wife, Agnes (née Syme, daughter of James Syme, professor of surgery in Edinburgh before Lister). Perhaps no less significant in the development of modern surgery, but less familiar, is Lister's work in the development of catgut as a suture material (p.95).

Although Lister dominates the book, some other remarkable figures emerge. In Aberdeen, Alexander Ogston did pioneering work in the field of microbiology, wherein he is credited with the first identification of *Staphylococcus aureus*. As a neurologist, I was inevitably fascinated by William Macewen's development of neurosurgery in Glasgow, including the credit of being the first to remove an intracranial tumour, an honour sometimes bestowed on Rickman Godlee (incidentally Lister's nephew and an early biographer).

Well written and handsomely illustrated, many of the images being photographs taken by the author, this book is to be recommended to anyone with an interest in the history of surgery. There is, perhaps inevitably, no patient perspective on the experience of surgery, to which end it might have been worth including material from WE Henley's (1849–1903) collection of poems *In Hospital* (1875; e.g. poem V, *Operation*) reflecting the many months (1873–5) he spent under Lister's care in Edinburgh Royal Infirmary.

Early in his career, in 1854, Lister was asked to take on the course of lectures due to be delivered by Dr Mackenzie in Edinburgh when the latter succumbed to cholera in the Crimea, a theatre of war which attracted many medical volunteers, including Spencer Wells, a pioneering ovariotomist who corresponded with Thomas Keith. Another such civilian volunteer[5] was Dr David Greig (1832–1890), a native of Dundee and an Edinburgh graduate (1853). During his time away (1854–6), Greig corresponded regularly with his family in Dundee, letters which only came to light during a recent house clearance, and which have now been published under the editorship of Douglas Hill.[6]

For many people, the Crimean War *is* Florence Nightingale, but although Greig travelled to Constantinople on the same vessel as Nightingale, the *Vectis*, and worked for a time at Scutari, she barely surfaces in his narrative. Accounts of Greig's medical duties feature somewhat less than travelogue, perhaps understandably considering the audience for his letters, but nonetheless he is clear about the origins of the ill health he saw:

People at home think we have nothing but sabre cuts and gunshot wounds, but that is a great mistake. Sickness which prevails in the Crimea is far worse than Russian bullets. (p.34)

... our poor men ... are suffering unknown hardships and being extirpated by degrees by sickness and not by wounds. (p.49)

Indeed, one of Greig's companions on the outward voyage, Dr Alexander Struthers, died of typhoid fever (pp.ix,40,50; cf. vii) within three months of their arrival, as did another friend, Dr Mason. Greig himself then fell ill with typhus (p.62). One can only imagine the anxiety of his family when receiving letters, from another doctor, informing them "that should our dear friend be taken away from us you may not be unprepared for the severe blow" (p.63).

After his recovery, Greig was present at the siege of Sebastopol (*sic*, in Greig's letters) in his role of "Assistant Surgeon". His work involved "trench duty", 24–hour spells at the Surgeon's hut every few days to attend to the wounded (e.g. pp.89–90, 107). This might on occasion involve surgery: "I had one amputation at the shoulder joint and another at the forearm" (p.94). Despite his Edinburgh training, Greig makes no mention of chloroform, perhaps a reflection of the notorious policy of Dr John Hall, Principal Medical Officer in the Crimea, who had advised against its use ("for however barbarous it may appear, the smart of the knife is a powerful stimulant; and it is much better to hear a man bawl lustily than to see him sink silently into the grave"), although of course there were those who did use it in this theatre of war.[7]

On the occasion of the fall of Sebastopol, Greig estimates seeing 2000 patients within 2–3 hours (p.123; at the conservative estimate, that would be 11 patients seen per minute). Trench duty might be avoided by travelling with the wounded, when the field hospitals were full, in ambulance carts to Balaclava (p.93). Perhaps surprisingly, only occasional cases of cholera are mentioned (pp.95, 157). Medical duties also required attendance at floggings, "in case the prisoner turns ill or faint" (pp.84, 142).

Toward the end of 1855, Greig was appointed Pathologist, a member of a pathological board (p.157) and hence exempted from regimental duties. "My duties now are something like a country practitioner ... [I] trot away to whatever regiment requires me to visit it ... I have to write out all my cases and enter them in a great big book" (p.161). With the making of peace and the gradual departure of the regiments, Greig was left with little to do (p.200). He eventually returned home, to set up practice in Dundee where he became surgeon to the Infirmary (although he does not appear in Jones's book). He died in 1890, following a return visit to Scutari, where he apparently contracted typhoid fever from which he later died (although this is not mentioned in his obituary[8]).

Greig's correspondence is a fascinating account of the experience of war at first-hand, with much incidental detail about matters of crucial personal importance (e.g. food, housing, the receipt of letters) which figure little if at all in official histories. This perspective may be at odds with reportage, and Greig is sometimes scathing about what he reads in the newspapers sent to him by his family, including *The Times* (pp.106,131,152).

One of David Greig's sponsors for the post in the Crimea was Professor James Young Simpson (1811–1870), presumably one of Greig's teachers in Edinburgh (pp.10,13). Morrice McCrae's biography of Simpson,[9] which appears to be the first scholarly biography devoted to Simpson to be published since the 1970s, examines his many medical interests, most notable of which was his pioneering role in anaesthesia, particularly the discovery of chloroform (David Waldie's bit part in the story is acknowledged, pp.117–9). Considering the long duration of drug development which is normative today, it is astonishing to consider the rapidity with which chloroform was introduced: first tested by Simpson and his assistants, Matthews Duncan and Keith, on 4 November 1857, Simpson used it in his obstetric practice on 8 November, announced the discovery to the Edinburgh Medico-Chirurgical Society on 10 November, and published observations in the *Lancet* on 21 November. Such was his consequent renown that he was even mentioned in a review by Dickens published in February 1848 (not cited by McCrae):

> Just as Queen Victoria ... bespeaks, towards the happy introduction of another approaching body, the services of ... Professor Simson [*sic*] of Edinburgh ...[10]

The dark side of chloroform (familiar from Stephanie Snow's work[11]) is also made apparent from the fact that Simpson' wife, Jessie (née Grindlay, born Toxteth Park, Liverpool), took to inhaling it (pp.147, 220) and may indeed have died from "chloroform syncope" (pp.232–3).

Simpson's life was, of course, more than simply chloroform: he maintained a large and lucrative clinical practice as well as his teaching commitments, penned many publications, not only addressing medical but also archaeological questions, and was obviously an important power broker in the vicious (and often libellous) Edinburgh medical scene of the day, James Syme (Lister's father-in-law) being a particular rival. His writings on cholera, "hospitalism", and medical reform are all covered at some length. Although based in part on previous biographies, the work has been informed by the author's reading of Simpson's extant correspondence held by the Royal College of Surgeons of Edinburgh.

Simpson's role in sponsoring doctors to go to the Crimean War is alluded to (p.178), as is Dr Richard Mackenzie who, unlike David Greig, did apparently take supplies of chloroform to the Crimea and used them despite Dr Hall's directives (p.125).

Although not mentioned in the context of the Crimea, "Dr Greig of Dundee" does appear, in January 1860, as one prepared to give a trial to Simpson's method of acupressure (p.205), designed to staunch intra- and post-operative blood loss and thereby reduce the risk of surgical fever which accounted for so many post-operative deaths during this period. The method, vigorously opposed by Syme, was later superseded entirely by Listerian antisepsis.

The various topics of relevance to Simpson are well contextualised making this a generally satisfying read, with good illustrations. The book is marred only by irritating errors of typography (e.g. Appendix II, p.247, has the same title as Appendix I, p.237; a 2004 biography of William Pitt is ascribed to "W Haig", which should surely be "W Hague"?; there is misordering of works in the Bibliography, pp.272, 273), inconsistencies (an attack on Simpson's discovery of chloroform is dated to March 1857, p.153, some seven months before the actual discovery on 4 November 1857, p.119), and frank errors, most egregiously the description of Erasmus Darwin as the father, rather than grandfather, of Charles Darwin (p.260n5). Hopefully these shortcomings might be corrected in a revised edition.

Acknowledgement

Adapted from: Larner AJ. *Medical Historian* 2010–2011;22:45–50.

References

1. Jones PF. *A surgical revolution. Surgery in Scotland 1837–1901*. Edinburgh: John Donald, 2007.
2. Florence AM. David Waldie and the chloroform scene in Liverpool. *The History of Anaesthesia Society Proceedings* 1997;21:30–34.
3. Gray TC. Whatever happened to Felix Yaniewicz? *J R Soc Med* 1978;71:292–299.
4. Florence AM. Some Liverpool firsts in medicine. *Medical Historian* 2008–2009;20:11–29.
5. Shepherd J. Civilian surgeons and hospitals in the Crimean War. *Medical Historian* 1989;2:27–30.
6. Hill D (ed.). *Letters from the Crimea. Writing home, a Dundee doctor*. Dundee: Dundee University Press, 2010.
7. Connor H. The use of chloroform by British Army surgeons during the Crimean War. *Med Hist* 1998;42:161–193.
8. Anon. David Greig, M.D., F.R.C.S.Edin., J.P. *BMJ* 1890;2:56.
9. McCrae M. *Simpson. The turbulent life of a medical pioneer*. Edinburgh: Birlinn, 2011.

10. Slater M. *The Dent uniform edition of Dickens' journalism. Volume 2: The amusements of the people and other papers. Reports, essays and reviews 1834–51.* London, JM Dent, 1996, p.88.
11. Snow S. Poison, myth and fear: the dark side of chloroform in Victorian Britain. *Medical Historian* 2007–2008;19:17.

8. Dickens and the workhouse

It was inevitable that the bicentenary of the birth of Charles Dickens (1812–1870) would be attended with a variety of publications to celebrate the writer's anniversary, notable amongst which is the biography by Claire Tomalin.[1] The breadth of Dickens's concerns, as reflected in his novels and journalism, was very extensive and included medical topics. At his death in 1870, the *Lancet* praised Dickens for his efforts to ameliorate conditions in workhouse infirmaries,[2] whilst the *British Medical Journal* noted the accuracy of his descriptions of certain medical conditions.[4] Hence, Dickens is of interest to historians of medicine.[4-6]

In his lecture to the Liverpool Medical History Society, delivered 18 April 2012, Sir Iain Chalmers mentioned in passing not only that he was born in Liverpool but also that he had trained in medicine at the Middlesex Hospital, an institution which is now no more than a "hole in the ground".[7] Although this is true of the main hospital, one part in fact does still remain, namely the old Annexe and Outpatient Department on Cleveland Street. This building is the focus of Ruth Richardson's book,[8] since it is her belief that this is the building which, in an earlier guise, namely the Cleveland Street Workhouse, inspired Dickens's descriptions of workhouse life in his novel *Oliver Twist, or, The Parish Boy's Progress* (1838). Dickens visited, and wrote about, other London workhouses in subsequent years, at Marylebone in 1850 (not identified as such in the original publication)[9] and at Wapping in 1860,[10] so evidently workhouses were a subject of continuing concern to him. His descriptions of the plight of epileptics in the workhouse have attracted recent attention.[11]

Some of Dickens's early years, 1815–1817 and 1829–1831, were lived at 10 Norfolk Street, which is now part of Cleveland Street and only a few doors away from the site of the workhouse. This early residence is apparently largely neglected in standard Dickens biographies, possibly because Dickens himself chose to say little about these particular social origins, as with his menial work in the blacking factory undertaken initially when his father was imprisoned for bankruptcy. Ruth Richardson suggests that during this time Dickens may have encountered other young employees, parish apprentices, with inside information about the Cleveland Street Workhouse. Furthermore, during his second period of residence in Norfolk Street, by which time his career as a short-hand writer was taking off, he may have learned more about the workings of the workhouse from local tradespeople, including his landlord, Mr Dodd.

As anyone familiar with Ruth Richardson's works would anticipate, much fascinating circumstantial evidence in support of these suggestions is adduced. There is much about the topography of this area of London, as well as about Dickens's early life there, the New Poor Law of 1834 and its workings, and the intersection of these factors, particularly what use Dickens may have made of his early experiences in his fiction, most particularly in *Oliver Twist*. For example, the author cites (p.260) the use of local street names for fictional characters in the book, to which I would venture to suggest a further addition, first noted when I worked at Queen Square in London: could Brownlow Mews, parallel to Doughty Street, whither Dickens moved in 1837, about the time he was writing *Twist*, have been the origin for the name of Oliver's protector, Mr Brownlow (the Mews acting as a Muse, as it were)? This Dickensian tendency to co-opt names extended beyond streets, for example both Pickwick and Bardell refer to modes of public transportation in and around London.[12]

The whole is compellingly written and beautifully produced and illustrated, in part with photographs taken by the author. The style is chatty and discursive, appropriate to a popular history, as encountered in the author's previous book on Henry Gray and his famous Anatomy.[13] However, Ruth Richardson cannot entirely forego the rigorous scholarship of the professional historian, so evident in her seminal work on *Death, dissection, and the destitute*[14] (the Anatomy Act of 1832 is briefly discussed here as well). She bemoans her lack of opportunity to pursue all the sources (e.g. reading articles in back issues of *The Dickensian*) and indicates where further work is needed, work which she would no doubt have done herself were it not for the demands of publication deadlines related to the Dickensian anniversary. The book is liberally, rather than densely, footnoted (the footnotes go briefly awry, at Chapter 9, p.258 n28). Nevertheless, because of the many lacunae in the historical record, this is in many ways a work of imagination, of informed speculation, rather than dry historical scholarship (count the number of usages of might have been/could have been/must have been/possibly). The thesis is not, and probably cannot be, proven.

The campaign to save the Cleveland Street Workhouse from the same fate as the Middlesex Hospital succeeded, at least in part because of the work documented in this book, so the author merits the congratulations of posterity for both this and her book, achievements which will further stimulate Dickens scholarship for years to come.

Acknowledgement

Adapted from: Larner AJ. *Medical Historian* 2011–2012;23:57–59.

References

1. Tomalin C. *Charles Dickens. A life*. London, Viking, 2011.
2. Anonymous. Charles Dickens. *Lancet* 1870;i:882.
3. Anonymous. Charles Dickens. *BMJ* 1870;i:636.
4. Dauber LG. Dickens and doctors: physicians in fiction of Charles Dickens. *NY State J Med* 1981;81:1522–6.
5. Andrews M. Dickens and the medical profession. *NZ Med J* 1985;98:810–3.
6. Cosnett JE. Dickens and doctors: vignettes of Victorian medicine. *BMJ* 1992;305:1540–2.
7. Chalmers I. The evolution of controlled trials before the middle of the 20th century. *Medical Historian* 2011–2012;23:23–4.
8. Richardson R. *Dickens & the workhouse. Oliver Twist & the London Poor*. Oxford: Oxford University Press, 2012.
9. Slater M (ed.). *Dickens' Journalism. Volume 2. The amusements of the people and other papers: reports, essays and reviews 1834–51*. London, JM Dent, 1996, pp.234–41.
10. Slater M, Drew J (eds.). *Dickens' Journalism. Volume 4. "The Uncommercial Traveller" and other papers 1859–70*. London, JM Dent, 2000, pp.41–51.
11. Larner AJ. Charles Dickens (1812–1870) and epilepsy. *Epilepsy Behav* 2012;24: 422–5.
12. Grossman JH. *Charles Dickens's networks. Public transport and the novel*. Oxford: Oxford University Press, 2012, pp.77, 228n67.
13. Richardson R. *The making of Mr Gray's Anatomy*. Oxford: Oxford University Press, 2008
14. Richardson R. *Death, dissection, and the destitute*. London: Routledge & Kegan Paul, 1987.

9. Memory: patient HM

It is an axiom of the neuropsychological understanding of brain function that an individual suffering from a dense anterograde amnesia (i.e. an inability to consolidate and store any new memories) could not narrate their own history, since they would have no memory traces to retrieve. Despite this, some imaginative and engaging attempts to portray anterograde amnesia have appeared, such as Christopher Nolan's film *Memento* (2000) and SJ Watson's novel *Before I go to sleep* (2011),[1] also filmed. (Many less credible movie portrayals of amnesia have also appeared.[2]) Both these literary and filmic conceits are acknowledged to have been based, at least in part, on the case of one patient with anterograde amnesia, a patient denoted in the medical literature as "HM", and revealed after his death in December 2008 to be Henry Gustave Molaison (1926–2008). The story of HM is told by the researcher, Suzanne Corkin,[3] who had the extreme good fortune ("Henry's case fell into my lap"; p.xiv) to study him for over forty years, after his initial description in the medical literature by Brenda Milner (with whom Corkin later worked) and William Beecher Scoville, the surgeon whose operation caused HM's amnesia.[4]

The basic facts of HM's life are well-known. He developed epilepsy at the age of ten. His seizures eventually became intractable to the anti-epileptic drugs then available. At age twenty-seven, in 1953, he underwent surgery to try to relieve his seizures using the relatively new and experimental technique of bilateral anterior temporal lobe resection, with some success in terms of seizure control, but with the unanticipated complication of a memory disorder which meant that he could lay down no new memories from the time of his surgery: "experiences slipped out of his consciousness seconds after they happened", hence he lived in the "permanent present tense" of the book's title (a patient with a similar dense amnesia is described by Oliver Sacks as having "lost … his moorings in time"[5,6]). HM never managed to live independently, but became an apparently willing research subject, a highly unusual but instructive case study which the practitioners of cognitive neuropsychology could probe to infer mental structure based on neuropsychological test performance. (A very good recent account of HM's importance to the understanding of memory is that of Moscovitch.[7])

HM's case showed unequivocally that the hippocampus, a structure in the medial temporal lobe which was largely removed in his surgery, was critical for memory function, specifically for the consolidation and storage of experiences (autobiographical memory) and facts (semantic memory). But memory is not a unitary function, and studies of HM also permitted a deeper understanding of the fractionation of memory functions. These may be broadly divided into declarative memory (Ryle's "knowing that") and non-declarative or procedural or implicit memory ("knowing how"). Corkin documents some of the many studies she and her collaborators undertook on HM, for example demonstrating retention of familiarity but loss of recollection, and preservation of (non-declarative) motor skill learning and priming, and some aspects of spatial memory, reflecting function in preserved brain areas outside the hippocampus. Contrary to some textbook accounts and simplistic teaching, HM also had a significant retrograde amnesia, in particular for autobiographical material, reflecting the importance of the hippocampus in the retrieval of such memories. The book's neuropsychological detail is leavened with information about Henry the man, his day-to-day life, his carers, his interests, his sayings, so giving a flavour of personality to the dry factual presentation contained in the academic publications concerning him.

Suzanne Corkin's account of the man she knew for 46 years is thus a hybrid: it probably has too much science for the popular reader wanting to know about HM, and not enough science for the cognitive neurologist wanting to know about memory function, a hybridity perhaps indicating an authorial desire to appeal to two markets (certainly the book has been reviewed in the broadsheet press). Because HM himself left no record – he "could not construct an autobiography as his life unfolded" (p.235) – the narrative becomes rather more concerned with the narrator and her work than the subject of the narration (as in other accounts of amnesic individuals, e.g. Clive Wearing[8]).

Corkin eventually became HM's "sole keeper" (p.206). She carefully guarded his anonymity for many years, some might say jealously guarded access to him since many research proposals to study HM were rejected by Corkin. Laudable though this regard may be, in this context I admit to having felt some disquiet about the publicity surrounding HM's death: a PBS film crew is on hand to document the journey of HM's brain to the airport to be despatched to San Diego for further study (p.299); another film crew has been hired to witness the slicing of the brain in San Diego several months later, a function to which several scientific luminaries (some with no interest in memory studies) have been invited (p.300). The book ends in December 2012, more than 4 years after HM's death, with still no final neuropathological diagnosis disclosed and the promised online access to the complete neuropathology resource not yet available (http://thebrainobservatory. ucsd.edu/hm, accessed 23/11/13). However, these quibbles aside, it is certainly true that "the man with no memory" will not be forgotten in the annals of clinical neuropsychology for the insights his personal tragedy afforded to the workings of memory function.

Having read Suzanne Corkin's book, I thought it might be redundant to consult the book by Luke Dittrich[9] on HM, a journalist rather than a clinician or scientist. However, I believe this book is in fact a critical counterpoint to Corkin's personal and scientific biography of her patient. Dittrich has (at least) two points of contact with HM, although he never met him during life: firstly, his mother was a childhood friend of Suzanne Corkin, and secondly it was Dittrich's maternal grandfather, William Beecher Scoville, who undertook the bilateral anterior temporal lobectomy operation in August 1953 which inadvertently led to Henry's amnesia.[4]

As this book's subtitle implies, there is far more here than just HM: for example, there are detours into the history of Phineas Gage and of Walter Freeman's lobotomy techniques. Using a different (neurosurgical) methodology to Freeman, William Beecher Scoville was, following Freeman, a keen proponent of lobotomy for mental illness ("psychosurgery") and it was this methodology that led him to propose the surgical approach to HM which had such unanticipated and revelatory results. The material on Scoville, drawing on family lore and interviews with some who knew him (Brenda Milner, Karl Pribram, Dennis Spencer), is, to my knowledge, not available elsewhere.

The "post-mortem" of Dittrich's book answers some of the questions left outstanding in Corkin's book. The long wait for publication of HM's neuropathology, previously noted, finally ended in January 2014, more than 5 years after HM's death.[10] The delay appears to have been occasioned, at least in part, by wrangling between Corkin and the pathologist (chosen by her), Jacopo Annese, concerning the final destination of HM's brain, with eventual recourse to legal action. The exact pathological findings, showing preservation of some parts of the hippocampus, were possibly also a bone of contention.

Dittrich also has issues with respect to Corkin's handling of HM and his affairs, which some might see as effective ownership of a precious scientific resource. She allowed no one to record or photograph HM, hence perhaps the jacket image of this book showing HM but with his face cut out. Dittrich also raises questions about the arrangements made for HM's conservatorship, with someone who was (possibly) not his next of kin. Corkin denied Dittrich's request to meet HM (as with all such requests), and in his interview with Corkin Dittrich portrays her as evasive and as stating that records of HM's neuropsychological assessments performed in her department were to be destroyed rather than archived. In light of this, it is perhaps unsurprising that this book was not published until after Suzanne Corkin's death in May 2016. An August 2016 *New York Times* article abstracted from Dittrich's book has drawn a vigorous rebuttal in defence of Suzanne Corkin from many scientists.[11]

Evidently, as with all historical accounts, those of HM are partial and contingent, and hence open to differences of interpretation. For those wanting to learn about HM I suggest that reading of both Corkin and Dittrich is necessary. The latter book suffers a little from lack of images and I would have liked inclusion of references to some of the medical literature cited, as well as a bibliography, but I guess this reflects its target audience (popular rather than scientific). The medical material is handled well, considering the non-clinical background of the author, although the use of "petit mal" to describe HM's partial seizures (pp.203, 208, 209, 210, 299) is jarring.

Acknowledgement

Adapted from: Larner AJ. *Medical Historian* 2014;24:81–83 and *Medical Historian* 2018;28:71–73.

References

1.   Watson SJ. *Before I go to sleep.* London: Doubleday, 2011.
2.   Ford SF, Larner AJ. Neurology at the movies. *Adv Clin Neurosci Rehabil* 2009;9(4):48–49.
3.   Corkin S. *Permanent present tense. The man with no memory and what he taught the world.* London: Allen Lane, 2013.
4.   Scoville W, Milner B. Loss of recent memory after bilateral hippocampal lesions. *J Neurol Neurosurg Psychiatry* 1957;20:11–21.
5.   Sacks O. The lost mariner. In: *The man who mistook his wife for a hat.* London: Picador, 1985, p.22–41 [at 22].
6.   Hunter KM. *Doctors' stories. The narrative structure of medical knowledge.* Princeton: Princeton University Press, 1991, p.164.
7.   Moscovitch M. Memory before and after H.M.: an impressionistic historical perspective. In: Zeman A, Kapur N, Jones-Gotman M (eds.) *Epilepsy and memory.* Oxford: Oxford University Press, 2012, pp.19–50.
8.   Wearing D. *Forever today. A memoir of love and amnesia.* London: Corgi, 2005.
9.   Dittrich L. *Patient H.M. A story of memory, madness and family secrets.* London: Chatto & Windus, 2016.
10. Annese J, Schenker-Ahmed NM, Bartsch H et al. Postmortem examination of patient H.M.'s brain based on histological sectioning and digital 3D reconstruction. *Nat Commun* 2014;5:3122 (doi: 10.1038/ncomms4122).
11. http://news.mit.edu/2016/faculty-defend-suzanne-corkin-0809 (accessed 24/02/17).

10. American Civil War

The many commemorations of the centenary of the outbreak of the 1st World War in the United Kingdom have understandably overshadowed the anniversary of another cataclysmic military conflict – the sesquicentenary of the end of the American Civil War (1861–5). A commemorative volume, edited by three academics from Liverpool,[1] contributes to this anniversary, focussing "on the wounded and on medical practice" (p.1). The book's launch coincided with a small but informative exhibition entitled *Life and Limb* which ran from April 16th to June 20th 2015 at 19 Abercromby Square, Liverpool (a US Library of Medicine travelling exhibition).

The book combines first-hand accounts of Civil War medicine and nursing, some written contemporaneously and some from the post-war perspective. In addition, each section of the book intercalates more extended pieces written by academics with an interest in the Civil War, such that the volume is part anthology and part commentary.

It features material from authors well known to posterity who became embroiled in the war, such as Louisa May Alcott, Walt Whitman, and Ambrose Bierce, as well as Stephen Crane although he was not born until after the war. In addition there are contributions from what might be termed "rank-and-file" combatants and practitioners. Notable clinicians active during and writing on the war include physicians such as Austin Flint (cardiology) and Silas Weir Mitchell (neurology; it has been previously argued that the "rise of the new specialism of neurology ..[had] .. roots in the clinical opportunities presented by the Civil War"[2]), and the surgeon Roberts Bartholow (incorrectly given here as "Bartholomew"; now recognised as a pioneer of electrical brain stimulation techniques akin to those used today in the treatment of some neurological disorders[3]).

The overriding medical image, as implied by the book's title, is that of amputation. It is estimated that some 60000 amputations took place during the War, as a consequence of trauma (the devastating effects of the Minié bullet) and of wounds becoming gangrenous. An ineluctable consequence was the boost to the manufacturers of limb prostheses, and examples of recommendations and testimonials for these products are included (pp.123,127). Weir Mitchell's work on phantom limbs, the sensation that all or more commonly part of an amputated limb was still present, is obviously also pertinent here. He recognised that this phenomenon must ultimately be mediated by the brain (p.148), but it was not until the latter part of the 20th century that the subject of phantom limbs once again captured significant medical attention, giving important insights into brain function and plasticity. [4]

The book is nicely presented and handsomely illustrated with both figures and plates. It bears similarities in form with David Seed's earlier edited anthology on *American Travellers in Liverpool* (Liverpool University Press, 2008). *Life and Limb* may find a welcome niche in the library of anyone with an interest in medical history and of the American Civil War in particular.

Acknowledgement

Adapted from: Larner AJ. *Medical Historian* 2016;26:83–84.

References

1.   Seed D, Kenny SC, Williams C (eds.). *Life and limb. Perspectives on the American Civil War*. Liverpool: Liverpool University Press, 2015.
2.   Scull A. The social history of psychiatry in the Victorian era. In: Scull A (ed.). *Madhouses, mad-doctors, and madmen. The social history of psychiatry in the Victorian era*. Philadelphia: University of Pennsylvania Press, 1981, pp 5–32 [at 17].

3. Cambiaghi S, Sandrone S. Robert [sic] Bartholow (1831–1904). *J Neurol* 2014;261:1649–50.
4. Ramachandran VS, Blakeslee S. *Phantoms in the brain. Human nature and the architecture of the mind.* London: Fourth Estate, 1998.

11. Lancaster

This slim volume[1] explores the medical history of the city of Lancaster during the 19th century, based on the concept that a "community of practice amongst a few medical professionals shaped Lancaster's medical landscape" (p.3–4).

Its eight chapters chart the evolution of various medical institutions, including the Dispensary, the Lancaster Medical Book Club, the House of Recovery, the Infirmary, and the Asylum, as well as examining the local consequences of the seminal advances of the era, in anaesthesia, germ theory, and antiseptic surgical practice. Although most medical practitioners of that era are now long forgotten, some had significant influence beyond the locality (and beyond medical practice), and two in particular are discussed at some length, Sir Richard Owen (1804–1892) and Sir William Turner (1832–1916), biographical vignettes which are based in part on papers published in the *Journal of Medical Biography.*[2,3]

Whilst some of these contributions might be considred as solely of parochial interest, this is decidedly not so for Lancaster Asylum, opened in 1816, which served the county of Lancashire. The large increase in admissions to this Asylum over the 19th century is discussed, and the relative merits of industrialisation and Irish immigration[4] as causes of this increase are presented. Of particular interest to this reviewer[5] is the discussion of the role of Samuel Gaskell and Edward de Vitre in transforming the administrartive regime at the Asylum to a more humane footing ("moral treatment") which was gradually adopted nationally, not least through Gaskell's role as a Commissioner in Lunacy in the 1850s and 1860s.

Edited by Quenton Wessels, an anatomist in Lancaster with an interest in local medical history, the book is nicely presented, but regrettably there are many typographical errors which, for me, detracted from the pleasure of reading, the impression being that the book would have benefitted from a careful proof-reading. Comparisons with contemporary developments in other cities, such as Liverpool, might also have been of interest, to help ascertain which changes were common to the era covered and which were particular to Lancaster.

Acknowledgement

Adapted from: Larner AJ. *Medical Historian* 2017;27:49–50.

References

1. Wessels Q (ed.). *The Medical Pioneers of Nineteenth Century Lancaster*. Berlin: epubli GmbH, 2016.
2. Wessels Q, Taylor AM. Anecdotes to the life and times of Sir Richard Owen (1804–1892) in Lancaster. *J Med Biogr* 2017;25:226–233.
3. Wessels Q, Correia JC, Taylor AM. Sir William Turner (1832–1916) – Lancastrian, anatomist and champion of the Victorian era. *J Med Biogr* 2016;24:500–506.
4. Cox C, Marland H. Itineraries of insanity: madness, migration and the Irish in Lancashire, c.1850–1900. *Medical Historian* 2011–2012;23:19–20.
5. Larner AJ. Dr Samuel Gaskell (1807–1886): a brief biography, and thoughts on his possible influence on Elizabeth Gaskell's writings. *Gaskell Society Newsletter* 2016;62:11–18.

12. Smallpox: Benjamin Jesty

The history of smallpox vaccination has attracted much attention over many years, not least because this discovery set in motion a process which eventually resulted in the global eradication of the disease, one of the undoubted pinnacles of medical success. The origins of smallpox vaccination are usually attributed to Dr Edward Jenner (1749–1823), a Gloucestershire doctor, but certainly his work did not occur in isolation, and others have argued in favour of Benjamin Jesty (1736–1816), a Dorset farmer, not least when Jenner was being remunerated for his troubles by Parliament in the early 1800s, not without contention. Whilst Jenner has found lasting and universal fame, Jesty has remained relatively obscure.

Patrick J Pead's book[1] is the culmination of more than 30 years of research on Jesty,[2,3] following a chance encounter with the subject's tombstone in Worth Matravers churchyard in 1985. Jesty's vaccination of his wife and two young sons in 1774 predated Jenner's first attempt by more than 20 years (1796), prompting Pead to conclude that Jesty should be called the "Grandfather of vaccination". The author has assiduously tracked down all the sources, contemporary and secondary, making this a medical detective story, which has resulted in a comprehensive text. One outcome of these labours has been the rediscovery of Jesty's portrait, last seen outside the Jesty family in 1888 and found in South Africa in 2004. Subsequently the portrait was repatriated and restored under the auspices of the Wellcome Trust in London, where it is now housed.

A disclosure: the author of this review originates from Cirencester in Gloucestershire where Jenner had some of his schooling, and hence has had a long-standing interest in (and admiration for) Jenner, his work, and his circle.[4-6] Hence, it was a relief to find that this book is no idle point scoring for Jesty vs. Jenner; the latter's work is carefully considered. The fascinating question as to whether or not Jenner knew of Jesty's work but chose not to discuss or acknowledge it in his own publications, remains shrouded in mystery.

Patrick Pead must be congratulated for producing a highly readable and well-presented text, copiously but unobtrusively referenced, and complemented by over 100 illustrations. To be sure, there are some very occasional errors, e.g. Saunders book on Jenner is dated as 1882, not 1982 (p.208); another Jenner biographer is given as "D Fisher" rather than "RB Fisher" (pp.221–3); and it is corneal, rather than retinal, transplants that have been associated on occasion with the subsequent development of Creutzfeldt-Jakob disease (p.100). Notwithstanding these minor lapses, which do not detract from the flow of the text, I would suggest that this is the work against which any future Jesty biography will require comparison.

Acknowledgement

Adapted from: Larner AJ. *Medical Historian* 2017;27:51–52.

References

1. Pead PJ. *Benjamin Jesty. Grandfather of vaccination.* Chichester: Timefile Books, 2016.
2. Pead PJ. Benjamin Jesty: new light in the dawn of vaccination. *Lancet* 2003;362:2104–2109.
3. Pead PJ. The origins of vaccination: history is what you remember. *J R Soc Med* 2014;107:7.
4. Larner AJ. Smallpox. *N Engl J Med* 1996;335:901.
5. Larner AJ. Jenner, on the intellect. *Adv Clin Neurosci Rehabil* 2003;3(2):29.
6. Larner AJ. Caleb Hillier Parry (1755–1822): clinician, scientist, friend of Edward Jenner (1749–1823). *J Med Biogr* 2005;13:189–194.

13. Roald Dahl

2016 marked the centenary of the birth of the writer Roald Dahl (1916–1990) whose stories for children remain extremely popular even 25 years after his death. In this book,[1] Tom Solomon, who, working as a house physician in Oxford, came to know Dahl during his final illness in 1990, recalls his interactions with the author and examines Dahl's medical interests, based largely around ailments suffered by himself and various family members, and speculates on the potential impacts of these experiences on Dahl's writing.

Before any further review, some important disclosures. I have worked in the same department as a colleague of this book's author for the past 17 years. One of the charities to which royalties from the book are directed is one of the hospitals where we both work. Moreover, I have previously written on the subject of Dahl and his medical portrayals and interests.[2,3]

Those unfamiliar with Dahl's life (although he did of course publish volumes of autobiography[4,5]), as opposed to his work, may be interested to learn of his medical interests, although these were previously covered in Donald Sturrock's official biography published in 2010 (in which Tom Solomon is mentioned).[6] The material is presented here within the context of young Dr. Solomon's late night conversations with his patient Dahl, largely in the pedagogic mode and with detours into the author's own current research interests. It must be acknowledged as possible that with the passage of more than 25 years some of these memories may have become semanticized, if not inadvertently fictionalised.

Following an accident in which Dahl's son suffered a brain injury requiring a shunt operation, a procedure notoriously liable to complication due to shunt blockage, Dahl attempted to develop a new type of shunt valve. Working with the neurosurgeon Kenneth Till and the engineer Stanley Wade, the Wade-Dahl-Till (or WDT) valve emerged. Dahl's daughter tragically died of encephalitis, prompting an interest in this condition. His first wife, the Oscar-winning actress Patricia Neal, suffered a stroke rendering her aphasic, for which Dahl arranged intensive speech and language therapy.

It is possible that these experiences may have influenced some of Dahl's creative writing. For example, the speech patterns of one of Dahl's most noted creations, *The BFG* (1982), may owe something to Patricia Neal's aphasia. Solomon spots the possibility that one of Dahl's schoolteachers, Captain Hardcastle, may have suffered from Tourette syndrome (p.15) but does not seem aware of a literary parallel in the character of "Captain Lancaster", also a teacher, who appears in Dahl's book *Danny the champion of the world* (1975).[2]

As a pilot in the RAF during World War II, Dahl suffered a crash in which he sustained a head injury. Solomon argues that this injury may have caused some frontal lobe brain damage and hence released Dahl's creative writing abilities. Certainly neurologists are familiar with occasional patients who develop previously unknown creative abilities following brain disorders. (Another possible, Liverpool-related, example is the painter Augustus John, after whom a pub is named on the University campus, whose creative abilities are said to have been released following a head injury.) However, I'm not sure this formulation is tenable for Dahl, since it is clear that he was writing even as a schoolboy. Moreover, I think another possible, and more plausible, formulation has been missed by Solomon, although he does present evidence which may support it (p.68).

I have previously suggested (2010–11, although this failed to get accepted for publication) that Dahl had some characteristics suggestive of an obsessive-compulsive spectrum condition, albeit without tics. For example, when writing in his famous hut at the bottom of the garden at Gypsy House, he had to have a particular type of paper, lined yellow American Legal, and both a particular brand (Dixon Ticonderoga HB) and an even number of pencils ("because odd numbers were unlucky"), supplied by his publishers in the USA. When, in 1980, his publishers became unable to supply this particular type of pencil, but something "very similar" instead, Dahl wrote to say that the substitute pencils "don't have erasers on top. They are too hard. And they are the wrong colour" (see Sturrock, 2010: pp.269,286,378,504).

Dahl's desire for routine and order is further exemplified in an account given by his daughter, Tessa:

> He had a routine. Every single day of his life was the same. He got up at the same time, he took the children to school, he made his thermos of coffee, he went up to the hut, he worked to a certain time, he listened to *The World at One* [a radio news programme], he had his Bloody Mary, he had his second Bloody Mary, he had his lunch, he had his nap, he watched the horse racing, he put on his bets, he got up, he took his coffee back to the hut. He was up there till about quarter to six. He'd start sniffing the scotch at six, then he'd either drive up to London or he'd have supper at home, then he'd take the dogs out they'd go out and pee and he'd go to bed. Imagine disrupting that … he'd been doing that for over twenty years (see Sturrock, 2010: 462–463; my ellipsis).

In a short story, *The Wish*, Dahl described a child who was terrified of stepping on the cracks in the pavement or the wrong colour in the carpet. Dahl's biographer states that, like this child, the author had a premonition of disaster (Sturrock, 2010: 367). He also speaks of "an obsessive need" that Dahl had to clarify the storyline of *Charlie and the Chocolate Factory* (1964) (Sturrock, 2010: 396).

Although these scattered references cannot establish a diagnosis in the way that a formal consultation may do (and of course I may be subject here to the American Psychiatric Association's 1973 "Goldwater rule", forbidding diagnosing at a distance), nonetheless they are suggestive of behaviours seen in the obsessive-compulsive spectrum. Most might be described as impulsions, to distinguish them from obsessions and compulsions, namely repetitive behaviours which, unlike compulsions, are performed not to avoid harm or reduce anxiety but to achieve a sense of rightness, completion, or satisfaction. These behaviours do not seem to have impaired Dahl's productivity as a writer, indeed they may have facilitated it, and I would suggest they represent a more compelling explanation of his creativity than a response to traumatic brain injury.

The volume has been nicely produced by Liverpool University Press, but with some variability in the approach to spelling (e.g. Oompa Loompas p.196, Oompa-Lumpas p.197; neoligisms and neogolisms for neologisms, p.151). Considering the author's current appointment it is strange that he omits to mention that Dahl's consultant, and Solomon's boss in 1990, David Weatherall, held a chair in Liverpool prior to his move to Oxford (p.187).

Acknowledgement

Adapted from: Larner AJ. *Medical Historian* 2018;28:67–70.

References

1. Solomon T. *Roald Dahl's marvellous medicine*. Liverpool: Liverpool University Press, 2016.
2. Larner AJ. Three historical accounts of Gilles de la Tourette syndrome. *Adv Clin Neurosci Rehabil* 2003;3(5):26–27
3. Larner AJ. Tales of the unexpected: Roald Dahl's neurological contributions. *Adv Clin Neurosci Rehabil* 2008;8(1):22. [Reprinted, abridged, as: Tales of unexpected [*sic*]: Roald Dahl's neurological contributions. *The Encephalitis Society Newsletter* 2008;Autumn (number 44):12].
4. Dahl R. *Boy. Tales of childhood*. London, Puffin; 1984.
5. Dahl R. *Going solo*. London, Puffin; 2001.
6. Sturrock D. *Storyteller. The life of Roald Dahl*. London, Harper; 2010.

14. Metabiography?

Joseph Lister (1827–1912) is generally acknowledged as one of the most significant figures in medical history for his development of antiseptic surgery from the 1860s onwards. A testament to his enduring influence was the publication of many articles on the man and his work to mark the centenary of his death in 2012. He has attracted many previous biographers, a list to which Lindsey Fitzharris now adds her name.[1]

Lister's story is well-known: from Quaker roots he excelled at London University before surgical training and research in Scotland, where, coming under the influence of Pasteur's doctrines, he studied putrefaction in wounds and its prevention by means of antiseptic procedures, prompting epochal changes in surgical practice which faced initial resistance but which eventually gained universal acceptance.

This biography is nicely written, reads easily (for those untroubled by visceral detail), and has attracted reviews in the Sunday supplements, but to my knowledge tells us little about Lister which is new. I don't know if there is a specific name for the form of biography which is built largely or exclusively on previous biographies ("metabiography", perhaps?) but I think this may be an example.[2] Certainly the majority of the notes allude to previous biographers such as Rickman Godlee, Cameron, and Fisher. I'm not certain if any original research was undertaken to inform the book, although the acknowledgements note a "brilliant research assistant, whose tireless work in the archives around London helped bring color to Lister's story" (p.268).

Colour and immediacy may be generated by an omniscient narrator imputing the protagonist's mental states. This approach (e.g. Lister "remembered", "recognised", "made a split-second decision"), which owes much to theory of mind (our developmentally programmed belief that we can interpret or impute the mind states of others), troubles me in a work of biography, as probably not objective (unless there is a contemporary primary source which can be referenced, in which the protagonist specifically states "I remembered, recognised, made a split-second decision") and hence unjustifiable. I accept this is how many biographies are now written,[3] and is probably not an issue to many readers.

This book may serve as a readable introduction to Lister and his work. Disappointingly there are no illustrations and no bibliography.

Acknowledgement

Adapted from: Larner AJ. *Medical Historian* 2018;28:75–76.

References

1. Fitzharris L. *The butchering art. Joseph Lister's quest to transform the grisly world of Victorian medicine.* London: Allen Lane, 2017.
2. This comment betrayed my ignorance of the subject at the time of writing. Metabiography is a growing academic discipline, see, for example, Ní Dhúill C. *Metabiography. Reflecting on biography.* London: Palgrave Macmillan, 2020.
3. This is now generally referred to as biographical fiction, or biofiction.

15. Robert Burton: *The Anatomy of Melancholy*

Why read, and indeed review, a 400 year-old book?[1] Which was written by a man in holy orders, Robert Burton (1577–1640), rather than by a clinician or a scientist? And which does not apparently relate to a neurological subject? And which runs to over 1000 pages? Are there not enough contemporaneous documents for the clinical neurologist or neuroscientist to try to keep abreast of, without having recourse to ancient history?

And it is a tough assignment: it took me, admittedly a slow reader, about 7 months of occasional, opportunistic, linear reading to complete. Not only through the unfamiliarity of the conceptual frame, and the frequent recourse to Latin quotations (fortunately mostly translated), but also mechanically from manipulating this brick of a book in order to consult the editor's explanatory notes (which run to over 200 pages) to understand the breadth of cultural references, in addition to the author's own copious footnotes.

Some context is called for here, regarding both the timing and the methodology of the book. The first edition of *The Anatomy of Melancholy* appeared in 1621, hence this publication to coincide with the anniversary (which was also marked by an exhibition at the Bodleian Library in Oxford). Four further editions appeared during Burton's lifetime (1624, 1628, 1632, 1638) and a sixth edition was published posthumously in 1651. The writing of the *Anatomy* therefore spans the historical period of the reigns of King James I and King Charles I and extends to the cusp of the English Civil War, the horrors of which Burton was thankfully spared. The King James Bible (1611) was only 10 years old when the *Anatomy* first appeared and the publication of Shakespeare's First Folio (1623) had yet to occur, although some allusions to the playwright's works are included (likewise Ben Jonson). In the scientific world, Harvey's publication of his discovery of the circulation of the blood, *De Motu cordis* (1628), occurred during the years in which Burton was revising the *Anatomy*, but Harvey's time in Oxford (October 1642 to June 1646), which did much to establish the tradition of experimental physiology in the university,[2] postdates Burton's death. He was not therefore exposed to the new ideas about experimental method promulgated by Harvey and his successors in Oxford (e.g. Boyle, Hooke, Wilkins, Wren, Willis, Lower). Hence the absence of any reference, as far as I have noted, to Harvey in the *Anatomy* is unsurprising. Burton's intellectual world was still that of scholastic philosophy and of humoural pathophysiology, from which of course the notion of "Melancholia" derives.

Burton was evidently interested in the causes, symptoms, prognostics and cures of the various forms of melancholia which he identified (e.g. head melancholy, love melancholy, religious melancholy, the latter apparently his own innovation, but cf. Paulus Aegineta, 7th century CE[3]). Although authorial experience does creep in occasionally, this is essentially a summative work, technically a cento, "a patchwork of passages taken from other books and stitched together with an authorial commentary" (p.xxii). Or as Burton puts it: "what I say, is merely reading, … by mine own observation, and others' relation" (p.850). Whilst the citations from traditional medical authorities are thus to be expected (e.g. Hippocrates, Galen, Rhazes, Avicenna) many less familiar names also occur, and moreover keep company with references to the Bible (perhaps especially Ecclesiastes, Ecclesiasticus, and the Psalms), the Church Fathers (e.g. Augustine, here referred to as Austin, Jerome, Chrysostom), and most copiously from the writers of classical Latin antiquity (e.g. Terence, Seneca, Ovid, Horace, Virgil, Juvenal), upon whom Burton often calls for an apposite quotation. This emphasis of course reflects Burton's classical Oxford education in the late sixteenth and early seventeenth centuries, grounded in Latin and Greek authors. Moreover, his cosmology still accommodates the influence of the Devil, demons, and witches, in addition to natural causes.

What Burton's education had taught him about science is uncertain, but some passages are suggestive. He was obviously familiar with the workings of a camera obscura (p.413–4, although not named as such) although unclear about the mechanisms of vision: "Many excellent questions appertain to this sense, discussed by Philosophers: as whether this sight be caused *intra mittendo, vel extra mittendo, etc.*, by receiving in the visible species, or sending of them out" (p.161). Kepler is not amongst the "Philosophers" Burton references, so presumably he was unaware of Kepler's (1604) theory of vision which definitively established intromission over extromission or emission,[4] although elsewhere he alludes to Kepler's astronomical works (p.475–6). As for the brain, Burton still holds to the ancient ventricular localisation of cognitive faculties, mediated by animal spirits (p.157). In his characterisation of memory, which "lays up all the species which the senses have brought in, and records them as a good *Register*, that they may be forthcoming when they are called for by *Fantasy* and *Reason*" (p.162; italics in original) we may detect the conceptual confusions (encoding, storage) which continue to haunt this subject.

The hope or expectation that the *Anatomy* might contribute to our understanding of neurology founders, of course, on the rocks of anachronism. The year of the first edition of the *Anatomy* coincided with the birth of Thomas Willis (1621–1675), and hence the origin of the term "neurology" postdates Burton, first appearing long after his death in Willis's *Cerebri Anatome* (1664). This work was itself a product of the experimental methods developed in Oxford under the influence of Harvey, and it prompted the revision of ventricular to cortical localisation of faculties. Thomas Willis was admitted to Christ Church, Burton's Oxford college, in 1638, but I would imagine it unlikely that the teenager "batteller", or pupil-cum-lodger, in the house Canon Thomas Isles, and the sexagenerian sage ever met. Burton does not appear in either Hughes's biography of Willis,[5] or Dewhurst's transcriptions of Willis's Lectures.[6] Nevertheless, clinical neurologists may be interested to read some of the occasional case histories cited by Burton. Wearing our neurological (pattern-recognising) spectacles, the nuggets of clinical information contained therein may prompt us, even involuntarily, to hazard retrospective diagnoses. For example, could "a man shaking with the palsy" (p.379) have Parkinson's disease (two centuries before the eponymous description)? When "Theophrastus in Galen, thought he heard music" (p.414) was he experiencing musical hallucinosis? When the "old are ... so much altered as that they cannot know their own face in a glass" (p.276) are they demonstrating the "mirror sign" or the "phenomenon of the looking glass", a misidentification syndrome sometimes encountered in the context of cognitive decline? Of course, such diagnostic hypotheses can never be answered for want of further clinical information, so the epistemic case for retrospective diagnosis[7] cannot be established. Other snippets of information may, however, meet with the approbation of the modern neurologist: "such as are vertiginous, they think all turns round and moves, all err; when as the error is wholly in their own brains" (p.1024). And who will disagree with the injunction: "what should you pray for, except perhaps for a trustworthy doctor who can heal the brain?" (p.988)?

Burton's "melancholy" is generally equated with our category of depression, a disorder from which Burton himself may have suffered. Thankfully most neurologists no longer consider depression as something distinct ("psychiatric") and hence to be addressed by others, but an integral part of many (so-called) neurological conditions including neurodegenerative disorders, epilepsy, multiple sclerosis, and some examples of functional disorders. In addition to its many symptoms, Burton may also have recognised the possible relation of depression to creativity, citing Aristotle to the effect that "All geniuses are melancholics, and the greatest men in the arts and sciences ... are nearly all melancholics" (p.409, note c). It has been suggested that Burton's copious writing was a diversionary exercise from his own melancholy, perhaps an early example of what may now be termed "scriptotherapy". His other recommendations for melancholy may also be considered to have a modern flavour: diet, air, exercise, "they must not be left solitary, ... never idle, never out of company" (p.1062). As for therapeutics, many are discussed, mostly botanical in origin (the year 1621 also saw the founding of the Oxford Botanical Garden, which Burton commends as "now in *fieri*"; p.624). One of the fictional works of non-fiction which one most wishes had actually been written is the study of Robert Burton entitled *Borage and Hellebore* by Nicholas Jenkins, the protagonist of Anthony Powell's sequence of twelve novels *A Dance to the Music of Time*. The *Anatomy* informs particularly the tenth instalment, *Books do furnish a room*, as well as the penultimate paragraph of the whole novel sequence.[8] Powell is one of many writers to have engaged with and been inspired by Burton's work.

What is Burton's legacy? He has a monument in the north transept of Christ Church cathedral but none, to my knowledge, in Oxford's medical heritage.[9] But the *Anatomy* endures. "Some write such great Volumes to no purpose, take so much pains to so small effect" (p.1007). I would argue that this conclusion is not one could level at Burton's *Anatomy*. Whatever shortcomings or objections there might be to the creation or construction of a literary canon (or canons), there are generally reasons why works may be characterised as canonical, not least their transhistorical and transcultural relevance, despite the absence of new empirical research which we expect from today's publications. To immerse oneself in the *Anatomy* may serve to remind us of the transience of own culture and our explanatory schemata, and that our own cherished researches and ideas will likely turn to dust. Mood disorder is part of the human condition, which clinicians will always encounter and often be called upon to address, and indeed may experience as a consequence of their work: *Qui medice vivit, misere vivit* [He who lives by medicine lives miserably] (p.229).

Acknowledgement

Adapted from: Larner AJ. *The Anatomy of Melancholy* revisted after 400 years. *Brain* 2022;145:2617–8.

References

1. Gowland A (ed). *The Anatomy of Melancholy. Robert Burton.* London: Penguin Classics, 2021.
2. Frank RG Jr. *Harvey and the Oxford physiologists. A study of scientific ideas and social interaction.* Berkeley: University of California Press, 1980.
3. Arikha N. *Passions and tempers. A history of the humours.* New York: Harper Perennial, 2008, p.60.
4. Lindberg DC. *Theories of vision from Al-Kindi to Kepler.* Chicago and London: The University of Chicago Press, 1976.
5. Hughes JT. *Thomas Willis 1621–1675. His life and work.* London: Royal Society of Medicine Press, 1991.
6. Dewhurst K. *Willis's Oxford Lectures.* Oxford: Sandford Publications, 1980.

7. Muramoto O. Retrospective diagnosis of a famous historical figure: ontological, epistemic, and ethical considerations. Philos Ethics Humanit Med 2014; 9: 10.

8. Spurling H. *Invitation to the dance. A handbook to Anthony Powell's A Dance to the Music of Time.* London, Arrow Books, 2005, p.216–7.

9. Fitzherbert Jones R. *Oxford's medical heritage. The people behind the names.* Oxford: University of Oxford Medical Informatics Unit, 2014.

Index

www.ingramcontent.com/pod-product-compliance
Lightning Source LLC
Chambersburg PA
CBHW070239200326
41518CB00010B/1618